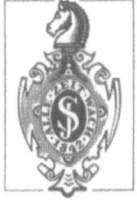

The Genetics of Diabetes Mellitus

Edited by
W. Creutzfeldt J. Köbberling J. V. Neel

In cooperation with J. H. Edwards S. S. Fajans
W. Fuhrmann D. R. Gamble G. C. Gerritsen
K. D. Hepp R. J. Jarrett G. Jörgensen H. Keen
U. Langenbeck H. Mehnert P. G. Nelson J. Nerup
Ruth Østerby D. A. Pyke D. L. Rimoin
Christa Schade K. Schöffling Nancy E. Simpson
W. Stauffacher R. Tattersall

With 64 Figures and 74 Tables

Springer-Verlag
Berlin Heidelberg GmbH

Prof. Dr. Werner Creutzfeldt
PD Dr. Johannes Köbberling
Medizinische Klinik und Poliklinik der Universität, Humboldt-
allee 1, D–3400 Göttingen, Germany

Prof. Dr. James V. Neel
Department of Human Genetics, 1137 E. Catherine Street,
Ann Arbor, MI 48104, USA

ISBN 978-3-540-07651-3   ISBN 978-3-642-66332-1 (eBook)
DOI 10.1007/978-3-642-66332-1

Library of Congress Cataloging in Publication Data. Main entry under title: The Genetics
of diabetes mellitus. Includes index. 1. Diabetes – Genetic aspects. I. Creutzfeldt, Werner.
II. Köbberling, Johannes, 1940– . III. Neel, James Van Gundia, 1915– . (DNLM: 1. Diabetes
mellitus – Familial and genetic. WK810 G329) RC660.G43 616.4′62′ 071 76–8475

© by Springer-Verlag Berlin Heidelberg 1976
Originally published by Springer-Verlag Berlin Heidelberg 1976
Offsetprinting and Binding: Beltz Offsetdruck, Hemsbach/Bergstr.

Foreword

On February 21 and 22, 1975, an International Workshop on the "Genetics of Diabetes Mellitus" was held in Göttingen, West-Germany. This workshop had been organized by the Department of Medicine, University of Göttingen, and was generously sponsored by the Deutsche Forschungsgemeinschaft. Some forty geneticists and clinicians from Europe and North America, working in the field of diabetes both in man and laboratory animals, participated. The 25 lectures presented at the workshop are now assembled for publication. Some of the animated discussion which followed the presentations has been included in the final papers by the speakers.

Some lectures summarize the recent literature, others present data from recent research. Thus, a comprehensive and modern review of the theoretical and practical problems related to the genetics of diabetes are offered by this volume.

The confusion about the mode of inheritance of diabetes mellitus during the last two decades can only be resolved by joint discussions between geneticists interested in diabetes and clinical diabetologists interested in genetics. Knowledge of modern genetics and of the heterogeneity of diabetes mellitus are necessary in order to disentangle the complex scene. Optimistically, the publication of this work on the genetics of diabetes will help to achieve this aim and to establish the concept of genetic heterogeneity of diabetes mellitus.

The editors are grateful to Springer-Verlag, Heidelberg, for the prompt publication of these proceedings and to the Farbwerke Hoechst AG, Frankfurt (M), for their contribution to the printing costs.

W. Creutzfeldt
J. Köbberling
J. V. Neel

Contents

List of Contributors

AMHERDT, M.: Institut d'Histologie et d'Embryologie, University of Geneva, Geneva (Switzerland)

ANDERSEN, ORTWED O.: Medical Department E, Frederiksberg, Hospital, Copenhagen (Denmark)

BLANKS, M. C.: Diabetes and Atherosclerosis Research, The Upjohn Comp. Kalamazoo, MI 49001 (USA)

CREUTZFELDT, W.: Medizinische Universitätsklinik Göttingen, Humboldtalle 1, D–3400 Göttingen (Germany)

CHRISTY, M.: Medical Department F, Gentofte Hospital, Hellerup, Copenhagen (Denmark)

DULIN, W. E.: Diabetes and Atherosclerosis Research, The Upjohn Comp. Kalamazoo, MI 49001 (USA)

EDWARDS, J. H.: The Infant Development Unit, Queen Elizabeth Medical Centre, Birmingham (England)

EGEBERG, J.: Anatomy Department B, University of Copenhagen (Denmark)

FAJANS, S. S.: Division of Endocrinology and Metabolism University Hospital, Ann Arbor, MI 48104 (USA)

FLOYD, J. C.: Division of Endocrinology and Metabolism University Hospital, Ann Arbor, MI 48104 (USA)

FUHRMANN, W.: Institut für Humangenetik der Universität, Am Schlangenzahl 29, D–6300 Gießen (Germany)

GAMBLE, D. R.: Public Health Laboratory, West Park Hospital, Epsom, Surrey (England)

GERRITSEN, G. C.: Diabetes and Atherosclerosis Research, The Upjohn Comp., Kalamazoo, MI 49001 (USA)

HEPP, K. D.: Städt. Krankenhaus München-Schwabing, Kölner Platz 1, D-8000 München 40 (Germany)

JARRETT, R. J.: Department of Medical, Guy's Hospital Medical School, London SE1 9RT (England)

JÖRGENSEN, G.: Institut für Humangenetik der Universität, Nikolausberger Weg 5 a, D-3400 Göttingen (Germany)

KEEN, H.: Department of Medicine, Guy's Hospital Medical School, London SE1 9RT (England)

KIKKAWA, R.: Medizinische Universitätsklinik, Inselspital, Ch-3010 Bern (Switzerland)

KÖBBERLING, J.: Medizinische Universitätsklinik, Humboldtallee 1, D-3400 Göttingen (Germany)

LANGENBECK, U.: Institut für Humangenetik der Universität, Nikolausberger Weg 5 a, D-3400 Göttingen (Germany)

LYNGSØE, J.: Medical Department T, Bispelbjerg Hospital, Copenhagen (Denmark)

MEHNERT, H.: Städt. Krankenhaus München-Schwabing, Kölner Platz 1, D-8000 München 40 (Germany)

NEEL, J. V.: Department of Human Genetics, 1137 E. Catherine Street, Ann Arbor, MI 48104 (USA)

NELSON, P. G.: Diabetic Clinic, King's College Hospital, Denmark Hill, London SE5 9RS (England)

NERUP, J.: Medical Department F, Gentofte Hospital, Hellerup, Copenhagen (Denmark)

ORCI, L.: Institut d'Histologie et d'Embryologie, University of Geneva, Geneva (Switzerland)

ØSTERBY, RUTH: University Institute of Pathology, Kommunehospitalet, Aarhus C (Denmark)

PEK, S.: Division of Endocrinology and Metabolism, University Hospital, Ann Arbor, MI 48104 (USA)

PLATZ, P.: Tissue Typing Laboratory, Rigshospitalet, Copenhagen (Denmark)

POULSEN, J. E.: Steno Memorial Hospital, Gentofte Copenhagen, Copenhagen (Denmark)

PYKE, D. A.: Diabetic Department, King's College Hospital, London SE5 9RS (England)

X

RIMOIN, D. L.: Devision of Medical Genetics, UCLA School of Medicine, 1000 West Carson Street, Torrance, CA 90509 (USA)

RYDER, L. P.: Tissue Typing Laboratory Rigshospitalet, Copenhagen (Denmark)

SCHADE, CHRISTA: Zentrum der Inneren Medizin, Universitätskliniken, Theodor-Stern-Kai 7, D–6000 Frankfurt/Main 70, (Germany)

SCHÖFFLING, K.: Zentrum der Inneren Medizin, Universitätskliniken, Theodor-Stern-Kai 7, D–6000 Frankfurt/Main 70 (Germany)

SCHMIDT, F. L.: Diabetes and Atherosclerosis Research, The Upjohn Comp. Kalamazoo, MI 49001 (USA)

SIMPSON, NANCY E.: Department of Paediatrics, Queen's University, Kingston, Ontario (Canada)

STAUFFACHER, W.: Medizinische Universitätsklinik, Inselspital, CH–3010 Bern (Switzerland)

SVEJGAARD, A.: Tissue Typing Laboratory Rigshospitalet, Copenhagen (Denmark)

TATTERSALL, R.: General Hospital, Nottingham NG1 6HA (England)

TAYLOR, C. I.: Division of Endocrinology and Metabolism University Hospital, Ann Arbor, MI 48104 (USA)

THOMSEN, M.: Tissue Typing Laboratory Rigshospitalet, Copenhagen (Denmark)

1. Diabetes Mellitus – A Geneticist's Nightmare

J. V. NEEL

Early Genetic Studies: Simple Hypotheses

It would be difficult to establish who first remarked on the familial
nature of diabetes mellitus. With the advent of Mendelism to medicine,
during the 1920s and early 1930s various investigators (e.g., Wright,
Cammidge, Macklin, Lawrence, White) interpreted particular pedigrees
in terms of either dominant or recessive inheritance, an approach implying major genetic heterogeneity in the disease. A standard difficulty with this approach is that when an affected individual married to
a normal person produces affected and normal children, this can be interpreted either as resulting from simple dominant inheritance or else
from the "pseudodominance" seen in the marriage of a person homozygous
for a recessive gene to a heterozygous, phenotypically normal carrier
of that gene; half of the children of this latter marriage will be affected just as in true dominant inheritance. In a common, familial disease, individual pedigrees can be found illustrating almost any mode
of inheritance.

It was, then, a significant advance when in 1933 Allan (1) and Pincus
and White (32-34) presented methods for pooling groups of pedigrees
and then testing them for adherence with a variety of simple genetic
hypotheses. Allan discounted dominant inheritance as a general explanation because of the many pedigrees in which a diabetic patient reported unaffected parents but, estimating the frequency of the assumed
recessive gene from the square root of the frequency of diabetics in
the population, escaped the trap of pseudodominance and observed (without statistical tests) that the proportions of affected from various
types of matings were such that "it seems possible diabetes may be
transmitted as a recessive unit character". Unfortunately, in addition
to some statistical difficulties, the frequency he assumed for diabetes
mellitus in the population of adults who have expressed their genotype
(1.4%) was well below what we now know to be the case, the resulting
spuriously low estimate of gene frequency thus invalidating much of his
analysis.

Pincus and White first established clearly, through the use of nondiabetic controls, that diabetes mellitus was by history significantly
more frequent in the parents and siblings of diabetics than of controls. They then concluded that dominant inheritance as a general explanation was unlikely on the basis of the frequent absence of the disease in both the parents of affected individuals. In order to test for
agreement with the ratios expected in recessive inheritance, they made
the questionable assumption that all "potential" diabetics develop the
disease by the ninth decade (see Genotype-Environment Interaction below). This assumption permitted them to obtain from the observed age-
specific data a genotype prevalence, but only with the further assumption that "ordinary" life table expectancies apply to diabetics before

1

they present themselves to the physician. They also attempted to correct for the influence of the ascertainment bias on their ratios, by
an adjustment which was, however, inappropriate to their situation.
Despite these obvious problems in analysis, the results appeared to
agree with the hypothesis of recessive inheritance.

Recognizing the inadequacy of histories, these investigators also obtained either 2-hour postprandial blood sugars or glucose tolerance
tests on 169 "close", nondiabetic relatives of known diabetics and
125 controls. Relatives of diabetics were judged abnormal in14.5% of
the postprandial levels and 25.3% of the tolerance tests in that they
exceeded any of the control values. On the hypothesis that diabetes
mellitus is a recessive disease, the three types of marriages that
produce diabetics (normal x normal, diabetic x normal, and diabetic
x diabetic) should be, with some error, because of the incomplete penetrance, Dd x Dd, Dd x dd, and dd x dd, respectively. Given the Mendelian expectation of diabetes mellitus from these marriages (1/4, 1/2,
1) then the _percentage_ of diabetic offsprings, even with incomplete
penetrance, should be in the ratio 1:2:4; the observed ratios were
1:2.6:3.7 in the small series on which the above-mentioned tests were
performed. These papers are truly remarkable for the effort made to
come to grips with the various complications in the study of the genetics of diabetes and the shortcomings of the data.

The next three decades witnessed several more extensive studies based
on the pedigree approach. Levit and Pessikova in 1934 (23) observed
a similar frequency of diabetes in the parents and the siblings of diabetics, and concluded from this that their data were best explained
if most diabetes mellitus were due to a dominant gene which usually
failed to find expression. Harris in 1950 (14), in addition to con-
firming in general the findings of Pincus and White, observed that the
siblings of early-onset diabetics were more likely to develop diabetes
in childhood or early adult life than those of late-onset diabetics.
He suggested as a "useful working hypothesis" that "many of the late-
onset mild cases could be regarded as heterozygous for a gene which,
in homozygous form, gives rise to the early onset homozygous form."
Steinberg and Wilder in 1952 (45) (see also 48), in a collection of
pedigree data whose shortcomings they carefully enumerated, also observed a good approximation to this 1:2:4 ratio of diabetic children
from the appropriate marriages in their material. In dominant inheritance, after suitable adjustment for age differences, the frequency
of disease should be the same in the siblings as children of an affected individual, a circumstance they did not observe in their data. They
point out that it is an essential consequence of Harris' hypothesis
that there be more diabetes in the parents of juvenile-type diabetics
than adult-type; this was also not found in their data. They therefore
favored simple recessive inheritance as accounting for the bulk of
diabetes mellitus.

Quite aside from the complications introduced into these studies by
the factors mentioned, these early investigations suffered from two
other defects, one recognized by the investigators, one not. The first
was the dependence (aside from a portion of the Pincus-White study)
on the pedigree approach, when diabetes is so frequently an undiagnosed disease. The second was the assumption that the diabetic state
was a discrete or qualitative trait, clearly to be differentiated
from normal, to which one could apply the analytic techniques appropriate to a qualitative trait. In the last 30 years, two types of
observations have made it clear this is not the case. In the USA and
elsewhere, periodic health appraisal programs and community surveys
utilizing a standard or modified glucose tolerance test agree in dem-

2

onstrating that the mean of the 1- or 2-hour postprandial value increased significantly with age (15,30,31,37,50). When either of these
values (depending on the study) was plotted against the number of
persons in the survey presenting it, the resulting histogram was, for
all age classes, unimodal but skewed to the right. There was no bimodality in the data, i.e., no clear division into persons with normal
tolerance and with impaired tolerance. It is important to point out
that in these studies known diabetics did not receive a modified glucose tolerance test. The various ways in which the data are presented
and the inability of diabetologists to agree on a standard definition
of diabetes renders it impossible to make a clear statement regarding
the frequency of undiagnosed diabetes in the older age groups. However, on the criteria employed in the study of Wilkerson and Krall
(50) ("consistent one to one and one-half hour postprandial venous
blood sugar of 170 mg. per one hundred cubic centimeters of blood or
above or a capillary blood sugar of 200 mg. or more per one hundred
cubic centimeters plus glucosuria"), 5.1% of Caucasoid persons aged
55-64 and 7,2% of persons aged 65-74 would be adjudged to have overt
or chemical (latent) diabetes mellitus. From the study of Petrie *et
al*. (31), the comparable figure was 5.0% for persons aged 50-59 years,
6.2% for persons aged 60-69 years, and 7.3% for persons over 69.

Multifactorial Hypotheses

Family studies, largely of adult-onset type diabetes mellitus, then
began to employ glucose tolerance tests as a matter of course, and
soon it became clear that within the immediate (first-degree) relatives of diabetics, not only was there a far higher proportion of
diabetics than a family history would reveal, no matter how careful,
but also that in the first-degree relatives of diabetics, as in the
general population, there was no clear tendency to bimodality in the
distribution of the 1/2-, 1- or 2-hour values obtained on a glucose
tolerance test (18,28,49). In the studies of Neel *et al*. (28), this
was also true after the administration of a standard dose of cortisone
acetate. Both the survey and the family data thus made it clear that
until more is known about the consequences of an elevated blood sugar,
the diagnosis of diabetes mellitus is somewhat arbitrary; we follow
most recent investigators in regarding a glucose tolerance test yield-
ing a blood glucose value above 160 mg % at 1 hour, above 140 mg %
at 1 1/2 hours, or above 120 mg % at 2 hours as abnormal (i.e., indicative of chemical or latent diabetes mellitus), in otherwise healthy
and ambulatory individuals under the age of 50 years.

Stimulated by this demonstration that there was a unimodal continuum
in the impairment of glucose metabolism, a number of investigators now
began to explore the possibility that the majority of cases of diabetes mellitus had a multifactorial basis, comparable to the assumed basis for stature or intelligence (17,18,26,28,39,40,49). This possibility had in fact been raised in 1925 by Hansen (13) and again in 1934
by Hogben (quoted in 21). Furthermore, Lamy *et al*. (20) suggested in
1961 that the phenotype might usually be the result of a main gene
with modifiers but that if sufficient modifiers were present, the main
gene was unnecessary; the latter is equivalent to multifactorial inheritance. In the usual sense,multifactorial inheritance in this context implies the action of genes with approximately additive effects
occurring at two or more loci. However, these additive effects on the
phenotype may result from a variety of different primary effects. Furthermore, given the data on the effect of cultural changes on the frequency of diabetes (see below), it would appear that the responsible
genes are influenced in their manifestations by many extraneous factors.

When the genetic contribution to a trait is thought to be multifactorial, the magnitude of the genetic contribution is expressed in terms
of "heritability", defined as the ratio of that part of the genetic
variation which is simply additive to the total phenotypic variation
exhibited by the trait, and when the point at which a disease is diagnosed represents an arbitrary cut-off point in a continuun of liability, as is the case for diabetes mellitus, we can speak of a "threshold character". The special statistical problems in estimating heritability for threshold characters have been addressed by Falconer (8,
9), who from data from Birmingham, England, estimates the heritability
of diabetes mellitus, with age disregarded, as about 38%, and from
data from Canada, about 48%. By comparison, similar estimates for
congenital pyloric stenosis, clubfoot, and peptic ulcer yielded values of 79, 68, and 37%, respectively. Similar values were obtained
whether the estimates were based on the values in the siblings, parents, or children of the diabetic proband.

Simpson (41), applying the same type of analysis to a more extensive
set of Canadian data (overlapping with the first), obtained essentially the same overall estimate as Falconer, and from details of the
analysis concluded that " early and late ages at onset are different
genetically". In a later treatment using data obtained in Edinburgh,
Smith *et al.* (44) explored in detail the effect of basing the estimate
of the heritability of diabetes mellitus on different classes of relatives. Different estimates of heritability were obtained using different classes of relatives (siblings, 56%; parents, 52%; children,
19%; uncles and aunts, 38%), and the details of the analysis suggested
that "early-onset and late-onset diabetes are largely the same genetic disease". Since similar methods of analysis are employed in the
studies of Simpson and Smith *et al.*, one must conclude that the data
sets vary. Whether this is related to the nature of the disease or
to environmental differences between the study areas is not clear,
but the problems in dealing with the genetics of diabetes were by no
means solved by the introduction of the heritability concept.

Although it would appear that the mathematical precision of modern
genetics would surely permit discrimination between two genetic models
as different as a monogenic recessive and multifactorial additive,
Edwards (5,6) has stated the situation succinctly: "the numerical similarities of the two models persist up to high levels of penetrance so
that even models based on indefinitely large numbers of hereditary factors or genes can very closely simulate the consequences of single-factor inheritance". In this connection, Barrai and Cann (2), reanalyzing
Simpson's data with a sophisticated computer analysis, were unable to
differentiate between the two hypotheses in a material of 204 sibships
ascertained through a juvenile diabetic.

Diabetes in the Amerindian

A relatively high frequency of diabetes mellitus has been reported
in various Amerindian groups (7). Two recent studies report that in
the Pimas and Seminoles respectively the distribution of blood glucose values at 2 hours postprandial to a 75g carbohydrate load is bimodal (7,38,46). The findings in male Pima Indians aged 35-74 are
reproduced in Figure 1. Elston *et al.* (7) have argued that their data, based on Seminoles living in Florida and Oklahoma, are compatible
with the hypothesis that there is a principal gene governing serum
glucose levels which, for the Oklahoma data, if a recessive has a
frequency of 0.41 and if a dominant is 0.09. It is further argued
that the incidence of abnormal tests is higher in Oklahoma than in
Florida Seminoles because "there is a major gene (probably from found-

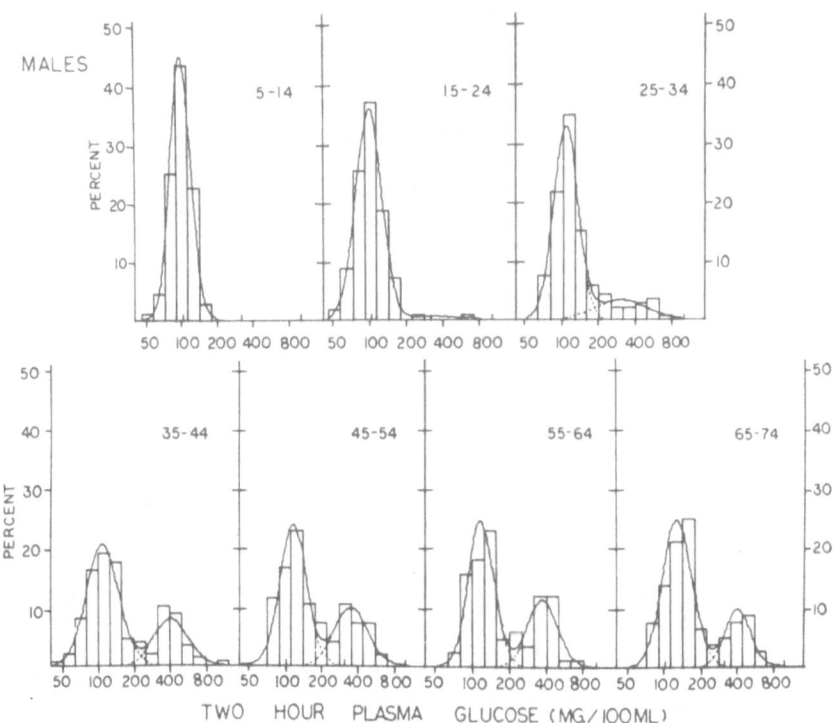

Fig.1. Distribution of plasma glucose levels in Pima Indians 2 hours after 75-g carbohydrate load (after Rushfort *et al.* 1971)

er effect) segregating there that is either rare or non-existent in Florida. "This argument overlooks the fact that the average Oklahoma Seminole is some 10 lbs heavier than his Florida kinsman; the differ- ence between the two populations can be adequately explained by the weight difference. Furthermore, as is apparent from Figure 1, in the Pima population the nadir of bimodality occurs at about 250 mg%. At the higher ages, about half of the persons in the left-hand mode - as well as all the individuals in the right-hand mode - have values patho- gnomonic of chemical or latent diabetes. There does not appear to have been an effort to exclude manifest diabetics from the study. The reviewer suggests that unless one wishes to redefine diabetes mellitus for the Amerindians, the second mode does not correspond to a geno- type, as is assumed in the analysis that yields a gene frequency, but is composed of the more severe diabetics in the population, who in the absence of control of their disease have moved to an equilibrium with their disease bounded, at the upper extreme, by a glucose level inconsistent with sustained survival. Otherwise stated, a physiologic explanation of that bimodality is much more convincing than a genetic one.

The Heterogeneity of the Disease

That diabetes mellitus is really a collection of diseases is an old concept. For instance, in his Croonian lectures of 1908, Garrod (12) wrote: "In diabetes mellitus, under which name we probably include more than one morbid condition attended by persistent glycosuria, the metabolic derangements, primary and secondary, dominate the clinical picture." Even while testing the data for adherence to one hypothesis or another, most investigators left open the possibility that the entity was etiologically heterogeneous. Indeed, it is well established that there are a number of rare genetic syndromes in which diabetes mellitus occurs with striking frequency: for example, the Alstrom syndrome; ataxia telangiectasia; Werner's syndrome; the syndrome of photomyoclonus, deafness and neuropathy; etc. (reviewed in 36). However, for several of these it is by no means clear whether the diabetes mellitus is a primary manifestation of the genotype or unrelated, i.e., the development of diabetes mellitus in the Lawrence-Moon-Biedl syndrome might well be encouraged by the obesity of the disease and have the same genetic basis as diabetes mellitus in other fat people (not all persons with the Lawrence-Moon-Biedl syndrome are obese or diabetic). We may take it as established, that this type of heterogeneity exists, but the rare syndromes probably account, in round figures, for less than 1% of diabetes mellitus. The question has been, is there recognizable heterogeneity within the remaining 99% of the disease.

The chief efforts to establish a case for heterogeneity in the larger group have, beginning with Harris (14, see also (39)) involved juvenile-onset as opposed to adult-onset diabetes mellitus. Several studies have revealed that, as was the case for adult-onset diabetes mellitus, the frequency of chemical diabetes was also substantially increased among the first-degree relatives of patients with juvenile-onset diabetes mellitus (3,16,18,42). Recently, Lestradet *et al.* (22) and Tattersall and Fajans (47) have conducted genetic studies of early-onset diabetes in which a clear distinction has been drawn between probands whose diabetes mellitus, although of early-onset, clinically behaves as late-onset or maturity-type diabetes - ketosis-resistant, requiring little or no insulin - and probands whose diabetes mellitus is the ketosis-prone, highly insulin-dependent type. The familial patterns exhibited by the two types are clearly different, there being substantially less diabetes mellitus in the families of the juvenile-onset type than in the families of the adult-onset type. The recent study of MacDonald (25), demonstrating an equal incidence by history of adult-onset diabetes mellitus among ancestors of juvenile diabetics and nondiabetics, must be considered confirmatory of the Tattersall-Fajans findings, and if confirmed illustrates once again for students of human genetics the dangers of relying on the anamnestic approach to a ubiquitous and poorly defined disease. It will be most interesting to see this type of approach extended to older age groups.

In parallel with these developments Gamble *et al.* (10,11) have implicated the Coxsackie viruses, especially Type B4, as a precipitating cause of early-onset diabetes, and important work with experimental animals is underway. Further, Nerup *et al.* (29) have recently reported that in a series of diabetics, there was a disproportionate representation of two histocompability types, HL-A 8 and W 15, the increase being "found almost exclusively in insulin dependent diabetics." Finally, there is the recent evidence associating juvenile-type diabetes with the autoimmune diseases and the preliminary evidence that this type of diabetes mellitus itself may in some cases have characteristics of an autoimmune disease (reviewed in 24). There is thus growing reason to suspect that early-onset, insulin-requiring diabetes is often a delayed response to a viral infection, a response which of course might have a genetic basis. Furthermore, the fact that everyone who contracts these diseases does not subsequently develop diabetes mellitus also suggests the operation of a genetic factor and, in fact, the co-dominant inheritance of the HL-A types would, given the above-mentioned association, predict a familial pattern.

Table 1. Possible points of genetic intervention in the pathogenesis of diabetes mellitus. (The author is indebted to Dr. Stefan Fajans for helpful discussions in this regard)

---

1. Decreased output of normal insulin
   a) Decreased number or affinity of beta-cell receptor sites to glucose or amino acids, i.e., insufficient stimulus
   b) Decreased net synthesis of proinsulin
   c) Abnormal or deficient "excision enzyme"
   d) Defective release of insulin from beta cell
   e) Degeneration of beta cell

2. Production of abnormal insulin molecule

3. Production of insulin antagonist
   a) Antibody in nature
   b) Hormonal in nature

4. Abnormal insulin transport

5. Abnormal cellular receptors of insulin (including inability to dissociate insulin complexes)
   a) Decreased number
   b) Decreased function

6. "Obesity factor"

7. Abnormal rate of insulin degradation by target cells

Since, however, juvenile-type diabetes mellitus is a small fraction of all diabetes mellitus - perhaps 3-5% - the evidence for heterogeneity still applies to a small minority of diabetes mellitus. However, when one contemplates the many routes or combinations of routes by which an impaired glucose tolerance test might result - as shown in Table 1 - certainly there is abundant reason to be prepared for heterogeneity in the remaining 95-97% of the disease. Furthermore, the concept of heterogeneity is by no means inconsistent with multifactorial inheritance; the cumulation of genetic defects which results in diabetes mellitus in one person may not be the same in another. However, until each of these possible pathogenic routes is subject to examination, it will be difficult to advance the concept of heterogeneity greatly.

The Offspring of Conjugal Diabetics

The literature contains numerous studies of the occurrence of diabetes mellitus among the offspring of diabetic parents (reviewed in 35). The particular genetic significance of such children is that if diabetes mellitus, except for the rare types mentioned earlier, were due to homozygosity for the same recessive gene, then all of the children from such a marriage should be affected sooner or later. However, the projections for the percentage of children ultimately to be affected involve a number of assumptions difficult to defend in detail. Furthermore, since the various series usually involve no more than a few hundred children, there are the usual errors of estimate, so that a series compatible with an ultimate frequency of 100% may also be compatible with only 75% developing the disease (28). It must not be forgotten that with multifactorial inheritance with a threshold effect, one expects a very high proportion of the children of two affected persons to be affected, such a high proportion that most data could not distinguish between results consistent with this expectation and with a 100%

expectation. Since, finally, even if two parents were diabetics for different genetic reasons an offspring with such bilateral inheritance might well be abnormal, it seems unlikely the results of this approach can yield a decisive test of the genetic basis of the disease.

The Genotype-Environment Interaction

There is abundant evidence concerning the role of the environment, broadly defined, in the expression of the diabetic predisposition (19). For example, although proper base-lines from Amerindians living under truly primitive conditions are still lacking, it seems clear that the recently altered life style of the acculturated Indian of the USA has been accompanied by a great increase in diabetes mellitus, along with obesity and hypertension. Chemical diabetes seems to be increasing in the Eskimo as his way of life alters (27). Recent immigrants to Israel from Yemen and Kurdistan had significantly less diabetes mellitus than long-established immigrants from these areas (4). Furthermore, monozygous twins discordant for diabetes supply evidence for the role of environmental factors in the etiology of the disease, although the evidence is limited by their generally similar way of life. Studies on the familial patterns of glucose tolerance in groups such as those mentioned above, before and after some major cultural transition, would be highly desirable.

Given all these facts, it is scarcely surprising that the results of studies in two different countries may appear to differ significantly. Studies on the genetics of diabetes mellitus which somehow factor out dietary and socioeconomic factors are of course highly desirable but difficult in the extreme. Furthermore, if the environment is changing across generations, this fact may also introduce such inconsistencies into the data as to doom the effort from the start. Under these circumstances, if the juvenile-onset, juvenile-type of diabetes mellitus really is frequently a sequel to infectious disease, one would expect the familial pattern of this type of diabetes mellitus to be more constant from country to country than that of adult-onset type, simply because the agents which have been implicated are more uniformly distributed than life styles. Incidentally, if environmental factors are changing rapidly, this creates severe difficulties for the derivation of simple empiric risk figures to be used in the genetic counseling of diabetics, since the risk figures derived from one generation may not be applicable to the next.

Why the Slow Progress?

It will be seen, then, that exact knowledge of the inheritance of the predisposition to diabetes mellitus has scarcely advanced in the past 40 years. This is in striking contrast to the exciting developments elsewhere in human genetics. The reason is clear: The phenotype of analysis is probably heterogeneous (in addition to the rare entities), has an unknown basis, and is not clearly defined; and is of variable age of onset and influenced in its manifestations by environmental variables. These factors have permitted competent geneticists to reach such widely different conclusions that one wonders if they were all talking about the same disease, and at this point perhaps it is clear why the historical approach has been pursued in this presentation. Contrast the slow pace here with the really amazing developments in cytogenetics and somatic cell genetics or in the biochemical genetics of traits wherein the genetic lesion can be identified clearly, as in the hemoglobinopathies. In 1965 in a discussion of the genetics of diabetes mellitus the author referred to it as a "geneticist's nightmare." Nothing that has happened in the past 10 years calls for a reevaluation of that description.

References

1. Allan, W.: Heredity in diabetes. Ann. Int. Med. 6, 1272 (1933)

2. Barrai, I., Cann, H.M.: Segregation analysis of juvenile diabetes mellitus. J. Med. Genet. 2, 8 (1965)

3. Burkeholder, J.N., Pickens, J.M., Womack, W.N.: Oral glucose tolerance test in siblings of children with diabetes mellitus. Diabetes 16, 156 (1967)

4. Cohen, A.M.: Effect of environmental changes on prevalence of diabetes and of artherosclerosis in various ethnic groups in Israel. In: The Genetics of Migrant and Isolate Populations, Goldschmidt, E. (ed.). Baltimore: Williams & Wilkins, 1963, p. 127

5. Edwards, J.H.: The simulation of Mendelism. Acta Genet. (Basel) 10, 63 (1960)

6. Edwards, J.H.: The genetic basis of common disease. Am. J. Med. 34, 627 (1963)

7. Elston, R.C., Namboodiri, K.K., Nino, H.V., Pollitzer, W.S.: Studies on blood and urine glucose in Seminole Indians: Indications for segregation of a major gene. Am. J. Hum. Genet. 26, 13 (1974)

8. Falconer, D.S.: The inheritance of liability to certain diseases, estimated from the incidence among relatives. Ann. Hum. Genet. 29, 51 (1965)

9. Falconer, D.S.: The inheritance of liability to diseases with variable age of onset with particular reference to diabetes mellitus. Ann. Hum. Genet. 31, 1 (1967)

10. Gamble, D.R., Taylor, K.W., Cumming, H.: Coxsackie virus and diabetes mellitus. Brit. Med. J. 4, 260 (1973)

11. Gamble, D.R., Kinsley, M.L., Fitzgerald, M.G., Bolton, R., Taylor, K.W.: Viral antibodies in diabetes mellitus. Brit. Med. J. 3, 627 (1969)

12. Garrod, A.E.: Inborn errors of metabolism. Lecture 1. Lancet 2, 1 (1908)

13. Hansen, S.: Über die Vererbung des Diabetes mellitus. Acta Med. Scand. 62, 85 (1925)

14. Harris, H.: The familial distribution of diabetes mellitus: a study of the relatives of 1241 diabetic propositi. Ann. Eug. 15, 95 (1950)

15. Hayner, N.S., Kjelsberg, M.O., Epstein, F.H., Francis, T., Jr.: Carbohydrate tolerance and diabetes in a total community, Tecumseh, Michigan. Diabetes 14, 413 (1965)

16. Hunter, S., McKay, E.: Intravenous glucose-tolerance test in parents of diabetic children. Lancet 1, 1017 (1967)

17. Jörgensen, G.: Zur Genetik des idiopathischen Diabetes mellitus. Deutsch. Med. J. 17, 609 (1966)

18. Keen, H., Track, N.S.: Age of onset and inheritance of diabetes: importance of examining relatives. Diabetologia 4, 317 (1968)

19. Labhart, A.: Endogene und exogene Faktoren des Diabetes: Heredität, Adipositas, Zivilisation. Helv. Med. Acta 32, 349 (1965)

20. Lamy, M., Frézal, J., Rey, J.: Hérédité du diabète sucré. J. Ann. Diabet. Hôtel Dieu 2, 5 (1961)

21. Lawrence, R.D.: Heredity in diabetes mellitus and renal glycosuria. In: Chances of Morbid Inheritance, Blacker, C.P. (ed.). Baltimore: Wm. Wood 1934, p.332

22. Lestradet, H., Battistelli, F., Ledoux, A., Combier, E.: L'hérédité du Diabète Sucré Etude Effectuée à Partir de 1000 Familles d'Enfants Diabétiques et de 1000 Familles Témoins. Nouv. Presse Med. 1, 2543 (1972)

23. Levit, S.G., Pessikova, L.N.: The genetics of diabetes mellitus. Trudy Med. Genet. Inst. Gorky 3, 132 (1934)

24. MacCuish, A.C., Irvine, W.J., Barnes, E.W., Duncan, L.J.P.: Antibodies to pancreatic islet cells in insulin-dependent diabetics with coexistent auto-immune disease. Lancet 2, 1529 (1974)

25. MacDonald, M.J.: Equal incidence of adult-onset diabetes among ancestors of juvenile diabetics and nondiabetics. Diabetologia 10, 767 (1974)

26. Miyao, S.: Diabetes mellitus and inheritance. Bull. Inst. Const. Med. Kumamoto Univ. 18, 1 (1967)

27. Mouratoff, G.J., Scott, E.M.: Diabetes mellitus in Eskimos after a decade. J. Am. Med. Ass. 226, 1345 (1973)

28. Neel, J.V., Fajans, S.S., Conn, J.W., Davidson, R.T.: Diabetes mellitus. In: Genetics and the Epidemiology of Chronic Diseases. Public Health Service Publication No. 1163. Neel, J.V., Shaw, M.W., Schull, W.J. (eds.). Washington: Government Printing Office, 1965, p. 105

29. Nerup, J., Platz, P., Andersen, O.O., Christy, M., Lyngsøe, J., Poulsen, J.E., Ryder, L.P., Nielsen, L.S., Thomsen, M., Svejgaard, A.: HL-A antigens and diabetes mellitus. Lancet 2, 864 (1974)

30. O'Sullivan, J.E., Williams, R.F., McDonald, G.W.: The prevalence of diabetes mellitus and related variables: a population study in Sudbury, Massachusetts. J. Chron. Dis. 20, 535 (1967)

31. Petrie, L.M., McLaughlin, C.D., Hodgins, T.E.: Mass screening for lowered glucose tolerance. Ann. Int. Med. 40, 963 (1954)

32. Pincus, G., White, P.: On the inheritance of diabtes mellitus. I. An analysis of 675 family histories. Am. J. Med. Sci. 186, 1 (1933)

33. Pincus, G., White, P.: On the inheritance of diabetes mellitus. II. Further analysis of family histories. Am. J. Med. Sci. 188, 159 (1934)

34. Pincus, G., White, P.: On the inheritance of diabetes mellitus. III. The blood sugar values of the relatives of diabetics. Am. J. Med. Sci. 188, 782 (1934)

35. Rimoin, D.L.: Inheritance of diabetes mellitus. Med. Clin. N. A. 55, 807 (1971)

36. Rimoin, D.L., Schimke, R.N.: Genetic Disorders of the Endocrine Glands. St. Louis: C.V. Mosby, 1971

37. Rush, T., Tupper, C.J.: Two-hour postprandial glucose determinations in a periodic health appraisal program. Geriatrics 15, 630 (1960)

38. Rushfort, N.B., Bennett, P.H., Steinberg, A.G., Burch, T.A., Miller, M.: Diabetes in the Pima Indians. Diabetes 20, 756 (1971)

39. Simpson, N.E.: The genetics of diabetes: A study of 233 families of juvenile diabetics. Ann. Hum. Genet. 26, 1 (1962)

40. Simpson, N.E.: Multifactorial inheritance: a possible hypothesis for diabetes. Diabetes 13, 462 (1964)

41. Simpson, N.E.: Heritabilities of liability to diabetes when sex and age at onset are considered. Ann. Hum. Genet. 32, 283 (1969)

42. Sisk, C.W.: Application of one-hour glucose tolerance test to genetic studies of diabetes in children. Lancet 1, 262 (1968)

43. Smith, C.: Discrimination between different modes of inheritance in genetic disease. Clin. Genet. 2, 303 (1971)

44. Smith, C., Falconer, D.S., Duncan, L.J.P.: A statistical and genetical study of diabtes. II. Heritability of liability. Ann. Hum. Genet. 35, 281 (1972)

45. Steinberg, A.G., Wilder, R.M.: A study of the genetics of diabetes mellitus. Am. J. Hum. Genet. 4, 113 (1952)

46. Steinberg, A.G., Rushfort, N.B., Bennett, P.H., Burch, T.A., Miller, M.: Nobel Symposium 13: The Pathogenesis of Diabetes Mellitus. Cerasi, E., Luft, R. (eds.). New York: John Wiley & Sons 1970, p. 237

47. Tattersall, R.B., Fajans, S.S.: A difference between the inheritance of classical juvenile-onset and maturity-onset type diabetes of young people. Diabetes 24, 44 (1975)

48. Thompson, M.W., Watson, E.M.: Inheritance of diabetes mellitus: analysis of family histories of 1,631 diabetics. Diabetes 1, 268 (1952)

49. Thompson, G.S.: Genetic factors in diabetes mellitus studied by the oral glucose tolerance test. J. Med. Genet. 2, 221 (1965)

50. Wilkerson, H.L.C., Krall, L.P.: Diabetes in a New England town. J. Am. Med. Ass. 135, 209 (1947)

2. The Genetics of Diabetes Mellitus – A Review of Family Data

N. E. SIMPSON

Some of the more recent approaches to the etiology of diabetes mellitus which may lead to new genetic hypotheses may turn the "geneticists' nightmare" of Neel *et al*. (42) into a dream. In this chapter, an attempt will be made to describe historically the development of genetic thought derived from family data on diabetes and thereby set the stage for more exciting things to be discussed later in this volume.

Ancient Reports

The ancient Hindu physicians were the first known to recognize that diabetes might be determined from inheritance or environment. Both Charaka and Sushruta wrote of the hereditary nature of diabetes in their Samhitase (9,56). It appears that there is considerable uncertainty as to when Sushruta and Charaka lived but it was probably in the period from 1000 B.C. to 500 A.D. (32). There is also uncertainty as to whether Sushruta or Charaka came first. The original Sanskrit writings are lost and it was after several revisions that the Sanskrit versions were translated into English. In the sixth lesson of the Charaka Samhita (9) it is said: "A person suffering from congenital Prameha owing to the fact of his birth from a father afflicted with Mahumeha cannot be cured for the primary defect in the seed"; Prameha being a general word for "diseased flow of urine" and Mahumeha the word for "honey urine" (32). Sushruta in his Samhita (56) went even further and taught of the Prameha: "This disease may be ascribed to two causes, such as the congenital (Sahaja) and that attributable to the use of injudicious diet. The first type (Sahaja) is due to a defect in the seeds of one's parents and the second is originated from the use of unwholesome food."

It was many centuries after the Hindu writings before other students of diabetes wrote of the hereditary nature of the disease, for example, Rondoletius in 1574 (48) wrote "I saw it three times in a daughter and her father, as if to say the disease were hereditary, or I may better say, because they were of the same temperament, namely, bilious"; Morton on 1696 (40) reported a family in which four of seven siblings were diabetic, and Naunyn in 1906 (41) stated that 18% of relatives of his diabetic patients had diabetes.

In the early part of this century other reports of single families with more than one diabetic followed (reviewed in 65). It is interesting to note at this point that Allen and Mitchell (2) discussed the testing of glucose tolerance in relatives and the role of infectious or toxic agents which might be accidental causes, in view of the recent work with viruses and diabetes (5,12,13,19). It was not until insulin had been in use for about a decade that pooling of data from large numbers of families began. By this time, Mendel's concept of the gene as the unit of heredity was firmly established and it was the vogue to pool data of phenotypes from

pedigrees and try to fit observed ratios into recessive, dominant or
X-linked recessive patterns of inheritance.

Pooled Family Data

In the beginning of the fourth decade of this century, pooled family
studies were reported. Cammidge (7,8) was the father of genetic heterogeneity and suggested dominant inheritance for mild diabetes and recessive inheritance for severe insulin-dependent diabetes. Pincus and
White (45) and Allan (1) in the same year and later Hanhart (22) proposed
the recessive hypothesis and genetic homogeneity. Pincus and White (45)
recognized the problem of a variable age at onset and introduced a statistical correction. Soon to follow were Levit and Pessikova (30) who
thought their data suggested a dominant mode of inheritance. Penrose
and Watson (44) proposed X-linked recessive inheritance but later re-
tracted their hypothesis to the autosomal recessive one.

Around the turn of the half-century, pedigree studies using more sophisticated statistical approaches continued to support the single gene
hypotheses. Harris (25,26) modified Cammidge's heterogeneity hypothesis;
homozygosity for early-onset and heterozygosity for late-onset for a
gene at the same locus, an hypothesis which was later taken up by Lamy *et
al.* (29). Hanhart (23,24) continued to support the recessive hypothesis
along with Steinberg and Wilder (55), Thompson and Watson (60), and
Grunner (21). Von Kries (62) upheld dominance and Barker *et al.* (3) supported the X-linked recessive hypothesis using evidence from a single
large family. Steinberg (53) at this time was by far the most influential,
and convincingly reanalysed the data of Harris (26), Lamy *et al.* (29)
and Von Kries (62) to show that their data fit the recessive hypothesis.
By the beginning of the seventh decade of this century the recessive
hypothesis was commonly interpreted as follows: "if both of your parents
are diabetic you have a 100% chance of developing the disease; if one
of your parents is a diabetic you have a 50% chance; and if neither parent is affected but you have an affected sib your risk is 25%," all
three risks being qualified by if you live long enough or if your genes
are fully penetrant, based, of course, on the single recessive gene
hypothesis.

Statistical Approaches

A variety of statistical approaches for analysing family data on diabetes
began to appear in the seventh decade. Lilienfeld (31) discredited the
method of Steinberg by applying it to data for the trait "medical student." He found that the data fit the single gene recessive hypothesis
with reduced penetrance because the trait occurred in the ratio 1:2:4
among the children from the three mating types of neither, one, and both
parents being doctors, respectively. One different approach was to use
the K-ratios developed by Penrose (43) and modified by Edwards (14). The
K-ratios are familial/population frequencies in first-degree relatives
which Simpson (49) corrected for age by using weighted means calculated
from data for each decade of life. Her data for first-degree relatives
of a clinical subgroup (early-onset, insulin-dependent, ketotic diabetics)
collected by questionnaire did not fit an autosomal single-gene hypothesis and suggested a multifactorial hypothesis for which the K-ratio for
sibs (there were not enough data for children and parents) was close to
that expected for multifactorial inheritance. Later, a sample including
intermediate and late-onset and a new sample of early-onset diabetics
collected by questionnaire by Simpson (50) was analyzed in the same manner,
to show that the familial/population frequency was greater in the early-

onset group (onset less than 20 years) than in either the intermediate-onset group (20-39 years) or the late-onset group (40 years and over) and rather by default multifactorial inheritance was again suggested (50). In the meantime, Barrai and Cann (4) using another statistical method of analysis; the maximum likelihood segregation analysis of Morton (37,38) on the early-onset data of Simpson (49) showed a fit with the recessive hypothesis albeit with low penetrance (about 25%). These authors admitted, however, that the low penetrance might be due to the effects of other genes. On the other hand, a Working Party (64) reported similar findings to those of Simpson (50) using the same analysis of K-ratios on different data collected by interview from Birmingham, England. It should be pointed out that "multifactorial inheritance" in relation to K-ratios was defined as an unspecified number of genes with small additive effects normally distributed with an arbitrarily chosen abrupt threshold beyond which an individual was defined as a "diabetic." Although both the Birmingham study (64) and the Canadian study (50) found that their K-ratios did not fit single gene hypotheses and were closer to the K expected for a multifactorial hypothesis they did not fit the latter particularly well either and the "bad fit" for any of the hypotheses could have been equally well explained by "genetic heterogeneity." In fact, this explanation was invoked to some extent from the results of both of these studies, which indicated that the familial/population frequency (K) decreased as the age of the index case increased. Mimura (34), using a similar analysis to that of Steinberg, in a small study of mostly late-onset diabetics also showed that his data did not fit a single gene hypothesis.

More recently Falconer (18) has estimated heritabilities of liability to diabetes from the Birmingham (64) and Canadian (50) data. It should be emphasized that this type of analysis is not designed to distinguish the type of inheritance but rather assumes that the multifactorial hypothesis as defined above is already proved and attempts to estimate the contribution to the trait or disease by the additive genetic variance in relation to the total phenotypic variance. Similar calculations had been performed by Simpson (51) and Smith et al. (52). They are reported in detail elsewhere in this volume (see Chapter 10, p. 88).

Finally, an additional attempt at distinguishing the type of inheritance has been made by Goodman and Chung (20). They have taken the Canadian data (51) and reanalyzed them using Morton's et al. (39) complex segregation analysis designed to discriminate between a generalized two-allele single locus model and a multifactorial one. For the rank 1 hypotheses the penetrance was assumed to be 100% and the frequency of sporadic cases was estimated from the data for the particular single gene hypothesis by an iterative process to give the best fit for the expected segregation ratio or the number of sporadic cases was assumed to be zero (no phenocopies) and the penetrance was estimated in a similar manner as for the frequency of sporadic cases. For the rank 2 hypotheses both the penetrance and the number of sporadic cases were similarly estimated simultaneously. As can be seen in Tables 1-3 for each of the three age groups (early, middle and late) the data fit several hypotheses although some better than others. For early onset the heritability is so high (99%) as to suggest a single gene hypothesis but when the penetrance was assumed to be 100% the data only fit the recessive hypothesis with an estimate of sporadic cases of 78%. On the other hand, when no sporadic cases were assumed the data fit the three single gene hypotheses equally well with about 15% penetrance for the recessive and additive hypotheses and about 8% for the dominant hypothesis. For the rank 2 hypotheses, the data fit only the dominant hypothesis with estimates for penetrance being about 13% and the number of sporadic cases being about 47%. The last hypothesis may not be unreasonable; the proportion of sporadic cases may indeed be

Table 1. Complex Segregation Analysis for Diabetes when Onset Age is 0-19 years

	Hypotheses	x^{2a}	D.F.	Estimated Gene Frequency
Rank 1	Recessive			
	100% penetrance	58.1	63	.013
	no phenocopies	13.0	63	.075
	Additive			
	100% penetrance	–	–	–
	no phenocopies	12.3	63	.005
	Dominant			
	100% penetrance	–	–	–
	no phenocopies	12.2	63	.005
Rank 2	Dominant	13.3	62	.002
	Multifactorial [.99][b]	21.22	63	

[a]x^2 for maximum likelihood. [b]Heritability.
Modified from Goodman and Chung (28).
Rank 1 = either penetrance or the proportion of sporadic cases was estimated (see text).
Rank 2 = penetrance and the proportion of sporadic cases was estimated (see text).

Table 2. Complex Segregation Analysis for Diabetes when Onset Age is 20-39 Years

	Hypotheses	x^{2a}	D.F.	Estimated Gene Frequency
Rank 1	Recessive			
	100% penetrance	50.7	78	.001
	no phenocopies	30.3	78	.139
	Additive			
	100% penetrance	49.4	78	.019
	no phenocopies	34.1	78	.140
	Dominant			
	100% penetrance	–	–	–
	no phenocopies	34.4	78	.016
Rank 2	Recessive	27.3	77	.066
	Dominant	28.0	77	.003
	Multifactorial [.81][b]	28.6	78	

[a,b]See footnotes, Table 1.

Table 3. Complex Segregation Analysis for Diabetes when Onset Age is $\geq$ 40 Years

	Hypotheses	x^{2a}	D.F.	Estimated Gene Frequency
Rank 1	Recessive			
	100% penetrance	198.1	86	.076
	no phenocopies	98.9	86	.316
	Additive			
	100% penetrance	190.1	86	.012
	no phenocopies	123.6	86	.068
	Dominant			
	100% penetrance	–	–	–
	no phenocopies	144.6	86	.065
Rank 2	Recessive	92.8	85	.251
	Additive	88.6	85	.029
	Dominant	91.2	85	.026
	Multifactorial [.66][b]	98.04	86	

[a,b]See footnotes, Table 1.

about 50% (see Chapter 12, p.106) and the dominant gene may be the HL-A types which predispose to the early-onset of diabetes in some families but not all of the individuals with the specific HL-A type develop the condition (see Chapter 12, p.106). For the middle and late groups, a number of single gene hypotheses fit as well the multifactorial one. Lack of a good fit could result from inadequacies in the data which have been discussed and appreciated (50) but perhaps more importantly, from the fact that diabetes is likely determined by more than one gene; not all diabetics have the same genes for the disease and there may well be different environmental agents responsible for its manifestation. Such a hypothesis might be better stated as "genetic heterogeneity" rather than "multifactorial" which has a precise meaning to the geneticist.

Genetic Studies Designed to Identify the Diabetic Genotype

Many investigators have been convinced that no amount of sophistication of statistical methods is going to solve the genetics of diabetes and we must get around the lack of precision of the diagnosis in some way. From the foregoing section the statistical approach has certainly not been very fruitful to date. Since diabetics have impaired glucose tolerance, this was the natural place to look first and indeed, Fajans and Conn (17) and more recently Taylor *et al.* (58) and Köbberling *et al.* (28) found that impaired glucose tolerance had a much higher frequency among the relatives of diabetics than in controls. These findings stimulated inves- tigations of glucose tolerance; some studied glucose tolerance in chil- dren of conjugal diabetics using various modifications of the glucose tolerance test (oral, intravenous, and steroid-induced) and considered the age of their children and projected an expected frequency among the children if they lived to be elderly. For example, West (63) and Post (46) considered that 100% of the children would have impaired glucose tol- erance if they lived long enough; compatible with the recessive hypothesis whereas others found that the projected frequency fell short of the 100%. Cooke *et al.* (11) predicted 25% eventually, Kahn *et al.* (27) predicted 30% by 85 years of age and Tattersall and Fajans (57) 60% by age 60. These findings could be interpreted to support either the multifactorial hypo- thesis or could be explained by genetic heterogeneity.

Family studies of glucose tolerance in ethnic groups other than white have supported the various genetic hypotheses. Steinberg *et al.* (54) again supported the recessive hypothesis from a study of glucose toler- ance in Pima Indians from North America. In this ethnic group, in which there is a high frequency of impaired glucose tolerance, when a maximum likelihood method of classifying genotypes from a bimodal distribution of glucose tolerance was used and these corrected data subjected to gene- tic analysis, the data fit the recessive hypothesis. Using a similar approach, Elston *et al.* (16) concluded that impaired glucose tolerance in Seminole Indians of Oklahoma was best explained by the hypothesis of recessive inheritance although the data also fit a dominant allele hypo- thesis. The data for Seminole Indians in Florida, however, did not fit any mendelian hypothesis (16). On the other hand, Neel *et al.* (42), Thompson (59) and Mimura *et al.* (35,36) analyzed family data on glucose tolerance in Caucasians in the United States, Britain, and Japan , and proposed a multifactorial hypothesis. Braunsteiner *et al.* (6) using tolbutamide tolerance tests on parents of early-onset patients concluded that parents were heterozygous and the children homozygous for a gene at the same locus, a hypothesis earlier proposed by Harris (26). The hypotheses from studies of the inheritance of "impaired glucose tolerance" did not agree with each other any better than those from studies of clinical diabetes.

Attempts to identify the genotype more directly have utilized studies of the destruction, production, or rate of release of insulin. Vallance-Owen (61) proposed that a high level of synalbumin, the insulin antagonist, represented the diabetic genotype and that high levels were dominantly inherited, whereas Ehrlich and Martin (15) thought that adult diabetics were heterozygous for a gene for increased synalbumin, and juvenile diabetics were homozygous for the same gene. Few people, however, were able to reproduce the synalbumin assay.

Genetic Heterogeneity

More and more evidence is accumulating that there is genetic heterogeneity for diabetes. If there are different genes which determine the susceptibility of diabetes, it is not surprising that attempts to establish a pattern of inheritance from pooled data consisting of many families have failed. There have always been "lumpers" and "splitters" when trying to classify disease (33). Joslin exerted a strong influence as a "lumper" but more recently Clarke (10) and many others have advocated clinical subdivisions of diabetes. Some attempts were made to subdivide the data by age at onset and clinical severity in the genetic studies which have been described but better ways of looking for genetic heterogeneity are at last emerging and will be discussed below.

References

1. Allan, W.: Heredity in diabetes. Ann. Intern. Med. 6, 1272 (1933)

2. Allen, F.M., Mitchell, J.W.: A case of hereditary diabetes. Arch. Intern. Med. 25, 648 (1920)

3. Barker, O.B., Commons, R.R., Shelton, E.K.: Sex-linked juvenile diabetes mellitus. J. Clin. Endoc. 2, 608 (1951)

4. Barrai, I., Cann, H.M.: Segregation analysis of juvenile diabetes mellitus. J. Med. Genet. 2, 8 (1965)

5. Boucher, D.W., Notkins, A.L.: Virus-induced diabetes mellitus. I. Hyperglycemia and hypoinsulinemia in mice infected with encephalomyocarditis virus. J. Exper. Med. 137, 1226 (1973)

6. Braunsteiner, H., Hansen, W., Jung, A., Seiler, A.: Latent diabetes in the parents of juvenile diabetics. German Med. Monthly 11, 227 (1966)

7. Cammidge, P.J.: Diabetes mellitus and heredity. Brit. Med. J. 2, 738 (1928)

8. Cammidge, P.J.: Heredity as a factor in the aetiology of diabetes mellitus. Lancet 1, 393 (1934)

9. Charaka Samhita: Lesson VI, part XXXVII. Translated into English by Kaviratna, A.C. Calcuta: Charkravarti and Kaviratna, 1905, p. 1206

10. Clarke, C.A.: Genetic aspects of diabetes. In: Diabetes mellitus. Duncan, L.J.P. (ed.). Edinburgh: Pfizer Medical Monographs 1966, Vol. I, p. 103

11. Cooke, A.M., Fitzgerald, M., Malins, J.M., Pyke, D.A.: Diabetes in children of diabetic couples. Brit. Med. J. 2, 674 (1966)

12. Graighead, J.E., Higgins, D.A.: Genetic influences affecting the occurrence of a diabetes mellitus-like disease in mice infected with the encephalomyocarditis virus. J. Exper. Med. 139, 414 (1974)

13. Graighead, J.E., Steinke, J.: Diabetes mellitus-like syndrome in mice infected with encephalomyocarditis virus. Amer. J. Path. 63, 119 (1971)

14. Edwards, J.H.: The simulation of mendelism. Acta Genet. 10, 63 (1960)

15. Ehrlich, R.M., Martin, J.M.: Presence of synalbumin antagonist in siblings of diabetic children. Diabetes 15, 400 (1966)

16. Elston, R.C., Namboodiri, K.K., Nino, H.V., Pollitzer, W.S.: Studies on blood and urine glucose in Seminole Indians: indications for segregation of a major gene. Amer. J. Hum. Genet. 26, 13 (1974)

17. Fajans, S.S., Conn, J.W.: An approach to the prediction of diabetes mellitus by modification of the glucose tolerance test with cortisone. Diabetes 3, 296 (1954)

18. Falconer, D.S.: The inheritance of liability to disease with variable age of onset with particular reference to diabetes mellitus. Ann. Hum. Genet. (Lond.) 31, 1 (1967)

19. Gamble, D.R., Kinsley, M.L.: Viral antibodies in diabetes mellitus. Brit. Med. J. 3, 627 (1969)

20. Goodman, M.J., Chung, C.S.: Diabetes mellitus: discrimination between single locus and multifactorial models of inheritance. Clin. Genet. 8, 66-74 (1975)

21. Grunnet, J.: Heredity in diabetes mellitus. Opera ex Domo Biological Hereditariae Humanae. Universitatis Hafniensis 39. Copenhagen: Munksgaard, 1957

22. Hanhart, E.: Nachweis der ganz vorwiegend einfach rezessiven Vererbung des Diabetes mellitus. Erbarzt 6, 5 (1939)

23. Hanhart, E.: Neue Beiträge zur Kenntnis der Vererbung des Diabetes mellitus. Helv. Med. Acta 14, 243 (1947)

24. Hanhart, E.: Neue Forschungsergebnisse über die Vererbung des Diabetes mellitus sowie Anhaltspunkte für seine primäre Genee in Strammhirn. Arch. Julius Klausstift. 25, 586 (1950)

25. Harris, H.: Incidence of parental consanguinity in diabetes mellitus. Ann. Eugen (Lond.) 14, 293 (1949)

26. Harris, H.: Familial distribution of diabetes: a study of relatives of 1241 diabetic propositi. Ann. Eugen (Lond.) 15, 95 (1950)

27. Kahn, C.B., Soeldner, J.S., Gleason, R.E., Rojas, L., Camerini-Davalos, R.A., Marble, A.: Clinical and chemical diabetes in offspring of diabetic couples. New Engl. J. Med. 281, 343 (1969)

28. Köbberling, J., Appels, A., Köbberling, G., Creutzfeldt, W.: Glucose tolerance tests in 727 first-degree relatives of maturity-onset diabetics. Germ. Med. Monthly 14, 290 (1969)

29. Lamy, M., Frézal, J., de Grouchy, J.: Résultats d'une enquête sur l'hérédité du diabète sucré. Extr. Rev. Franc. Etude Clin. Biol. 2, 907 (1957)

30. Levit, S.G., Pessikova, L.N.: The genetics of diabetes mellitus. Trudy Med. Genet. Inst. Gorky 3, 132 (1934)

31. Lilienfeld, A.H.: Methodological problem in treating the recessive genetic hypothesis in human disease. Amer. J. Public Health 49, 199 (1959)

32. Major, R.H.: A History of Medicine. Springfield, I 11. Chas. C. Thomas, 1954, Vol.I

33. McKusick, V.A.: The nosology of genetic disease. In: Medical Genetics. A Hospital Practice Text. McKusick, V.A., Claiborne, R. (eds.). New York: H.P. Publishing, 1973

34. Mimura, G.: The mode of inheritance of diabetes mellitus in Japan. Kumamoto Med. J. 15, 154 (1962)

35. Mimura, G., Oshiro, S., Koganemaru, K., Haraguchi, Y., Jinnouchi, T., Hashiguchi, H.: Studies on the heredity of diabetes mellitus in Japan. I. Inheritance of the fasting blood sugar value in Uto and Tomiai inhabitants. Kumamoto Med. J. 17, 45 (1964)

36. Mimura, G., Oshiro, S., Koganemaru, K., Haraguchi, Y., Jinnouchi, T., Hashiguchi, J.: Studies on the heredity of diabetes mellitus in Japan. II. Inheritance of the fasting blood sugar value and the blood sugar value two hours after meals in Uto and Tomiai inhabitants. Kumamoto Med. J. 17, 50 (1964)

37. Morton, N.E.: Segregation analysis in human genetics. Science 127, 79 (1958)

38. Morton, N.E.: Genetic tests under incomplete ascertainment. Amer. J. Hum. Genet. 11, 1 (1959)

39. Morton, N.E., Lew, R.: Complex segregation analysis. Amer. J. Hum. Genet. 23, 602 (1971)

40. Morton, R.: Opera Medica. Donatum Donati, Amstelodami 1696, p. 22

41. Naunyn, B.: Der Diabetes mellitus. 2 Vienna: A.A. Holder, 1906

42. Neel, J.V., Fajans, S.S., Conn, J.W., Davidson, R.T.: Diabetes mellitus. In: Genetics and the Epidemiology of Chronic Disease. U.S. Public Health Service Publication, 1163, 105 (1965)

43. Penrose, L.S.: The genetical background of common diseases. Acta Genet. 4, 257 (1953)

44. Penrose, L.S., Watson, E.M.: A sex-linked tendency in familial diabetes. Proc. Amer. Diabetes Assoc. 5, 163 (1945)

45. Pincus, G., White, P.: On the inheritance of diabetes mellitus. I. An analysis of 675 family histories. Amer. J. Med. Sc. 186, 1 (1933)

46. Post, R.H.: An approach to the question, does all diabetes depend upon a single genetic locus? Diabetes 11, 56 (1962)

47. Rimoin, D.L.: Inheritance in diabetes mellitus. Med. Clin. N. Amer. 55, 807 (1971)

48. Rondeletius, G.: Methodus curandorum omnium morborum corporis humani in tres libros distincta, 1574

49. Simpson, N.E.: The genetics of diabetes: a study of 233 families of juvenile diabetics. Ann. Hum. Genet. (Lond.) 26, 1 (1962)

50. Simpson, N.E.: Multifactorial inheritance: a possible hypothesis for diabetes. Diabetes 13, 462 (1964)

51. Simpson, N.E.: Heritabilities of liability to diabetes when sex and age at onset are considered. Ann. Hum. Genet. (Lond.) 32, 283 (1969)

52. Smith, C., Falconer, D.S., Duncan, L.J.P.: A statistical and genetical study of diabetes. Ann. Hum. Genet. (Lond.) 35, 281 (1972)

53. Steinberg, A.G.: Heredity in diabetes mellitus. Diabetes 10, 269 (1961)

54. Steinberg, A.G., Rushfort, N.B., Bennett, P.H., Burch, T.A., Miller, M.: On the genetics of diabetes mellitus. In: Pathogenesis of Diabetes Mellitus. Cerasi, E., Luft, R. (eds.). Milano: Casa Editrice "Il Ponte", 1970

55. Steinberg, A.G., Wilder, R.M.: Genetics of diabetes. Amer. J. Hum. Genet. 4, 113 (1952)

56. Sushruta Samhita, 2nd. ed. Translated into English by Bhishagratna, K.K. Varanasi, India: The Chowkhamba Sanskrit Series, Vol. II, p. 372

57. Tattersall, R.B., Fajans, S.S.: Prevalence of diabetes and glucose intolerance in 199 offspring of 37 conjugal diabetic parents. Diabetes 24, 452 (1975)

58. Taylor, K.W., Sheldon, J., Pyke, D.A., Oakley, W.G.: Glucose tolerance and serum insulin in the unaffected first-degreee relatives of diabetics. Brit. Med. J. 4, 22 (1967)

59. Thompson, G.S.: Genetic factors in diabetes mellitus studied by the oral glucose tolerance test. J. Med. Genet. 2, 221 (1965)

60. Thompson, M.W., Watson, E.M.: The inheritance of diabetes mellitus, an analysis of the family histories of 1631 diabetics. Diabetes 1, 268 (1952)

61. Vallance-Owen. J.: The inheritance of essential diabetes mellitus from studies of the synalbumin insulin antagonist. Diabetologia 2, 248 (1966)

62. Von Kries, I.: Beitrag zur Genetik des Diabetes mellitus. Z. Kont-Lehre 31, 406 (1953)

63. West, K.M.: Response to cortisone in prediabetes glucose- and steroid-glucose tolerance in subjects whose parents are both diabetic. Diabetes 9, 379 (1960)

64. Working Party of the College of General Practitioners: The family history of diabetes. Brit. Med. J. 1, 960 (1965)

65. Wright, I.S.: Hereditary and familial diabetes mellitus. Amer. J. Med. Sci. 182, 484 (1931)

3. The Genetics of Diabetes Mellitus – A Review of Twin Studies

U. LANGENBECK and G. JÖRGENSEN

Twin studies are "the most general method for examining the problem, if and how much phenotypic differences in man are caused by genetic differences" (45). Classic twin research started in 1924 with the work of Siemens (32) and had its heyday in the 1930s. Presently, some human geneticists seem to be rather tired of twin research, or, as C. Smith (36) states: "Different authors collect their data in different ways, present their results in different forms, use different methods of analysis, and use different forms of genetic interpretation. Thus the results and their interpretations are usually not comparable in different studies, and often they are not meaningful in genetic terms." We have the impression that the situation is a little better.

Specifically it will be shown that analysis of discordance in monozygotic (MZ) twins should yield further insights into the mechanisms of pathogenesis of diabetes mellitus by defining the parts played by heredity and environment, respectively. It was found quite early that diabetes mellitus shows familial aggregation. The earliest reports on diabetes mellitus in twins were those of May (24), Curtis (5), Peck (28), Pannhorst (27), Umber (44), Watson (47), White et al. (48,49), Steiner (39), and Hermann and Jentsch (16).

These studies, covering the period 1914-1937, demonstrated the importance of genetic factors in the causation of diabetes mellitus, concordance being considerably higher in monocygotic (MZ) than in dicygotic (DZ) twins.
The first large unselected twin series, which was made up from a group of 85,000 diabetics, was that of Hildegard Then Bergh from Munich (42). In 1938 she reported on 46 MZ and 87 DZ, of which 36 MZ and 50 DZ could be studied clinically and with an oral glucose tolerance test. Clinical or absolute concordance was observed in 17/36 MZ and 9/50 DZ twin pairs. Concordance after glucose load was found in 30/36 MZ and 18/50 DZ twin pairs.

Interestingly, Then Bergh found no discordance after glucose load in MZ twins aged over 43 years. She interpreted this observation as being due to complete manifestation of the hereditary trait ("absolute heredity") in MZ twins (43).
Whereas Then Bergh's study gained wide recognition in the USA through a small letter of a correspondent in the Journal of the American Medical Association (3), another German twin study also published in 1938, namely that of Lemser (19), went by almost unnoticed. He found concordance in 9/12 MZ and 3/14 DZ. The work of Lemser is particularly interesting through his attempt to analyze the environmental peristatic factors leading to the expression of the hereditary trait or the prevention of its expression in MZ twins. A main factor according to his observations was the number of pregnancies.

More recent studies could not find such a relation, possibly due to the
reduced number of pregnancies in our times. Lemser (18-20) also studied
the time of discordance in MZ twins pairs. Of 13 concordant MZ pairs 7
became concordant in the same year, 11 within 4 years, 12 within 10 years,
and all of them within 13.5 years. One MZ pair with juvenile diabetes
was found discordant for 11 years, also with respect to glucose tolerance.
This observation lead Lemser to ask: "Can the hereditary trait *(Erbanlage)*
for diabetes remain dormant?" (18), a question in which there is renewed
interest as a result of the recent twin studies from the King's Hospital
London (23,40,41). In Table 1 the major classic twin studies are combined.

Table 1. Concordance rates for overt diabetes (uncorrected)

	Ref.	MZ	DZ
Then Bergh, 1938	(42)	17/36	9/50
Lemser, 1938	(19)	9/12	3/14
White and Pincus, 1946	(49)	16/33	2/63
Harvald and Hauge, 1963	(14, 15)	36/76	22/238
Gottlieb and Root, 1968	(11)	9/30	2/60
		87/187	38/425
		±46.5%	=8.9%

The ratio of concordance in monocygotic compared to dicygotic twins is
about 4.9, a value in the range encountered in diseases with alleged
multifactorial inheritance. Clearly more criteria are needed to settle
this important question. It has been demonstrated by C. Smith (34,35)
that twin studies may yield estimates of heritability of liability to
disease which should conform with estimates from family studies if the
model of a multifactorial system with additive components is to apply.

In two studies (8,33) heritability (h^2) was found to decrease at higher
ages of onset. This observation and the observed differences in concordance rates of MZ twins with early- and late-onset diabetes (11,14,41,42)
cannot be brought into accordance with a model of multifactorial inheritance. Reported heritabilities and observed concordance rates for late-
onset diabetes require incredibly high incidences in the general population (cf. 34).

It may well be that within the multifactorial system for diabetes some
recessive genes work together with genes of additive action. The slight
increase in consanguinity observed by Harris (13) and Lestradet *et al.*
(21) among parents of juvenile diabetics could well be used in favor
of such a hypothesis. (Recessive genes in polygenic systems have been
brought to light by Morton *et al.* (25) through analysis of interracial
crosses). Alternately, we can conclude that diabetes in MZ twins is
something special and different.

A last classic aspect of twin studies in diabetes mellitus is the observation of Tattersall and Pyke (41) that familial incidence of juvenile
diabetes is higher in families of concordant MZ twins than in those of
discordant twins. This situation was theoretically envisioned by Luxenburger (22) in 1935 and could mean that in discordant MZ pairs diabetes
has a predominantly exogenous cause.

An important environmental factor for the etiology of juvenile diabetes is also suggested by the biochemical discordancies in clinically discordant juvenile diabetic MZ twins (11,38,40).

Presently under discussion is a viral hypothesis (9,4).
The association of juvenile diabetes with the tissue antigens HL-A 8 and W 15 (26) also speaks in favor of an infectious hypothesis.

The situation could be somewhat similar to tuberculosis in MZ twins where the prognosis of discordant tuberculosis is much better than for the concordant one (7), obviously because a more resistant genotype is involved in the former.

From these data it may be predicted that the association of HL-A 8 and W 15 antigens and diabetes mellitus will be found more pronounced in MZ twins concordant for juvenile diabetes than for juvenile diabetes in general.

Future twin research should be carried out having in mind the working hypothesis of genetic heterogeneity of diabetes mellitus. Several lines of evidence indicate that insulin-dependent and insulin-independent forms of diabetes are at least partially different in etiological and genetic terms. Among others the family studies of Köbberling (17), the studies of tissue antigens (26), and the twin studies of Tattersall and Pyke (41) must be mentioned in this context. Yet, the heterogeneity is not absolute as has been shown in the statistical analysis of C. Smith et al. (37). Unfortunately, their most realistic "related model" cannot be treated mathematically. In more general terms such a model may be called "overlapping multifactorial systems" implying that some factors are common to both early- and late-onset diabetes. Clearly, genetic syndromes with glucose intolerance should not be included in a twin series.

If under these premises it turns out that late-onset diabetes almost always runs concordant in MZ twins, as suggested by the data of Tattersall and Pike (41), twin studies will not be able to add new information as to the causation of late-onset or insulin-independent diabetes.

But at least in juvenile, insulin-dependent diabetes the potentially powerful instrument of analysis of discordance in MZ twins should yield relevant data for a causal analysis of diabetes mellitus. Physiologic and biochemical analyses of discordance in MZ diabetic twins have been reported by Cerasi and Luft (2), Pyke et al. (29,31), Wahren et al. (46), Gottlieb et al. (11,12), Daweke et al. (6), Goecke and Grote (10), and Bivens and Feldman (1).

The main problem which emerged from these studies is how long MZ juvenile diabetic twins can remain discordant and whether or not discordant twin siblings are so-called prediabetics. A solution to this question has important implications for possible preventive measures, a fact realized by Lemser in 1938 (20).

References

1. Bivens, C.H., Feldman, J.M.: Metabolic and endocrine studies in identical diabetic twins. Arch. Int. Med. 134, 639 (1974)

2. Cerasi, E., Luft, R.: Insulin response to glucose infusion in diabetic and nondiabetic monozygotic twin pairs. Genetic control of insulin response? Acta endocrinol. 55, 330 (1967)

3. Correspondent: The genetic aspects of diabetes mellitus. J. A. M. A 112, 1091 (1939)

4. Graighead, J.E., Higgins, D.A.: Genetic influences affecting the occurrence of a diabetes mellitus-like disease in mice infected with the encephalomyocarditis virus. J. Exp. Med. 139, 414 (1974)

5. Curtis, W.S.: Diabetes in twins. J. Amer. Med. Ass. 92, 952 (1929)

6. Daweke, H., Grote, W., Gries, F.A., Liebermeister, H.: Zur Genetik des Diabetes mellitus: Glucosetoleranz, Seruminsulin und freie Fettsäuren bei eineiigen Zwillingen. Dtsch. Med. Wschr. 95, 983 (1970)

7. Diehl, K., v.Verschuer, O.: Zwillingstuberkulose. Jena: Gustav Fischer, 1933. Cited by F. Vogel, 1961

8. Falconer, D.S.: The inheritance of liability to diseases with variable age of onset, with particular reference to diabetes mellitus. Ann. Hum. Genet. (Lond.) 31, 1 (1967)

9. Gamble, D.R., Taylor, K.W., Cumming, H.: Coxsackie viruses and diabetes mellitus. Brit. Med. J. 4, 260 (1973)

10. Goecke, T., Grote, W.: Metabolic research in MZ twins with diabetes mellitus. Progress report (abstract). Acta genet. med. gemell. 23, 45 (1974)

11. Gottlieb, M.S., Root, H.F.: Diabetes mellitus in twins. Diabetes 17, 693 (1968)

12. Gottlieb, M.S., Soeldner, J.S., Kyner, J.L., Gleason, R.E.: Oral glucose-stimulated insulin release in nondiabetic twin siblings of diabetic twins. Diabetes 23, 684 (1974)

13. Harris, H.: The incidence of parental consanguinity in diabetes mellitus. Ann. Eugen. 14, 292 (1947-1949)

14. Harvald, B., Hauge, M.: Selection in diabetes in modern society. Acta med. Scand. 173, 459 (1963)

15. Harvald, B., Hauge, M.: Hereditary factors elucidated by twin studies. In: Genetics and the epidemiology of chronic diseases. Neel, J.V., Shaw, M.W., Schull, W.J. (eds.). Washington, D.C.: U.S. Dept. HEW, 1965, p.61

16. Hermann, M., Jentsch, F.-R.: Über das Auftreten von Diabetes mellitus (konkordant) und Ostitis fibrosa (diskordant) bei einem eineiigen Zwillingspaar. Erbarzt 4, 48 (1937)

17. Köbberling, J.: Studies on the genetic heterogeneity of diabetes mellitus. Diabetologia 7, 46 (1971)

18. Lemser, H.: Kann eine Erbanlage für Diabetes latent sein? (Zwillingsbeobachtungen) Erbarzt 5, 33 (1938)

19. Lemser, H.: Zur Erb- und Rassenpathologie des Diabetes mellitus. I. Über den Einfluß von Erbe und Umwelt beim Diabetes mellitus. Arch. f. Rassen- u. Gesellschaftsbiol. 32, 481 (1938)

20. Lemser, H.: Untersuchungsergebnisse an diabetischen Zwillingen. Münchener Med. Wschr. 85, 1811 (1938)

21. Lestradet, H., Battistelli, F., Combier, E., Giron, B.J.: L'hérédité du diabète insulinodépendant. Nouv. Presse Méd. 3, 1077 (1974)

22. Luxenburger, H.: Untersuchungen an schizophrenen Zwillingen und ihren Geschwistern zur Prüfung der Realität von Manifestationsschwankungen. Zschr. Ges. Neurol. Psychiat. 154, 351 (1935)

23. Malins, J.M., Cassar, J., Pyke, D.A.: Diabetes in a pair of identical twins. Diabetes 19, 878 (1970)

24. May, O.: The significance of diabetic family history in life insurance. Lancet I, 679 (1914)

25. Morton, N.E., Chung, C.S., Mi, M.P.: Genetics of interracial crosses in Hawaii. Monographs in Human Genetics. Basel, New York: S. Karger, 1967, Vol. III

26. Nerup, J., Platz, P., Andersen, O.O., Christy, M., Lyngsøe, J., Poulsen, J.E., Ryder, L.B., Thomsen, M., Nielsen, L.S., Svejgaard, A.: HL-A antigens and diabetes mellitus. Lancet 2, 864 (1974)

27. Pannhorst, R.: Zwillingsuntersuchungen bei Diabetes mellitus. Dtsch. Med. Wschr. 60, 1950 (1934)

28. Peck, F.B.: Diabetes in twins. J. Mich. St. Med. Soc. 32, 359 (1933). Cited by H. Harris, 1947-1949

29. Pyke, D.A., Taylor, K.W.: Glucose tolerance and serum insulin in unaffected identical twins of diabetics. Brit. Med. J. 4, 21 (1967)

30. Pyke, D.A., Cassar, J., Todd, J., Taylor, K.W.: Glucose tolerance and serum insulin in identical twins of diabetics. Brit. Med. J. 4, 649 (1970)

31. Pyke, D.A., Tattersall, R.B.: Diabetic retinopathy in identical twins. Diabetes 22, 613 (1973)

32. Siemens, H.W.: Die Zwillingspathologie. Ihre Bedeutung, ihre Methodik, ihre bisherigen Ergebnisse. Berlin: Springer, 1924

33. Simpson, N.E.: Heritabilities of liability to diabetes when sex and age at onset are considered. Ann. Hum. Genet. (Lond.) 32, 283 (1969)

34. Smith, C.: Heritability of liability and concordance in monozygous twins. Ann. Hum. Genet. (Lond.) 34, 85 (1970)

35. Smith, C.: Correlation in liability among relatives and concordance in twins. Further results. Human Heredity 22, 97 (1972)

36. Smith, C.: Concordance in twins: Methods and interpretation. Amer. J. Hum. Genet. 26, 454 (1974)

37. Smith, C., Falconer, D.S., Duncan, L.J.P.: A statistical and genetical study of diabetes. II. Heritability of liability. Ann. Hum. Genet. (Lond.) 35, 281 (1972)

38. Soeldner, J.S., Johansen, K., Gleason, R.E., Smith, T.M.: Serum insulin and growth hormone responses to four types of tests in young monozygotic twins with a juvenile diabetic twinmate (abstract). Diabetes 23, 350 (1974)

39. Steiner, F.: Untersuchungen zur Frage der Erblichkeit des Diabetes Mellitus. Dtsch. Arch. Klin. Med. 178, 497 (1936)

40. Tattersall, R.B., Pyke, D.A.: Discordant identical twins. IV. Diabetes mellitus. Practitioner 209, 569 (1972)

41. Tattersall, R.B., Pyke, D.A.: Diabetes in identical twins. Lancet 2, 1120 (1972)

42. Then Bergh, H.: Die Erbbiologie des Diabetes mellitus. Vorläufiges Ergebnis der Zwillingsuntersuchungen. Arch. Rassen- und Gesellschaftsbiol. 32, 289 (1938)

43. Then Bergh, H.: Zur Frage der psychischen und neurologischen Erscheinungen bei Diabeteskranken und deren Verwandten. Zschr. ges. Neurol. Psychiat. 165, 278 (1939)

44. Umber, F.: Diabetes bei drei eineiigen Zwillingspaaren. Dtsch. Med. Wschr. 60, 544 (1934)

45. Vogel, F.: Lehrbuch der allgemeinen Humangenetik. Berlin, Göttingen, Heidelberg: Springer, 1961

46. Wahren, J., Felig, P., Cerasi, E., Luft, R., Hendler, R.: Splanchnic glucose production and its regulation in healthy monozygotic twins of diabetics. Clinical Science 44, 493 (1973)

47. Watson, E.M.: Diabetes mellitus in twins. Canad. Med. Ass. J. 31, 61 (1934)

48. White, P., Joslin, E.P., Pincus, G.: The inheritance of diabetes. J. Amer. Med. Assoc. 103, 105 (1934)

49. White, P., Pincus, G.: Heredity in diabetes. In: The Treatment in Diabetes Mellitus. 8th ed. Joslin, E.P., Root, H.F., White, P., Marble, A., Bailey, C.C.. Philadelphia: Lea & Febiger, 1946, p. 56

4. Unsolved and Unsolvable Problems in Studying the Genetics of Diabetes

J. H. EDWARDS

The approximate nature of the relationship of curves and lines to natural phenomena is easily misunderstood by those who lack any experience with both things and numbers and, in biology, has led to a false exactitude, the basic realities being concealed, but not improved, by a baroque encrustation of numerical results implying an exactitude which is, in principle, both unattainable and irrelevant, and which has no basic relationship to the supporting structure.

The Gaussian curve, by definition, is the product of numerous small and independent sources of variation. Where the sources are not small (as in the effects of strong genetic determinants), or not independent (as in the transmission of genetic units in small numbers of blocks, the chromosomal segments), or where there is a non-linear effect of numerous independent units (as those defining environment and heredity), the conditions of summation are not fulfilled and, if the basis of summation is not satisfied, it is impossible to dissect the consequences of numerous events into distinct and additive causes.

If we draw a normal curve or, as in Figure 1, a family of three normal curves, and their sum, which is not a normal curve, we can at once see the way in which distributions of overlapping normal curves can lead to a composite curve which resembles a normal curve. In the limiting case of small differences the composite curve is normal. We can also see the beauty of these curves, a beauty rarely revealed as many textbooks and articles are illustrated by drawings with little pretence to normality. (I certainly claim no exemption from this indolent disregard for both truth and beauty). The shoulders of the curve are very straight - a point exploited by Gauss in his two-coil magnetometer in which the two distributions of magnetic fields with their centres two standard deviations apart provided a uniform magnetic field. It is unfortunate that those who search for antimodes in numerical distributions rarely appreciate that an antimode cannot be presented by extensive data unless the two distributions are this much distinct, although fortuitous antimodes are common in limited data.

We can approach the study of variation from the classical Gaussian viewpoint of defining plausible basic units and building them into a coherent and plausible whole, a view exemplified by the deductive approaches of Euclid, Descartes, Newton, Laplace, and Gauss, and, more recently, the molecular biologists, and usually termed the classical or Cartesian view. Or we can work backwards from consequences to determinants by the inductive or somatic approach which Gauss associated unfavourably with the scientific wanderings of Goethe, and which comprise a loosely knit federation of conventional approaches now associated with the hypothetico-deductive approach, statistical significance, and Karl Popper.

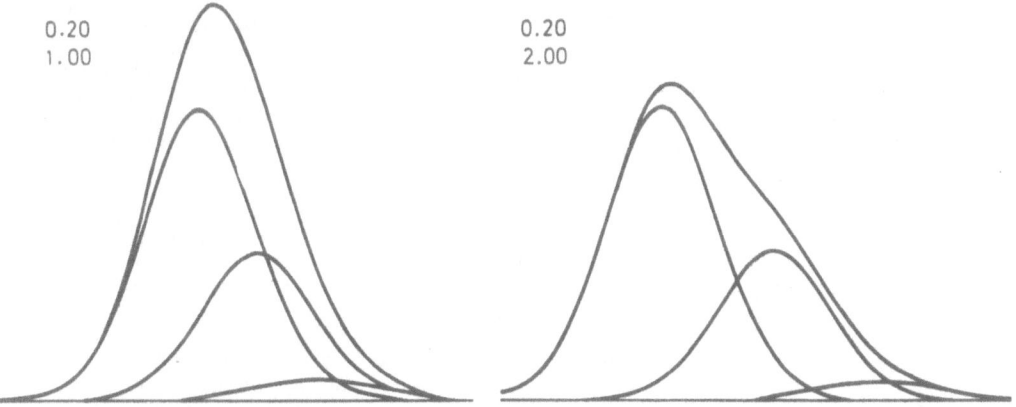

Fig. 1. Showing triplets of normal curves, with equally spaced mean, equal variance,
and areas proportional to the proportions of the genotypes for a diallelic locus
(lower number is distance between means, upper is proportion of rarer allele)

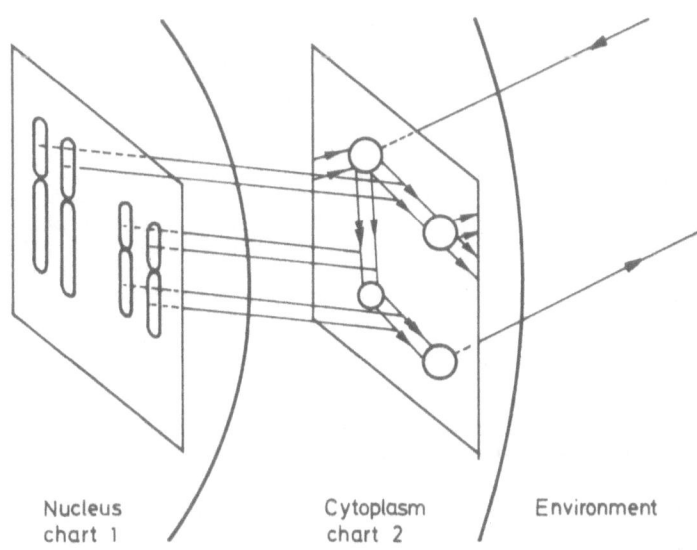

Nucleus	Cytoplasm	Environment
chart 1	chart 2	

Fig. 2. Diagram of structural and functional determinants of variation

These are extreme views and, while both are, in their extreme forms,
sterile, in that one cannot extend knowledge and the other cannot create
knowledge, they bound the spectrum of productive enquiry.

In 1975, we may approach the extent of relevant enquiry by genetical methods, with special reference to diabetes, by reference to a map on which
we must base our studies (Figure 2). The genetical map takes the form of
two related charts, the structural chart specifying the nature and position of the determinants, which are within the nucleus, or with a slight
exaggeration, are the nucleus, and the functional chart, normally termed

a metabolic map, which relates the catalytic or enzymatic pathways between metabolites. The enzymes are the product of genetic variation, and this variation explains adequately our inborn similarities and differences, in health and in disease. The environmental variation is, to a first approximation, based on the import and export of metabolites through the cell wall, and in multicellular organisms, most imports and exports are within, rather than between, organisms.

The map cannot be represented simply, for higher organisms do not seem to have any tidy or orderly arrangement between their structural determinants, neatly arranged in linear array and carried within the nucleus, and the functional or metabolic map, whose catalytic pathways are provided by enzymes coded by the genetic determinants.

Mapless surveying, although useful in basic decisions on short-term responses in animal and plant breeding, has not been useful in man so far, although it has led to serious confusion between data and inference in the field of education and educability, the present gravest manifestation of political biology.

It is not obvious how the various parameters which could specify the genetical basis of an organism with numerous genetic determinants of similar and weak effect, dispersed over very numerous chromosomes, and occupying an environment in which nutrition, exercise, and infection were not familiarly determined, would be of value to such practical matters as improving therapy or defining strategies in research. An unfortunate result of using such terms as high heritability is the belief that the common form of diabetes is a genetical or hereditary disorder.

If we reject this "black box" approach, and start to survey the land from the basis of our rough but well-founded charts, we may start at the structural map on the left of Figure 2. Genetical determinants which are necessary and sufficient, either alone or similarly partnered, reveal themselves by distinctive patterns. If the pattern of inheritance is associated with a distinctive clinical disorder, then there is little doubt of the reality of the condition. An extensive pedigree and a sound clinical judgment of congruity is sufficient without any numerical aid in dominant disorders. In recessive disorders the small number of cases found per afflicted family, usually one or two, imposes serious difficulties in the absence of convincing clinical similarities.

Given this structural map, which seems basic and conventional, we may ask how we can employ our surveying techniques to fill it in at an increased precision.

Firstly we may ask, can we dispense with both charts of Figure 2, the left and the right, and merely treat the cell as a "black box" and devise various measurements not related to its components, as in the so-called biometric approach. Surely, we may ask, a curve of such beauty as that of Gauss could be exploited in the study of variation. It certainly has been exploited, and a number of models, following Karl Pearson's concept of a diathesis as a group for whom the value of some normally distributed variants was beyond some arbitrary threshold, provides a simple and plausible model of any disease not capable of resolution in terms of such necessary or sufficient units of mechanism as a gene, a bacterium, or a toxin. Karl Pearson (5,7) did not approach biological activities in a Cartesian way.

In man the models are of interest in that they reveal how simple and acceptable models of disease, compounded of various environmental and genetical units, could lead to the sort of familial concentrations found in such diverse disorders as tuberculosis, malnutrition, and diabetes.

28

However, the similarity of the familial pattern of such diverse disorders reduces the prospect of any simple discrimination between extrinsic and intrinsic, or preventable and non-preventable. As I have tried to point out elsewhere, this is unlikely to be a useful procedure in man (1-4).

Can we study the similarities of relatives without the tedious need of surveying and measuring? A common measure of similarity is the ratio of the phenotypic correlation to the genotypic correlations, and is known as the heritability or h^2. Alternatively, we can use the additivity features, first described by Gauss, of squares of components of variation, and if we devise a model of an organism within its environment exposed to genetic influences g^2 and environmental influences e^2 we may write, where s^2 is the total variation

$$s^2 = g^2 + e^2,$$
$$h^2 = g^2/(g^2 + e^2).$$

This number is necessarily positive, but, since its value may be formally irrelevant to environmental influences in either prevention or therapy, its estimation is of little practical help.

In fact, in man, the familial or domestic environment, say d^2, is also correlated between relatives so that we have

$$s^2 = g^2 + d^2 + e^2 \text{ where } e^2 \text{ is the non-familial environment.}$$

Since g^2 and d^2 cannot readily be separated, it would be wiser to speak of familiarity, say f^2, than of heritability, and write $f^2 = g^2 + d^2$. Since familiarity associates those factors which it is the common aim of the clinicians, the epidemiologist, and the geneticist, to dissociate, it is not a particularly useful concept. The use of d^2 in this context should not be confused with its traditional use for dominance.

Can we not use extensive pedigree data to make more refined estimates? Here again we are in trouble, for whatever we do we will anticipate ending up with a regression of incidence on relationship, and the slope will give little help on familial environmental or familial genetical factors. Nor can such measures distinguish between genetic susceptibility to the influence of some virus or toxin which, in principle, could be evaded or countered.

This has, as yet, not been a very helpful approach, and there seems no reason to anticipate any advance in analytic method. The twin method has been helpful, in that any discrepancy in disease susceptibility in identical twins is likely to inform a careful observer. However, numerical measures of similarity of response do not seem to convey much. Since the pattern of inheritance of diabetes is far from obvious to the naked eye, excepting in various doubtless simple hereditary forms, and since numerical measures of similarity, or regressions of incidence on relationship have not helped much, further genetical enquiry is possible.

If we attempt to advance a simple model or map - the Cartesian approach which Gauss always employed - the various possible approaches can be enumerated and discussed. Basically, and, for simplicity, we reduce our organism to a single cell, or, if it seems plausible, say a relevant cell, such as a B-cell.

Chart 1 of Figure 2 gives us little guidance when the landmarks or orderly segregation are obscured. Segregational analysis might seem relevant but since the bulk of the information is in sibships and capable of specification by the three possible types of unordered pairs, there are but two degrees of freedom, and almost any model with two parameters will fit. We cannot work from Chart 1 alone, excepting by the recognition of varieties defined by simple inheritance.

If we turn our attention to Chart 2 we may look for associations between the disordered metabolic state of diabetes, which covers a substantial area on the metabolic map, and try to relate it to some simple genetically determined variant, such as an enzyme, or to some other genetic marker, such as a blood group. It seems reasonable to expect the variant enzymes intimately associated with those pathways, such as PGM_1, G 6 PO and 6 PG to be influential. There seem to be no reports of any association. A series of diabetic children from Birmingham studied at the Galton Laboratory showed no gross excess of the rarer phenotypes.

One approach to this problem is to study the susceptibility to diabetes of known heterozygotes, usually parents of rare recessives. This is a treacherous field as pregnancy predisposes to diabetes, so that women ascertained through children will necessarily be predisposed to diabetes, and this will be more extreme when sibships with two or more recessives are overrepresented. Further, almost all recessive disorders vary greatly by race, while diabetes varies greatly by the nutritional environment, and possibly also by race. In Britain an association of heterozygotes for phenylketonuria and cirrhosis, for Tay-Sachs' disease and diabetes, and for thalassaemia and rickets, could be predicted with some confidence.

Studies of red cell groups, although less obviously related to any part of the genetic map, have also been unrewarding; there is no strong association at the ABO locus. If an association had been found, the interpretation would have been difficult.

In the white cell studies associations have been found beyond doubt, although their nature is not yet clear. The HL-A region in man is carried on the sixth chromosome, and comprises at least two closely linked serologically defined loci, known as LA and FOUR, or, more usually outside Holland, as loci one and two, or SD1 and SD2. These are now known as HLA-A and HLA-B respectively. In addition there is at least one locus defined by lymphocytic interaction, and there are probably a series of loci in this region, which appears to define some regions on the cell surface associated with all forms of cell-cell interaction, including rejection of foreign cells both of the same species and of other species. This is an extremely variable system, so that only a few percent of individuals chosed at random are indistinguishable.

We may ask two questions of this association:
1. To what extent does this explain the familial association?
2. By what mechanisms could it be executed?

The extent of familial association is unlikely to be very high, although some individuals clearly have several fold the risk of others.

In general, to a close approximation, if we assume a series of alleles with risks of conferring diabetes of d_i and proportions p_i the incidence of diabetes in the population will be
$$Sp_i d_i$$
and in first-degree relatives of diabetics will be
$$\frac{1}{2}(1 + Sp_i d_i{}^2),$$
and this is unlikely to be large. At the ABO locus the predisposition to duodenal ulceration varies over a range of 1.4:1 or so, yet this explains only a few per cent of the familial predisposition.

What mechanism may we envisage? All that enters the cell enters through its surface, and, for cells deep in the body, entry through the gut, the lung, or elsewhere is necessary. The simplest suspect is a virus, for we have many examples of the parasites being so particular that they thrive differently in different tissues, some being completely destroyed.

While the most obvious examples involve nerve cells, no cell can be expected to be immune from all viruses. Further there is no doubt that diabetes may rarely occur after mumps, and may occur simultaneously in sibs, and even in parent and child. All that can be said is that association with the cell surface determinants is consistent with a viral cause. However, it is important not to associate a specific viral weakness with a genetical inadequacy. Viruses breed and mutate faster than men, and we may anticipate all permutations of surface determinants allow the entry of some viruses.

Finally, we may consider a further explanation. Olbers, the friend of Gauss, is best remembered for his paradox "Why is the sky black at night?" Why, we may ask, is the ground green by day? How can plants grow while surrounded by a wealth of animal life whose members are restrained by starvation? The answer, of course, is by poisoning most members of most species of potential eaters. These poisons are of all forms; many are degraded by cooking; others survive such unusual extraction procedures as the tea-pot and the cigar. Some such as ricin, are in two parts, a toxic protein which attacks within the cell, and a recognition protein, with which it is bound, which obtains entry to the cell by subterfuge or simulation, trailing its poisonous partner with it.

In a predominantly vegetarian species whose numbers were likely to have been restricted by starvation rather than predation, a very subtle interplay between plants trying to avoid being eaten, and man trying to eat everything edible, could be expected. The example of wheat and rust suggests that such dynamic stabilities, with wild but incomplete swings of population, can be dominated by single loci in both partners in this struggle in which total victory can be total defeat.

We have the example of wheat and rye which are toxic to 0.1% or so of the present population, causing celiac disease. Gut diseases are likely to be the first to be related to such mechanisms, and to be the first for which dietary treatment is possible. Even so, it is only possible because of the regenerative powers of the gut epithelium. If the B-cells were to be damaged in a similar way, prospects of recovery might be poor.

Whether it is a virus or a plant protein, we have, firstly, a genetic predisposition, and, secondly, a necessary extrinsic cause. There is no incongruity between genetical predisposition and preventable disease, and, at present, no reason to relate predisposition to diabetes to any general predisposition to disease, or to any limitation in the prospects of prevention, or, in mild and early cases, of therapy.

References

1. Edwards, J.H.: The simulation of mendelism. Acta genet. Statist. med. 10, 63 (1960)

2. Edwards, J.H.: The genetic basis of common disease. Amer. J. Med. 34, 627 (1963)

3. Edwards, J.H.: Familial predisposition in man, Brit. Med. Bull. 25, 58 (1969)

4. Edwards, J.H.: The nature of familial predisposition. In: IV Capri Conf., March 1970, on pathogenesis of diabetes mellitus. Acta Diabetologica Latina, 7, 360 (1970)

5. Pearson, K., Lee, A.: Mathematical contributions to the theory of evolution. Phil. Trans. R. Soc. A., 195, 79 (1900)

6. Pearson, K.: On the laws of inheritance in man, II. On the inheritance of the mental and moral characters in man and its comparison with the inheritance of the physical characters. Biometrika, 3, 131 (1904)

7. Pearson, K.: Tables for Statisticians and Biometricians. London: Cambridge University Press, 1914

5. Clinician's View and Questions on the Genetics of Diabetes Mellitus

H. Mehnert and K. D. Hepp

The idiom "diabetes mellitus, a geneticist's nightmare", introduced by Neel (1), has become one of the most cited statements in the field of genetics pertaining to diabetes. What does it mean for the clinician and the practitioner? One could even take this aspect further: the genetics of diabetes mellitus are worse than a nightmare for diabetologists; because it is tempting to speculate, and could lead to controversies among physicians, which probably would make doctors angry and patients confused. This in turn could lead to a loss of trust between the patient and his physician, who no matter how well informed, has only little working knowledge on some of the most important problems of diabetes mellitus and cannot answer every question that the patient is particularly interested in.

In the following, those questions on the heredity of diabetes are discussed which are most frequently asked by patients in the office or the hospital. In general, the interest of the diabetic in genetic problems is of a high level because his personal future and that of his family is involved and because the term "hereditary disease" has sinister and threatening overtones. The various forms of therapy in diabetes, although not optimal, have attained an excellent standard which ensures a fairly successful therapy for every diabetic. This applies to treatment with diet, with oral antidiabetic agents, and with insulin. The situation in diabetes therapy could be further improved by more intensified instruction of the patients. Already many hospitals, outpatient clinics and private practices provide teaching hours for diabetics, sessions which deal with many aspects of diabetes. The discussion of problems relative to heredity of the disease, marriage, and the founding of a family is of great importance for the patient. Here the physician will have to point out that diabetes is a hereditary disease. Our lack of knowledge in these matters at the moment can be summed up by the simple words: "diabetes runs in families." The following seven cases are thought to illustrate the most important genetic problems which confront the diabetologist in the counseling of his patients.

Case No. 1

During a teaching session the physician mentions that diabetes is a hereditary disease. This meets the immediate protest of a patient who does not want to have a "hereditary disease." He maintains that there was never any diabetes in his family. The doctor has to answer that the lack of diabetic family members in the past by no means proves that diabetes is not inherited. Even though only the half of all patients can report one or more diabetic family members, with more intensive epidemiologic investigation, the proportion is much higher. Fifty percent of the diabetics in a practice will still declare that no diabetes has been found in their family. Among these there are some who in spite of medical counseling believe that "their" diabetes is not due to a genetic defect but was caused by excitement, stress, or infection. The situation becomes especially critical for the doctor when another patient appears who states that he has indeed read in the newspaper about virus infections as the cause of diabetes mellitus. Depending on what the doctor has read about this work, he shall remain silent, he will contradict, or agree. In any case he will be less trustworthy in what he says. He has raised the first doubt in his patient.

Case No. 2

Although it is 30 years since World War II, the physicians are still faced with making decisions in court on the influence of war events on the etiology of diabetes. Certain enterprising attorneys advise their overweight clients who have become diabetic in the year 1975 to claim that diabetes was caused by several years captivity during the Second World War. Although such a connection between circumstances of war and the etiology of diabetes can also be negated on other grounds, the physician as a legal expert will always find the following interplay between the attorney and his client, on the one hand, and the medical expert, on the other side: Should the patient maintain that there is no diabetes in his family (as was said before, there is a probability of 50% which in practice may be inflated due to the tendency of the patient to forget any possible diabetic family members in this case), then the attorney will almost surely make the statement that this is with all certainty not a hereditary disease but an acquired one. This is usually countered by the medical expert by pointing out the relatively weak penetrance of the diabetic trait. However, sometimes the medical expert is just as wise as the attorney in stating that in view of the positive family history of many other patients, the genetic nature of diabetes is proven in the present case. But then how does the physician who uses such an argument explain the appearance of diabetic offspring in people who are not diabetic?

Case No. 3

A young diabetic girl wants to get married. She is 20 years old and has been diabetic for 2 years. Thanks to her cooperation in all questions of diet, in maintaining several insulin injections per day, and testing her urine sugar, she is in good control and apparently has no diabetic complications. Her future parents-in-law visit with her physician. They have been told by their own old family doctor that diabetic women have to expect diabetic children. The parents are desperate and want to prevent the marriage of their healthy son to the "sick girl." They ask the consulting physician of the diabetic about the pattern of inheritance of diabetes. The diabetologist is in a difficult situation; on the one hand, he has to contradict the apparently false opinion of their family physician and thus, whatever he will say, he may disturb the relationship between the doctor and his patients. This danger, however, is relatively small because the parents will rather believe their own trusted family physician than the diabetologist. It would certainly be simpler and without risk to dissuade the diabetic from a marriage, as the family physician has done, or to tell her that if married it would be best not to have any children. As a physician, one could in this case never make a "mistake", such as might become evident after a possible pregnancy with an infortunate end or later when diabetes becomes manifest in the child. In fact, of course, every pregnancy constitutes a certain hazard for mother and child and only the extent of the additional risks due to diabetes makes it necessary to deal with individual cases in a positive or negative sense. In any case the diabetic and the nondiabetic partner, not their parents should visit with the consulting physician of the diabetic to discuss future problems and the genetics of diabetes. The possibility that a child of a diabetic will become diabetic is relatively small. The healthy partner is greatly reassured upon hearing that the child of a diabetic mother has a probability of only about 1% of becoming diabetic during childhood as long as there is no additional familial factor. In any case the discussion between the diabetologist and the parents of the nondiabetic fiancé will be unsatisfactory: either one believes the family physician, which is most frequently the case, and thus hurts the diabetic, and the family physician will apparently never be wrong; or one believes the diabetologist with the result that the relationship between family physician and patient is now seriously disturbed.

Case No. 4

An unmarried pregnant diabetic consults with her physician. She wants to have the baby only if she can be sure that it does not become diabetic. However, no doctor can guarantee this. The possibility that the baby will not only be illegitimate but also diabetic may lead her to an abortionist. In such a case even convincing data showing that the probability is in fact very small that a child will develop diabetes during childhood will be of no help.

Case No. 5

Nondiabetic parents with or without a positive family history have two children who became diabetic at the ages of 3 and 5. The parents know about the bad prognosis when diabetes develops at such an early age and ask their doctor whether they will have to be faced with another diabetic child. Since the mode of inheritance is still obscure, the answer is especially difficult for the diabetologist. He cannot exclude the possibility of a third diabetic child in the family. The family physician would probably discourage them from having another child because he feels that with this history the risk of the disease in another child is high. His opinion will certainly be more convincing than that of the diabetologist who, on the one hand, cannot exclude a high risk, but on the other hand, would hope the parents had a nondiabetic child not only for idealistic reasons but also for a more material end, because the child could add his share to the upkeep of the family at a later point when the parents are old and both children are possibly ailing.

Case No. 6

A diabetic is married to a nondiabetic woman with a negative family history for diabetes. After a year of their marriage they are still without child and the woman develops a juvenile type diabetes. The couple are desperate; they visit the doctor and ask whether under these conditions they should have any children at all. One will find in most textbooks that doctors should discourage any diabetic couple from having children. The doctor would have done this, had he been confronted with this problem before their marriage. In a genetic sense we have the same situation as if the diabetes had been manifest before their marriage. From a human point of view, however, the whole thing has become much more complicated. We know the percentage of diabetic offspring is very high in such cases. It is, however, not 100% as it was often formerly quoted, due to misinterpretation of Steinberg's not entirely correct data. Accordingly, children of two diabetic parents were no longer called "prediabetics" but "potential diabetics," who could, but not in ev-

ery case, develop the disease. Another question in such a case is whether
one would not be in favor of a child for such a young diabetic couple,
not only because the child might not become diabetic, but in view of the
much greater probability that it may develop diabetes at a much later
age. It would be a better solution to adopt a child with respect to the
later support of the patients by the child. What parents, however, who
want their own child, will listen to such plans? The uncertainty about
the mode of inheritance will leave the diabetologist with a very unsatisfactory situation. Unsatisfactory for the parents who will sense his
insecurity and for the doctor who will have to admit that his answer is
not strictly scientific but will be influenced by the circumstances of
the individual case.

Case No. 7

One has to be especially afraid of the questions of those inquisitive
patients who look up the chapters on genetics of diabetes mellitus in
medical textbooks and handbooks on genetics. These patients very soon
will realize what degree of uncertainty there is among those physicians
and scientists who work in this area. A 22-year-old diabetic law student told us in the outpatient clinic that according to what he has
read about the studies of Siperstein's group, which he felt had proved
the independence of the development of vascular complications from the
metabolic situation, he was no longer willing to keep his diet and to
perform his own urine sugar controls. In his view, such studies have
proven the genetic basis and independent course of the microangiopathy.

Conclusions

In the preceding the difficulties in genetic counseling in practice
and hospital have been discussed. All cases are from personal observations, which of course are not encountered in every diabetic patient.
In view of our limited knowledge on the heredity of diabetes, one can
only give a rough estimate on the risk of becoming diabetic. Like most
diabetologists, we feel that the multifactorial mode of inheritance
should be the basis of our considerations. We use the tables of Simpson
(2), who on the basis of her extensive studies on 6600 diabetics has
provided convincing data. For us, as consultants, the most important
fact is that of a very low risk to become diabetic under the age of 20
years even if one parent, sibling, or child is a diabetic. An important
practical point in genetic counseling in the office and hospital is the
confirmation of the rate occurrence of diabetes in infants and juveniles.
Without trying to deemphasize the consequences of the diabetic condition in later years, the differences regarding therapy and prognosis
for early- and late-onset diabetes are evident. In genetic counseling
one can therefore rely on Simpson's numbers up to age 20 or at best,
age 40.

A special problem is caused by the statements of health politicians
who are fascinated by eugenics and on such ground agitate against the
founding of families by diabetics. Although such arguments can easily
be dispelled on professional and humanitarian grounds, the damage that
has been done in public for the diabetic can be great. In this respect
much hardship could be avoided, had the physicians more convincing
genetic data which would allow for comprehensible answers.

References

1. Neel, J.V., Fajans, S.S., Conn, J.W., Davidson, R.T.: Diabetes mellitus. In: Genetics and the Epidemiology of Chronic Diseases. Public Health Service Publication No. 1163. Neel, J.V., Shaw, M.W., Schull, W.J. (eds.). Washington: Government Printing Office, 1965, p. 105

2. Simpson, N.E.: Diabetes in the families of diabetics. Canad. Med. Ass. J. 98, 427 (1968)

6. Etiological and Promoting Factors in the Pathogenesis of Diabetes Mellitus

W. CREUTZFELDT

Despite the fact - known for centuries - that diabetes mellitus is a familial disease, the genetics of this disease are still poorly understood. The most important hindrance to a proper genetic study is the fact that the basic defect in diabetes is unknown. Therefore, no method exists for detecting individuals who possess the diabetic genotype but who have, as yet, no signs of abnormal carbohydrate metabolism (11). The clinical syndrome called diabetes is complex and any search for a common etiological factor may oversimplify the problem. However, many studies have shown that a subject with diabetes releases after glucose load too little insulin too late relative to a comparable but nondiabetic individual. Thus, an abnormality in the pancreatic B-cell appears central to the disease and the most simple definition of diabetes is absolute or relative insulin deficiency.

Absolute insulin deficiency can be produced by removal or destruction of the B-cells, by inactivation of insulin or by inhibition of insulin release. Relative insulin deficiency can be produced by inducing metabolic or endocrine patterns which increase the blood glucose either by glucose overproduction or by antagonism to the action of insulin at the tissue level. As a rule, diabetes due to relative insulin deficiency becomes manifest only if the B-cells are not or, after a period of increased insulin secretion, no longer able to produce enough insulin to overcome the high insulin requirement. This will be demonstrated by a simple scheme (Fig.1). Even in case of increased insulin requirement the B-cells can compensate by a higher rate of insulin secretion and replication (Fig. 1 B). Diabetes occurs if the B-cells are destroyed or are genetically unable to secrete or replicate normally even if the insulin requirement is normal (Fig. 1 C) or if genetically inferior B-cells cannot increase their secretion rate or replicate in case the insulin requirement increases (Fig. 1 D). This scheme can be applied to human diabetes as well as to experimental and spontaneous diabetes of animals.

For the better understanding of the pathogenesis of diabetes - both in animals and man - etiological factors and promoting or precipitating factors should be distinguished (5). Generally speaking all etiological factors refer to changes at the level of the B-cells or the availability of insulin to the body. These may be inherited or acquired. Research on these etiological factors is essential for the development of new treatments of diabetes.

Promoting or precipitating factors operate by increasing the insulin requirement of the body. Such promoting factors may be environmental, such as nutrition, or additional diseases.
Defining promoting factors is essential for the prevention of diabetes and may be of greater practical importance from the standpoint of public health.

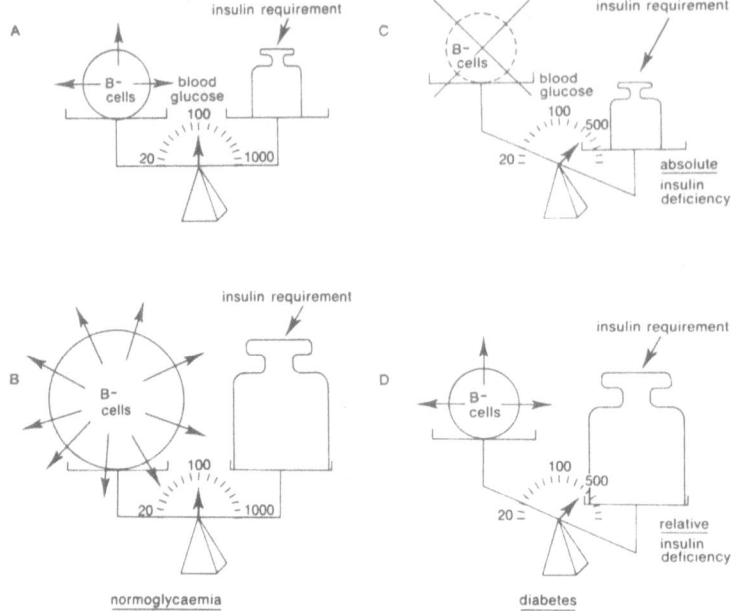

Fig. 1. Schematic illustration of role of etiological (decreased insulin secretion) and promoting factors (increased insulin requirement) involved in development of diabetes. A shift of the scale to the right means hyperglycemis (5)

In Table 1 are listed etiological factors leading to diabetes mellitus in animals and man. The different experimental methods of producing diabetes in animals by reducing or eliminating insulin from the circulation correspond to secondary diabetes in man. The listing of beta-tropic virus infection (7,1) in this group is preliminary, at least for the human situation, because it is not yet known if an inherited inferiority of the B-cells is a prerequisite for virus-induced diabetes in man.

By far the majority of all diabetics belong to the idiopathic group. The primary defect is located in the islets. Until recently only the insulin secreting B-cells were regarded as genetically defective. However, increasing data indicate that also the glucagon-producing A-cells are involved in the pathogenesis of idiopathic diabetes. We will discuss this later. Research on spontaneous diabetes in laboratory animals leads to the conclusion that some types of diabetes are mainly due to an inherited defect of the B-cells (2,6,12,14). These animals are similar to humans with idiopathic diabetes. However, only the Chinese diabetic hamster becomes spontaneously diabetic without having gone through a period of insulin hypersecretion correlated to obesity (14). In Table 2 are listed the promoting or precipitating factors leading to the manifestation of diabetes provided that the B-cells are reduced in number by pancreatic damage or that they are genetically inferior.

The conditions are very similar in animals and man. Any situation (either occurring spontaneously (10) or induced experimentally) which increases the insulin requirement may precipitate diabetes. These factors operate either by increasing blood glucose levels (i.e., glucose overproduction) or by decreasing the sensitivity of adipose, muscle or liver

Table 1. Etiological Factors (Spontaneous Manifestation of Diabetes)

A. ANIMALS
    1. Experimental diabetes
        pancreatectomy
        B-cytoxins
        inhibitors of insulin secretion
        injection of anti-insulin serum
        B-cytotropic virus infection

    2. Spontaneous diabetes (genetic)
        Chinese hamster (decreased insulin release,
                    increased glucagon release)
        spiny mice (decreased insulin release)
        db/db mice (decreased B-cell replication)
        NZO mice (decreased insulin release)

B. MAN
    1. Idiopathic diabetes (genetic)
        decreased insulin secretion and increased
           glucagon release
        decreased B-cell replication?
        autoimmunity (Schmidt's syndrome)

    2. Secondary diabetes
        pancreatitis
        carcinoma or trauma of the pancreas
        pancreatectomy
        virus infection?

Table 2. Promoting factors (manifestation of diabetes only if B-cells are defective)

A. ANIMALS
    1. Experimental
        glucose injection
        treatment with glucocorticoids, ACTH,
           growth hormone, glucagon
        gold-thioglucose-induced hyperphagia
        sucrose diet

    2. Spontaneous (genetic)
        obesity (ob/ob mice, KK mice)
        insensitivity of tissues (e.g., adipose,
           muscle, liver) to insulin

B. MAN
        Cushing's disease
        steroid or ACTH treatment
        acromegaly
        glucagonoma
        obesity (overfeeding)
        liver cirrhosis

tissue to insulin (i.e., glucose under-utilization). It is obvious that the exclusion of such promoting factors is the clue for the prevention of diabetes.

This has been most convincingly demonstrated by Gerritsen (9). Control of hyperphagia by restricted diet retarded or prevented the development of diabetes in prediabetic hamsters born of two ketonuric diabetic parents, while prediabetic siblings, fed ad libitum, developed glucosuria and ketonuria and died prematurely.

In a given case either in animals or in man a single etiological or promoting factor can be dominating or multiple factors are required until diabetes becomes manifest. If the genetic load is heavy (i.e., major B-cell deficiency) the promoting factors can be minor. If the genetic load is small, manifestation of diabetes occurs only in the presence of abundant promoting factors.

Cahill (1) has sketched a theoretical natural history of the B-cells in normal man, showing the transient increase in times of extra insulin need such as pregnancy, or, for a more prolonged period of time, in obesity (Fig. 2). Diabetics are unable to meet this need. The B-cell integrity decreases rapidly in the juvenile and slowly in the maturity-onset diabetes. A transient improvement or perhaps even remission may occur. According to this scheme B-cells lose their integrity during aging and the underlying hereditary defect would be an increased susceptibility to damage or possibly an earlier senescence of the B-cells. A virus would cause an early, rapid, and irreversible demise of the B-cells in this hereditary milieu. Otherwise advancing age, and particularly, an increase in insulin need, as in obesity, Cushing's disease, or acromegaly would unmask the B-cell deficiency.

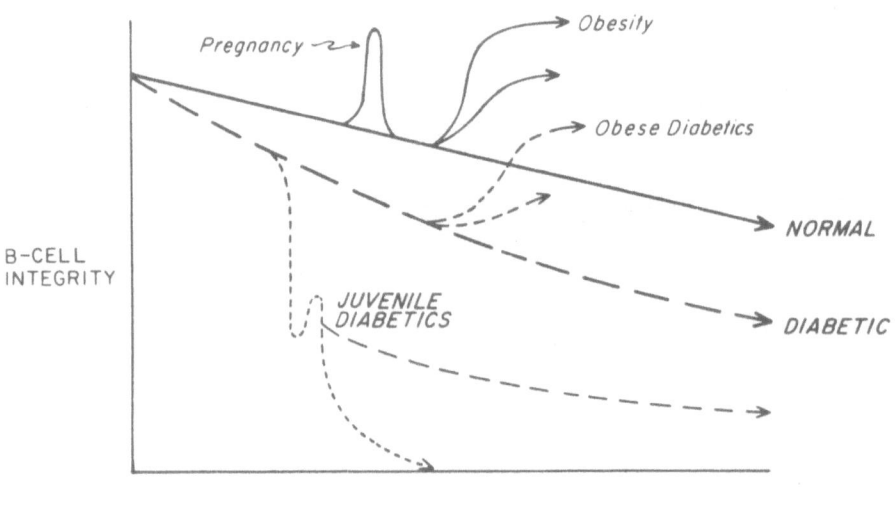

Fig. 2. B-cell integrity in normal man and in subjects with diabetes, showing increased need during pregnancy or obesity and deficiency in meeting this need in the diabetics (1). For details see text

Much work has been done to define the defect in the islet cells responsible for spontaneous diabetes mellitus in animals (14) and man (3). The molecular biology of the normal B-cell is far advanced. However, no common defect on the molecular level can yet be demonstrated. In Table 3 some findings are listed which could explain the fragility of the B-cells or the decreased insulin release in the respective diabetic animals and in man. The multiplicity of defects demonstrated so far may be disturbing for the geneticist who is looking for the basic defect in diabetes. And so are the recent observations on a defective cell function in spontaneous diabetes in man (15) and animals (6) which cannot be corrected by insulin injections as in experimental diabetes.

40

Table 3. Demonstrated defects in pancreatic islet cells of animals and man with spontaneous diabetes mellitus

1. Defect B-cell replication (db/db mice) (12)
2. Decreased insulin release 　　functional alteration or decrease of 　　　microtubular protein (spiny mice) (13) 　　decreased or absent cell-associated 　　　autonomic nerven endings (spiny mice) (14) 　　defect glucose receptor of B-cells (6,3) 　　　(Chinese hamster, man)
3. Increased glucagon release 　　defect glucose receptor of A-cells 　　　(Chinese hamster, man)　　　　　(6,15)

Based upon experimental evidence presented by different groups, Unger and Orci (16) have put forward the hypothesis that the complete diabetic metabolic syndrome is the consequence of deranged function of both the A- and B-cells. Relative insulin lack leads only to prolonged postprandial hyperglycemia (i.e., reduced rate of glucose disposal) while relative excess of glucagon leads to an inappropriately high rate of endogenous glucose production in relation to the prevailing glycemia. Normally, glucose stimulates insulin release and suppresses glucagon release. If the glucose receptor of the B-cell is defective, an increase of the blood glucose will not induce insulin release. If the glucose receptor of the A-cell is defective, an increase of blood glucose will not suppress glucagon release. Thus, the possibility has to be discussed that in idiopathic diabetes mellitus the glucose receptor of both the A- and B-cells is defective. This bihormonal-abnormality hypothesis is supported by the exciting recent experiments with the growth-hormone-release-inhibiting factor somatostatin (16). This tetradekapeptide inhibits, besides the release of many peptide hormones, insulin, and glucagon secretion. Complete suppression of insulin and glucagon secretion by somatostatin does not produce hyperglycemia in normals, reduces glycemia in diabetics receiving a fixed dose of exogenous insulin (8) and prevents hyperglycemia in the insulin-deprived state (16). This effect continues in the absence of the hypophysis, i.e., is independent of growth hormone (8).
These new observations make the search for the basic defect in diabetes mellitus and thus the life of the geneticist even more difficult. However, for the clinician they open up a new therapeutic field. Tentatively, I have listed in my tables on etiological and promoting factors in the pathogenesis of diabetes mellitus increased glucagon release under the etiological factors. But this is open for discussion.

In conclusion: Diabetes is defined as absolute or relative insulin deficiency. Etiological factors leading to diabetes are located in the B-cell, decreased insulin secretion, decreased B-cell replication or destruction of B-cells. Promoting factors operate by increasing the insulin requirement of the body. Normally, an increased insulin requirement is compensated by increased insulin production. However, if the B-cells are genetically deficient, diabetes becomes manifest. In the case of major B-cell deficiency the promoting factors are of minor importance and vice versa. Since the B-cell deficiency is genetically determined, prevention of diabetes has to be directed towards the promoting factors. This has been demonstrated convincingly in animals with spontaneous diabetes. It is possible that in idiopathic diabetes the glucose receptor not only of the B-cells but also of the A-cells is defective. Investigations with somatostatin support such a bihormonal-abnormality hypothesis.

References

1. Cahill, G.F.: Diabetes, insulin and future developments. In: Diabetes. Proceedings of the VIIIth Congress of the IDF. Malaisse, W.J., Pirart, J. (eds.). Amsterdam: Excerpta Medica, 1974, p. 53

2. Cameron, D.P., Opat, F., Insch, S., Lovell-Smith, C.J., Insch, J.G.T.: Studies of immunoreactive insulin secretion in NZO mice in vivo. Diabetologia 10, 649 (1974)

3. Cerasi, E.: Mechanisms of glucose-stimulated insulin secretion in health and in diabetes: some re-evaluations and proposals. The Minkowski Award Lecture 1974. Diabetologia 11, 1 (1975)

4. Graighead, J.E.: Viral lesions on the pancreatic islets of Langerhans. In: Diabetes. Proceedings of the VIIIth Congress of the IDF. Malaisse, W.J., Pirart, J. (eds.). Amsterdam: Excerpta Medica, 1974, p. 287

5. Creutzfeldt, W.: The relationship between etiological and promoting factors in the pathogenesis of diabetes mellitus in man and animals. Acta diabetol. lat. 7, 341 (1970)

6. Frankel, B.J., Gerich, J.E., Hagura, R., Fanska, R.E., Gerritsen, G.C., Grodsky, G.M.: Abnormal secretion of insulin and glucagon by the in vitro perfused pancreas of the genetically diabetic Chinese hamster. J. Clin. Invest. 53, 1637 (1974)

7. Gamble, D.R., Kinsley, M.L., Fitzgerald, M.G., Bolton, R., Taylor, K.W.: Viral antibodies in diabetes mellitus. Brit. Med. J. 1969, 3, 627

8. Gerich, J.E., Lorenzi, M., Schneider, V., Karam, J.H., Rivier, J., Guillemin, R., Forsham, P.H.: Effects of somatostatin on plasma glucose and glucagon levels in human diabetes mellitus. New Engl. J. Med. 291, 544 (1974)

9. Gerritsen, G.C., Blanks, M.C., Miller, R.L., Dulin, W.E.: Effect of diet limitation on the development of diabetes in prediabetic Chinese hamsters, Diabetologia 10, 559 (1974)

10. Iwatsuka, H., Taketomi, S., Matsuo, T., Suzuoki, Z.: Congenitally impaired hormone sensitivity of the adipose tissue of spontaneously diabetic mice, KK. Validity of thrifty genotype on the KK mice. Diabetologia 10, 611 (1974)

11. Johansen, K., Soeldner, J.S., Gleason, R.E.: Insulin, growth hormone and glucagon in prediabetes mellitus - a review. Metabolism 23, 1185 (1974)

12. Like, A.A., Chick, W.L.: Studies in the diabetic mutant mouse: I + II: Light microscopy, radioautography and electron microscopy of pancreatic islets. Diabetologia 6, 207 and 216 (1970)

13. Malaisse-Lagae, F., Ravvazola, M., Amherdt, M., Gutzeit, A., Stauffacher, W., Malaisse, W.J., Orci, L.: An apparent abnormality of the B-cell microtubular system in spiny mice (acomys cahirinus). Diabetologia 11, 71 (1975)

14. Renold, A.E., Rabinovitch, A., Wollheim, C.B., Kikuchi, M., Gutzeit, A.H., Amherdt, M., Malaisse-Lagae, F., Orci, L.: Spontaneous and experimental diabetic syndromes in animals. A re-evaluation of their usefulness for approaching the physiopathology of diabetes. In: Diabetes. Proc. VIIIth Congr. IDF. Malaisse, W.J., Pirart, J. (eds.). Amsterdam, Excerpta Medica, 1974, p. 22

15. Unger, R.H.: Alpha- and beta-cell interrelationship in health and disease. Metabolism, 23, 581 (1974)

16. Unger, R.H., Orci, L.: The essential role of glucagon in the pathogenesis of diabetes mellitus. Lancet I, 14 (1975)

7. Genetic Syndromes Associated with Glucose Intolerance

D. L. RIMOIN

The association of glucose intolerance with a number of distinct genetic syndromes due to mutations at different loci adds great support to the hypothesis that diabetes mellitus represents a heterogeneous group of disorders (66,69). Although these syndromes comprise only a small minority of the cases of diabetes mellitus, they illustrate the wide variety of pathogenetic mechanisms that can result in glucose intolerance. It must be stressed that the majority of these syndromes simply result in an abnormal glucose tolerance test without any of the clinical features of diabetes mellitus, but this is also true of a large percentage of the cases of so-called idiopathic diabetes mellitus. Thus, in defining the abnormality of carbohydrate metabolism in the various types of glucose intolerance, the presence or absence of clinical symptomatology and specific complications must be delineated, rather than lumping all types of glucose intolerance under the heading of diabetes mellitus. In this discussion, the term "diabetes" will be used only when the clinical syndrome, rather than uncomplicated glucose intolerance, is present. The more than 35 genetic syndromes associated with glucose intolerance will be discussed below and an attempt will be made to classify them either on the basis of the type of pathogenetic mechanism resulting in the abnormality in glucose tolerance or on the basis of the associated anomalies (Table 1).

Syndromes Associated with Pancreatic Degeneration

A number of single gene disorders can result in glucose intolerance as a result of structural degeneration of the pancreatic islets. Since in none of these disorders is glucose intolerance uniformly present, the question arises as to whether the pancreatic destruction simply uncovers an underlying genetic predisposition to diabetes mellitus or whether the presence or absence of glucose intolerance is simply correlated with the degree of islet cell loss.

Hereditary Relapsing Pancreatitis

This autosomal dominant disorder is characterized by recurrent episodes of severe abdominal pain beginning in childhood, eventually resulting in chronic pancreatitis, with severe fibrosis and inflammation of the pancreatic parenchyma with irregular calcific foci in small scattered nests of acini and islet cells (13,26,91). Diabetes mellitus is present in the majority of adults with hereditary pancreatitis. The diabetes is insulin-requiring, is frequently associated with ketosis, and appears to be secondary to the inflammatory destruction of the pancreas.

Table 1. Genetic syndromes associated with glucose intolerance

Syndromes associated with pancreatic degeneration

Hereditary relapsing pancreatitis
Cystic fibrosis
Polyendocrine deficiency disease
Hemochromatosis

Hereditary endocrine disorders with glucose intolerance

Isolated growth hormone deficiency
Hereditary panhypopituitary dwarfism
Pheochromocytoma
Multiple endocrine adenomatosis

Inborn errors of metabolism with glucose intolerance

Glycogen storage disease type I
Acute intermittent porphyria
Hyperlipidemias

Syndromes with nonketotic insulin resistant early-onset diabetes

Ataxia telangiectasia
Myotonic dystrophy
Lipatrophic diabetes syndromes

Hereditary neuromuscular disorders with glucose intolerance

Muscular dystrophies
Late-onset proximal myopathy
Huntington's chorea
Machado's disease
Herrmann's syndrome
Optic atrophy-diabetes mellitus syndrome
Friedreich's ataxia
Alstrom's syndrome
Laurence-Moon-Biedl syndrome
Pseudo-Refsum's syndrome

Progeroid syndromes with glucose intolerance

Cockayne's syndrome
Werner's syndrome

Syndromes with glucose intolerance secondary to obesity

Prader-Willi syndrome
Achondroplasia

Miscellaneous syndromes with glucose intolerance

Steroid-induced ocular hypertension
Mendenhall's syndrome
Epiphyseal dysplasia and infantile-onset diabetes

Cytogenetic disorders with glucose intolerance

Trisomy 21
Klinefelter's syndrome
Turner's syndrome

Cystic Fibrosis

The increase in longevity of patients with cystic fibrosis has been accompanied by a rise in the frequency of glucose intolerance. Indeed, abnormal glucose tolerance has been found in up to 75% of cystic patients (86). The frequency of diabetes mellitus increases with the age of the patient and the severity of the cystic fibrosis. A family history of diabetes is no more frequent in those cystics with diabetes mellitus than among those without diabetes (27). The abnormal glucose tolerance is usually not associated with ketoacidosis nor vascular complications, but this may be due to the early death of most patients. Handwerger *et al.* (27) found marked disorganization of the pancreas in which the fibrosis also disrupted the spatial relations of the islets. Several investigators have documented decreased insulin output following oral glucose, the degree of insuliopenia increasing with the severity of the glucose intolerance (27,32,56,79). Lippe *et al.* (46) have recently documented both impaired insulin and glucagon release in response to intravenous arginine (Table 2). Basal glucagon concentrations were normal and suppression of glucagon secretion by glucose was retained, in contrast to the increased glucagon secretion and lack of glucagon suppression by glucose in typical juvenile diabetics. Cystic fibrosis is inherited as an autosomal recessive trait.

Table 2. Plasma insulin and glucagon in gonadal dysgenesis (GD) and cystic fibrosis (C.F.)[a]

	Plasma insulin after glucose	Fasting Plasma glucagon	Glucagon rise after arginine	Glucagon suppression by glucose
Normal	N	N	N	N
Juvenile D.M.	↓↓	N–↑	N–↑↑	O
GD with N GTT	N–↑	↑	↑	N
GD with Abn. GTT	↑↑	↑	↑↑	O
Cystic Fibrosis	↓↓	N	↓↓	N

N = Normal; ↑ = increased; ↑↑ = markedly increased; ↓ = decreased; ↓↓ = markedly decreased; O = absent.

[a]from Lippe, B. and Sperling, M.: (56,57)

Polyendocrine Deficiency Disease (Schmidt's Syndrome)

Schmidt's syndrome is characterized by idiopathic Addison's disease, thyroiditis, and diabetes mellitus, frequently in association with hypoparathyroidism, pernicious anemia, and hypogonadism (8). It is thought to be an autoimmune disorder (see Chapter 12, p. 106). An autoimmune basis for diabetes mellitus has long been postulated, in view of the documented increased association of diabetes with pernicious anemia, thyroiditis, Addison's disease, and hypoparathyroidism and with its increased prevalence of organ-specific antibodies against the thyroid, adrenal, and gastric parietal cells (41). Although organ-specific antibodies against the pancreatic islets have not been found in typical diabetics, Bottazzo *et al.* (6) and MacCuish *et al.* (50) have both found islet cell antibodies in patients with diabetes who had associated autoimmune disease. Further evidence in favor of an autoimmune basis to some forms of diabetes include: (a) the presence of antipancreatic cellular hypersensitivity in 30% of diabetics as measured by the leukocyte migration technique; (b) blastogenic transformation of lymphocytes from untreated or new diabetics induced by prolonged culture of these cells with insulin or insulin beta chain antigen; (c) the presence of insulitis in some untreated young diabetics; and (d) the increased prevalence of HLA-8 in juvenile-onset insulin-dependent diabetics (50). Thus, there does appear to be an autoimmune form of diabetes mellitus and it has been postulated that the basic genetic defect in this disor-

der may be an immune defect possibly triggered by a viral infection (6).
There is a great deal of variability in the specific endocrine glands
affected in patients with this disorder as well as in the chronology of
their appearance. Gharib and Gastineau (23) have pointed out that in
cases of coexistant diabetes with Addison's disease, when the Addison's
disease precedes the diabetes, the diabetic syndrome is usually quite
mild, whereas in those patients in whom diabetes precedes the onset of
Addison's disease, the diabetes is of the severe, insulin-requiring,
ketoacidotic variety. Schmidt's syndrome has been reported in siblings
and concordant monozygotic twins (20).

Hemochromatosis

Abnormal glucose tolerance is present in over 50% of the patients with
hemochromatosis (73). The clinical features of the diabetes are quite
similar to typical maturity-onset diabetes and both retinal and vascular
complications have been reported. Although the heavy iron deposition
in the pancreas was originally thought to be totally responsible for the
glucose intolerance, both Balcerzak *et al*. (4) and Saddi and Feingold
(73) have recently provided evidence suggesting that the diabetes may
not be caused primarily by the iron overload. For example, the degree of
iron overload does not differ between those hemochromatotic patients
with diabetes (HD) and those without diabetes (HD⁻). The plasma insulin
response to oral glucose is increased in hemochromatotic diabetics; a
decrease would be expected if the glucose intolerance were solely due
to pancreatic islet destruction. The prevalence of diabetes is higher in
the parents of HD patients than in HD⁻ patients. Furthermore, the prevalence of diabetes among parents of HD patients is similar to that in parents of idiopathic diabetics and the prevalence of diabetes in the parents of HD⁻ patients is similar to that found in a control population.
On the basis of this evidence the authors have postulated that the diabetes mellitus in hemochromatosis is genetically determined per se and
that the pancreatic damage simply uncovers an underlying genetic consti-
tution. Furthermore, they suggest that the hemochromatotic gene in the
heterozygous state may contribute to the expression of diabetes (73).
Although simply uncovering an underlying genetic predisposition for diabetes may well be operative in numerous syndromes affecting the pancreas,
if this were the sole reason for the diabetes in hemochromatosis, the
prevalence of diabetes should not be as high as it is, as it would be
extremely unlikely that over 50% of the hemochromatotic patients were independently genetically predisposed to diabetes.

Hereditary Endocrine Disorders with Glucose Intolerance

There are a number of genetic syndromes associated with glucose intolerance in which the abnormality in carbohydrate metabolism appears to be
entirely secondary to a disturbance in the function of nonpancreatic
endocrine glands. In these disorders, the hormonal imbalance results in
a secondary effect on insulin secretion and/or insulin responsivness,
which is usually reversible following correction of the basic endocrine
disturbance. It must be stressed that the glucose intolerance in these
syndromes is a secondary phenomenon and not true diabetes mellitus.

Isolated Growth Hormone Deficiency (IGHD)

At least two forms of hereditary, isolated growth hormone deficiency
have been described, both of which are characteristically associated
with glucose intolerance (69). Type I IGHD is associated with insulinopenia following glucose and arginine stimulation as well as hyperres-

ponsiveness to exogenous insulin; all return to normal following growth hormone administration. This syndrome is inherited as an autosomal recessive trait. Type II IGHD is associated with hyperinsulinism in response to glucose and arginine and insulin resistance. This syndrome appears to be inherited as an autosomal dominant trait. It is quite likely that this classification does not fully delineate the heterogeneity of the isolated growth hormone deficiency syndromes, as families have been described with dominant inheritance and insulinopenia, and further delineation of this genetic heterogeneity must be accomplished (69). Although glucose intolerance is present in the majority of adults with IGHD, infants and young children with this syndrome frequently have episodes of hypoglycemia. Their insulin secretory capacity decreases with age, however, and glucose intolerance supervenes. The glucose intolerance, a feature of both types of IGHD, is not associated with any of the signs or symptoms of diabetes mellitus. Merimee et al. (54,55) have compared the glucose intolerance in type I IGHD cases to age-matched typical diabetics and have found that the glucose intolerance in IGHD is not associated with retinopathy or capillary basement membrane thickening. This glucose intolerance cannot be called "diabetes mellitus" as it is simply a chemical trait secondary to the effects of HGH deficiency on pancreatic insulin secretion. We have recently reported the results of an autopsy on a 78 year old man with IGHD type I who had glucose intolerance for many years (71). He was found to have severe generalized atherosclerosis, suggesting that HGH deficiency does not protect against middle and large vessel degenerative disease. Furthermore, he had marked fatty infiltration of the pancreas with an overall reduction in the number of islet cells, which may be related to the insulinopenic characteristic of this syndrome.

Hereditary Panhypopituitary Dwarfism

Although the majority of cases of panhypopituitary dwarfism are sporadic and presumably nongenetic, both an autosomal recessive and an X-linked recessive form of panhypopituitary dwarfism have been described (69). These individuals also frequently have glucose intolerance associated with insulinopenia, both of which return to normal following HGH therapy. The characteristics of the glucose intolerance will, of course, vary with the presence of other pituitary tropic hormone deficiencies, especially ACTH.

Laron Dwarfism

Laron dwarfism is an autosomal recessive disorder associated with elevated plasma concentrations of immunoreactive growth hormone and peripheral insensitivity to the metabolic effects of HGH. It is thought to be due to an inability to generate somatomedin from growth hormone (15, 43). The abnormality in carbohydrate metabolism in this syndrome is quite similar to that observed in IGHD type I with glucose intolerance and insulinopenia.

Pheochromocytoma

Hereditary pheochromocytoma may occur as an isolated disorder, or in association with medullary thyroid carcinoma, neurofibromatosis, or von Hippel-Lindau disease, all of which are inherited as autosomal dominant traits (69). In all forms of pheochromocytoma, glucose intolerance associated with decreased plasma insulin levels is a frequent finding, but the clinical symptoms of diabetes mellitus are usually not present (78, 85). The glucose intolerance and insulinopenia frequently return to normal following surgical ablation of the tumor or catecholamine blockade with phenoxybenzamine or phentolamine (85,92). Thus, the glucose intolerance associated with pheochromocytoma is due, at least in part, to catecholamine inhibition of insulin release via alpha adrenergic receptors. Peripheral resistance to the hypoglycemic effects of insulin also may be present, secondary to elevated free fatty acid concentrations, decreased tissue utilization of glucose, increased hepatic glycogenolysis, or decreased intestinal peristalsis and delayed absorption of glucose from the gut, all of which can be caused by excess catecholamines (85). Thus, the glucose intolerance of pheochromocytoma differs from diabetes mellitus, and is a simple chemical trait entirely secondary to excessive catecholamine secretion.

Multiple Endocrine Adenomatosis (MEA I) Syndrome

The dominantly inherited syndrome of multiple endocrine adenomatosis is characterized by hyperplasia or neoplasia of one or more endocrine glands, particularly the parathyroid, pancreatic islets, and pituitary and there is a high incidence of peptic ulcer disease (5,69). Although the usual disturbance in carbohydrate metabolism in this disorder is severe hypoglycemia secondary to an insulinoma, glucose intolerance may occur in these patients if they have eosinophilic adenomas of the pituitary or Cushing's disease in the absence of islet cell hyperplasia. In either case, the glucose intolerance is a simple chemical abnormality entirely secondary to the excess secretion of growth hormone or adrenocortical steroids.

Inborn Errors of Metabolism Associated with Glucose Intolerance

There are several inborn errors of metabolism which have been found to be associated with abnormal glucose tolerance. The relationship of the abnormality in carbohydrate metabolism to the basic metabolic error in these disorders has not been well clarified.

Glycogen Storage Disease Type I (von Gierke's disease)

This recessive disorder is caused by a deficiency of glucose-6 phosphatase which catalyzes the intracellular hydrolysis of glucose-6 phosphate to glucose. This enzyme deficiency results in an inability to maintain fasting plasma glucose levels from glycogen stores; fasting hypoglycemia in infancy is a prominent feature which improves with age. Abnormal glucose tolerance increasing in severity with age is a characteristic finding in this disorder (33). Insulinopenia both in the basal state and in response to glucose and arginine has been documented in adults, but prompt insulin responsivness has been found in affected children (47). Lockwood et al. (47) postulate that with increasing age, patients with von Gierke's disease develop decreased insulin output which results in improvement of the hypoglycemic tendency and a decrease in glucose tolerance.

Acute Intermittant Porphyria (AIP)

AIP is an inborn error of porphyrin metabolism which is inherited as an autosomal dominant trait. A variety of endocrine disturbances have been reported in this disorder, including inappropriate ADH release, paradoxical increases in plasma HGH in response to a glucose load, and isolated ACTH deficiency, all of which have been postulated to result from damage to the hypothalamus (88). Waxman et al. (87,88) have demonstrated a high prevalence of abnormal glucose tolerance in these patients, especially during acute symptomatic episodes. In some patients, the glucose intolerance was associated with excessive plasma insulin release. Unlike other patients with maturity-onset diabetes, high rather than low levels of plasma pyruvate and lactate followed a glucose load. The abnormalities in plasma glucose, pyruvate, and lactate were corrected by exogenous insulin administration. A high carbohydrate intake can block the induction of ALA synthetase and reverse the abnormality in porphyrin metabolism in this disease, and in fact, administration of a high carbohydrate intake and insulin can produce a dramatic decrease in the pain. The relationship of the basic defect in porphyrin metabolism to the glucose intolerance, however, is completely unknown.

The Hyperlipidemias

A number of genetic forms of hyperlipidemia have been found to be associated with a high prevalence of diabetes mellitus. These disorders are discussed in detail elsewhere in this volume by Fuhrmann (p. 138).

Syndromes with Non-Ketotic Insulin-Resistant Early-Onset Diabetes Mellitus

There are several genetic disorders associated with a peculiar form of nonketotic insulin-resistant diabetes with elevated plasma immunoreactive insulin concentrations. The pathogenesis of the abnormality in carbohydrate metabolism in these disorders and their relationship to each other is unknown.

Ataxia Telangiectasia

Ataxia telangiectasia is characterized by cerebellar ataxia, conjunctival and cutaneous telangiectasia, IgA deficiency, thymic hypoplasia, and frequent sinopulmonary infections. Schalch *et al.* (75) described an unusual form of diabetes in this syndrome and their observations have been confirmed and extended by McFarlin *et al.* (52). In both reports, over 50% of the patients studied with ataxia telangiectasia had an abnormal glucose tolerance, but this was rarely associated with glycosuria and never with ketosis. Fasting plasma insulin levels were elevated and there was excessive insulin secretion in response to glucose and tolbutamide. There was a blunted fall in blood glucose concentration in response to either endogenous or exogenous insulin, suggesting that the glucose intolerance is associated with peripheral insensitivity to insulin. Many of the patients with carbohydrate intolerance were also found to have liver dysfunction.

Myotonic Dystrophy

Myotonic dystrophy is an autosomal dominant disorder characterized by myotonia, progressive muscular atrophy, frontal baldness, cataracts, testicular atrophy, and decreased basal metabolic rate with normal thyroid function. Diabetes mellitus, impaired carbohydrate tolerance, or a flat glucose tolerance curve all have been documented on numerous occasions in these patients (10,14,34,44). Although fasting glucose concentrations are normal, abnormal glucose tolerance is frequent and is associated with marked hyperinsulinemia (25,34). Excessive insulin secretion also has been documented following intravenous glucose, arginine, tolbutamide, glucagon, and leucine (25,34). Thus, myotonic dystrophy

appears to be associated with markedly increased plasma insulin res-
ponsiveness to all stimuli. Both epinephrine infusion and fasting result
in normal suppression of insulin release, suggesting that insulin control mechanisms are normally operative (35). Although the glucose response to exogenous insulin is normal, myotonia dystrophia patients appear to have a blunted response to endogenous insulin since the excessive rise in plasma insulin concentrations is not accompanied by an
excessive fall in blood glucose. Peripheral unresponsiveness to insulin
or the secretion of a functionally defective insulin molecule have been
postulated, but further studies must be done to clarify the pathogenetic
mechanism involved in the abnormality of carbohydrate metabolism (35).
The glucose intolerance in myotonic dystrophy is not associated with
microangiopathy or any of the other diabetic complications and normal
capillary basement membrane thickness has been documented (12).

Lipoatrophic Diabetes Syndromes

A number of distinct syndromes have been described which are characterized by the absence of subcutaneous, intra-abdominal, and perinephric
fat, hyperlipidemia, insulin-resistant, nonketotic diabetes mellitus,
and a number of anomalies including acanthosis nigricans, genital hyperplasia, hepatomegaly, etc. These disorders of lipoatrophic diabetes are
described in detail elsewhere in this volume by Köbberling (p. 147).

Hereditary Neuromuscular Disorders Associated with Glucose Intolerance

A large number of distinct syndromes affecting the neuromuscular system
have been found to be associated with abnormal glucose tolerance. In
most of these syndromes, however, the glucose intolerance is present in
only a relatively small proportion of cases and is not associated with
the complications of diabetes mellitus. It is quite likely that in many
of these disorders the glucose intolerance is simply secondary to decreased muscle mass and inactivity, rather than to a basic defect in
carbohydrate metabolism. Indeed, abnormal glucose tolerance has been observed in 27-36% of patients with a variety of neuromuscular disorders
of diverse etiology, such as amyotrophic lateral sclerosis, late-onset
myopathy, muscular dystrophy, and chronic peripheral neuropathy (10).
There are, however, a number of syndromes discussed below in which the
diabetes mellitus is of the severe juvenile-onset variety and not simple
glucose intolerance.

The Muscular Dystrophies

There have been conflicting reports on the prevalence of abnormal glucose tolerance in individuals with progressive muscular dystrophy (69).
For example, Ionasecu and Luca (37) found abnormal glucose tolerance in
patients with both the facio-scapulo-humeral and Duchenne dystrophies,
and Herschberg et al. (30) observed impaired oral glucose tolerance,
intravenous glucose tolerance, and glucose response to glucagon infusion
in patients with Duchenne dystrophy. Danowski et al. (12) found abnormal glucose tolerance in 8 of 11 patients with the facio-scapulo-humeral
form of dystrophy, two of whom had basement membrane thickening, but all
of the 22 patients with Duchenne dystrophy studied had normal glucose
tolerance. The glucose intolerance in muscular dystrophy may well be
due to a delay in disposal of the glucose load as a result of decreased
metabolism of glucose in the diminished muscle mass and its decreased
ability to store glucose as glycogen, or to the relative inactivity,
lack of exercise, and/or poor nutrition of patients.

Late-Onset Proximal Myopathy

Swash *et al.* (<u>81</u>) described a sibship of 6 individuals all of whom had maturity onset diabetes and all but one of whom had senile cataracts. The four females in this sibship had a peculiar form of late-onset myopathy with a limb-girdle distribution, which had its onset after age 49 years, as well as bilateral Dupuytren's contractures. Although their two brothers had maturity-onset diabetes and one had cataracts, neither of the males had the myopathy nor Dupuytren's contracture; they were both over 60 years of age. The authors postulated that late-onset myopathy represents a distinct syndrome, but its relationship to glucose tolerance is obscure.

Huntington's Chorea

Abnormal glucose tolerance was observed in six of ten patients with Huntington's chorea by Podolsky *et al.* (<u>62</u>). These patients had hyperinsulinism following an oral glucose load as well as in response to intravenous arginine. Symptoms of diabetes mellitus, glycosuria, and vascular complications were not present. The only factor that was correlated with glucose intolerance was the duration of the Huntington's chorea. Although these patients were not wasted, it is likely that their abnormal glucose tolerance was due to decreased muscle mass and decreased physical activity similar to that which has been postulated in muscular dystrophy.

Machado Disease

Nakano *et al.* (<u>58</u>) described a large pedigree in Massachusetts with a dominantly inherited form of mild ataxia; all had descended from William Machado, a native of the Portugese Azores. The ataxia characteristically occurs late in life, is slowly progressive, and is associated with nystagmus, mild dysarthria, depressed or absent tendon reflexes, distal muscle atrophy, and sometimes contractures and fasciculations. All six affected individuals studied had diabetic oral glucose tolerance curves. Indeed, every person studied who had an abnormal neurological exam had elevated blood glucose levels, whereas all neurologically unaffected family members studied had normal blood glucose concentrations. The neurologic symptoms, however, were not secondary to diabetic neuropathy as treatment of the diabetes did not affect the ataxia. The pathogenesis of the abnormal glucose tolerance and its relationship to the ataxia is unknown, but it may well be due to the decreased muscle mass and inactivity.

Herrmann's Syndrome

Herrmann *et al.* (<u>28</u>) described a family in which 14 members of five generations had all or part of a syndrome consisting of light-sensitive seizures (photomyoclonus), progressive nerve deafness, nephropathy, progressive neurologic deterioration with dementia, and diabetes mellitus. The diabetes was of the mild adult-onset variety unasssociated with ketosis. At autopsy, both renal tubular epithelial cells and central nervous system neurones were found to be distended by PAS-positive lipid material. The authors postulated that this constellation of abnormalities represents a distinct lipid storage disease, inherited as an autosomal dominant trait.

The Optic Atrophy-Diabetes Mellitus Syndrome

The autosomal recessive syndrome of optic atrophy and juvenile diabetes mellitus was first recorded as a familial trait by Wolfram (94) in 1938, when he described four of eight siblings who developed juvenile diabetes between the ages of 5 and 10 years and thereafter primary optic atrophy. This family was subsequently reported by Cooper et al. (11) in 1950 who noted that one of these patients had developed ataxia, gynecomastia, and testicular atrophy. Six years later, a further report described the development of complete blindness, neurogenic bladder, and hearing loss in several of these siblings (84). Numerous other reports describing the association of optic atrophy and diabetes mellitus in siblings have been published since then, but a great deal of confusion exists in the literature as to how many syndromes exist with this combination of abnormalities (70,71). It is now well accepted that there is an autosomal recessive syndrome associated with optic atrophy, diabetes mellitus, and neurosensory deafness. The optic atrophy is of the primary variety and is characterized by white discs and in some instances, peripheral retinal pigmentation as well. The diabetes mellitus is of the severe juvenile-onset variety and frequently precedes the other symptoms. Bilateral neurosensory deafness has more recently been considered to be an integral component of this syndrome; it begins as a high frequency hearing loss and may remain quite mild. Indeed, in many affected patients, the hearing loss was not suspected until audiograms were performed.

A number of other associated abnormalities have been described in certain families including ataxia, autonomic dysfuntion with a neurogenic bladder, sideroblastic anemia, and hyperalaninuria (38). In view of the progression with time of simple optic atrophy and diabetes mellitus to the full-blown syndrome with neurosensory hearing loss, atonic bladder and ataxia in the original family described by Wolfram (11,84,94), it is quite likely that all of these anomalies are the result of a single pleiotropic mutant gene and represent one distinct syndrome. Furthermore, many of the cases of so-called Friedreich's ataxia, the Laurence-Moon-Biedl syndrome, Refsum's syndrome, and other neurodegenerative diseases which have been described in association with diabetes mellitus, also have had optic atrophy and it is quite likely that many of these cases have the optic atrophy-diabetes mellitus syndrome (19).

Several families also have been reported in which optic atrophy and juvenile diabetes mellitus have occurred in association with vasopressin-sensitive diabetes insipidus (57,65). Although this had been considered to represent a distinct autosomal recessive syndrome, Ikkos et al. (36) have reported a family in which three siblings had juvenile diabetes mellitus, optic atrophy, and mild perceptive deafness, one of whom also had diabetes insipidus. Furthermore, perceptive deafness, neurogenic bladder, and hyperalaninuria have been described in other individuals with diabetes insipidus, optic atrophy, and diabetes mellitus (60). Thus, it is quite likely that diabetes insipidus is simply another pleiotropic effect of a single mutant gene.

Thus, optic atrophy in association with juvenile diabetes mellitus appears to be inherited as an autosomal recessive trait with marked variability in the expression of the associated features. These include diabetes insipidus, perceptive deafness, ataxia, neurogenic bladder, and sideroblastic anemia. Careful examination of other families with this association of anomalies will be required to completely document whether this variable association of anomalies represents the pleiotropic effects of one mutant gene or whether genetic heterogeneity does really exist. Furthermore, the relationship of diabetes mellitus to optic atrophy and to other components of this syndrome is completely unknown.

Friedreich's Ataxia

Friedreich's ataxia is an autosomal recessive, spino-cerebellar degenerative disorder characterized by ataxia, dysarthria, nystagmus, diminished or absent tendon reflexes, impaired position and vibratory sensation, scoliosis, and pes cavus. The coexistence of Friedreich's ataxia and diabetes mellitus has been documented in over 70 patients and multiple siblings with both of these disorders have been described in at least 14 families (62). The diabetes mellitus is usually of the juvenile ketosis prone, insulin-requiring variety. An atrophic pancreas with a decreased number of islets has been found on autopsy (27). Thoren (82) studied glucose tolerance in 50 cases of Friedreich's ataxia and found a diabetic curve in 18%. The mean age of onset of diabetes in his series was 30 years, well after the patients were incapacitated from the neurologic disorder. Intravenous glucose tolerance tests were performed in 18 of nondiabetics, one of whom was abnormal; thus, diabetes and/or an abnormal glucose tolerance test was observed in 20% of his cases. Five of the cases, two of whom were siblings, also had optic atrophy. Indeed, optic atrophy was found in 5 of 12 cases of Friedreich's ataxia with diabetes mellitus but in only 1 of 44 cases without diabetes mellitus. Hewer and Robinson (30) found that only 8% of their series of 118 patients with Friedreich's ataxia had diabetes, and the combination of ataxia and diabetes was limited to a few sibships.

It is quite likely that many of the cases of "Friedreich's ataxia" and diabetes mellitus have the optic atrophy-diabetes mellitus syndrome, especially those cases in whom optic atrophy was demonstrated. Furthermore, many of the cases of Friedreich's ataxia with abnormal glucose tolerance without the symptoms of diabetes mellitus, may simply represent a chemical abnormality secondary to muscle wasting and inactivity. Thus, the real incidence of diabetes mellitus in true cases of Friedreich's ataxia is unknown and when the combination of ataxia and diabetes mellitus is encountered an attempt should be made to rule out optic atrophy, perceptive deafness and the other features of the optic atrophy-diabetes mellitus syndrome.

Alstrom's Syndrome

In 1959 Alstrom *et al.* (1) described an inbred kindred in which two siblings and their cousin were affected with a syndrome consisting of retinal degeneration resulting in profound childhood blindness, severe nerve deafness, obesity, and diabetes mellitus. Several other families with this syndrome have since been described and the number of associated anomalies has been expanded to include slowly progressive chronic nephropathy, acanthosis nigricans, baldness, hyperuricemia, hypertriglyceridemia, scoliosis, and hyperostosis frontalis interna (24,39,89). Affected males may also have small testes, low plasma testosterone, and elevated gonadotropin levels in the presence of normal sexual development. Thus, the typical patient with Alstrom's syndrome is an obese child with profound blindness and moderately severe nerve deafness, who, in adulthood, develops signs of carbohydrate intolerance and slowly progressive renal disease. The obesity may disappear as the patient ages. Carbohydrate intolerance is known to have been present in 8 of 10 cases reported with the Alstrom's syndrome (27). Indeed, a normal GTT has been reported in only one patient with this disorder. Goldstein and Fialkow (24) carefully studied carbohydrate metabolism in two of their patients with the Alstrom syndrome and found moderate carbohydrate intolerance, basal hyperinsulinemia, a delay in the initial rise in serum insulin followed by an elevated peak insulin response, and a greater than normal total insulin secretory response, i.e., insulin responses similar to those of typical maturity-onset diabetes.

Neither of their patients, however, were obese at the time of the study.

Thus, the Alstrom syndrome appears to be a distinct autosomal recessive disorder which resembles both the Laurence-Moon-Biedl syndrome and the optic atrophy-diabetes mellitus syndrome. It can be distinguished from the former by the absence of mental retardation and polydactyly and from the latter by the infantile obesity and mild maturity-onset nature of the glucose intolerance. There obviously exists a great deal of clinical overlap between the various neurologic syndromes with diabetes mellitus and it is most important to recognize this genetic heterogeneity and not simply lump all of these disorders into one broad diagnostic category.

Laurence-Moon-Biedl Syndrome

The Laurence-Moon-Biedl syndrome is characterized by retinitis pigmentosa, polydactyly, obesity, hypogonadism, and mental retardation. In the majority of patients reported with this syndrome, diabetes has not been listed as a prominent feature. A number of authors, however, have included diabetes mellitus or abnormal glucose tolerance as a common feature of this syndrome (18,39,76). Diabetes mellitus or an abnormal glucose tolerance test was found in 8 of 57 cases by Klein and Amman (39). Several of these cases were siblings, and one case also had optic atrophy. Furthermore, one case reported by Fraccaro and Gastaldi (18) as an example of the Laurence-Moon-Biedl syndrome associated with carbohydrate intolerance also had retinal degeneration with optic atrophy, juvenile diabetes mellitus, diabetes insipidus, and ataxia, much more suggestive of the optic atrophy-diabetes mellitus syndrome than the Laurence-Moon-Biedl syndrome (19). It is quite possible that many of the patients reported as having the Laurence-Moon-Biedl syndrome and diabetes mellitus had other entities, such as Alstrom's syndrome or the optic atrophy-diabetes mellitus syndrome. Furthermore, mild carbohydrate intolerance in these individuals may be simply secondary to the obesity and not an integral part of the disorder.

Pseudo-Refsum's Syndrome

A number of individuals have been reported with diabetes mellitus in association with Refsum's syndrome, a disorder characterized by retinitis pigmentosa, chronic polyneuritis, ataxia, and an increased CSF protein, associated with phytanic acid accumulation. It is quite likely, however, that most of these individuals did not have Refsum's syndrome, but some other disorder because they were either clinically atypical or found not to have phytanic acid accumulation (37). Furukawa et al. (22) reported a family in which multiple members in several generations had distal neurogenic muscular atrophy, ataxia, retinitis pigmentosa, and late-onset diabetes mellitus. Most of the patients in the family, however, had only one or two of these symptoms, but the authors postulated that this represented a new autosomal dominant disorder. It is quite possible that this family had one of the many other neurologic syndromes associated with ataxia and diabetes mellitus and that true Refsum's syndrome is not associated with abnormal carbohydrate tolerance in the majority of cases.

Progeroid Syndromes Associated with Glucose Intolerance

Several distinct genetic disorders associated with the appearance of premature aging have been reported to have a high prevalence of glucose intolerance. Not all patients with these syndromes, however, have been found to have true abnormalities in glucose tolerance and the possibility exists that carbohydrate intolerance may be at least partially secondary to their decreased muscle mass and relative inactivity. Welsh has also described a Mexican family in which four siblings had an unusual progeroid syndrome associated with early onset of somatic growth, partial alopecia without graying of the hair, a birdlike appearance of the face, total or partial absence of the clavicles, bell-shaped thorax, severe acroosteolysis, and coxa valga. One of the siblings had a definitely abnormal glucose tolerance test, whereas the two others studied had borderline glucose tolerance tests. The relationship of the glucose intolerance to this apparent autosomal recessive disorder is not known.

Cockayne's Syndrome

The Cockayne's syndrome is characterized by growth retardation with loss of adipose tissue beginning in mid- to late infancy. These children develop a markedly cachectic appearance with premature aging, mental retardation, microcephaly, deafness, retinal degeneration, intracranial calcification, and atrophic skin with cutaneous photosensitivity. Abnormal glucose tolerance has been reported in several patients with this syndrome, whereas in other patients it has been found to be normal (51,59,77). Elevated plasma insulin secretion and a blunted glucose response to insulin have been reported in patients with both normal and abnormal glucose tolerance, suggesting a peripheral unresponsiveness to insulin, which is compensated for by increased pancreatic insulin reserve (21). The metabolic features of this syndrome, however, have not been completely characterized and further studies are required to delineate the significance and pathogenesis of the carbohydrate intolerance in this recessice disorder.

Werner's Syndrome

This autosomal recessive disorder is characterized by the appearance of premature aging with symmetrical growth retardation, absence of the adolescent growth spurt, graying of the hair, atrophy and hyperkeratosis of the skin, generalized loss of hair, alterations of the voice, cataracts, ulcerations of the skin of the feet, atrophy of the extremities, soft tissue and vascular calcifications, generalized osteoperosis, hypogonadism, and severe arteriosclerosis and atherosclerosis. Abnormal glucose tolerance is present in approximately 50% of the cases and is considered to be an integral part of this syndrome (16). Most of the patients with glucose intolerance, however, have no symptoms related to the hyperglycemia and both ketoacidosis and diabetic microangiopathy are rare. The glucose concentration achieved following an oral glucose load, however, may be well over 400 mg %. In many of those patients, the glucose intolerance can be controlled by diet alone, or by oral hypoglycemic agents; exogenous insulin may be relatively ineffective in controlling the hyperglycemia. Epstein et al. (16) demonstrated increased plasma immunoreactive insulin concentrations following both intravenous glucose and tolbutamide in association with diabetic-like glucose responses. Although it has been suggested that this syndrome is associated with a defect in the utilization of carbohydrate similar to that in lipoatrophic diabetes, all of the features of the glucose intolerance in Werner's syndrome are quite similar to those found in the obese form of maturity-onset diabetes (16,17,96). The relationship of the glucose intolerance, however, to the muscle atrophy and relative inactivity of these patients has not been defined.

Syndromes with Glucose Intolerance Secondary to Obesity

In addition to the Laurence-Moon-Biedl syndrome, the glucose intolerance often found in the Prader-Willi syndrome and occasionally in achondroplastic dwarfism appears to be secondary to the obesity that is associated with these syndromes. In both instances, the glucose intolerance is usually mild, associated with relative hyperinsulinism, and unaccompanied by ketoacidosis or the vascular complications of diabetes mellitus.

Prader-Willi Syndrome

This syndrome is characterized by obesity, short stature, acromicria, and mental retardation. Generalized hypotonia is present in infancy and may lead to feeding difficulties and respiratory distress. The hypotonia usually decreases in severity after 2 to 4 months of age. Toward the end of the first year of life, they develop an insatiable appetite and resultant obesity; in fact, witholding of food frequently produces a rage reaction. A mild maturity-onset type of diabetes mellitus with insulin resistance and absence of ketosis frequently develops in late childhood or adolescence; but diabetes mellitus has been described as early as 2 years of age, as has the typical juvenile-onset form of the disease (<u>42,63,74,95</u>). Loriden *et al.* (<u>48</u>) found that the degree of glucose intolerance and the insulin hypersecretion in the Prader-Willi syndrome were compatible with that of children with simple obesity and postulated that the glucose intolerance in this syndrome was entirely secondary to their obesity.

Although the polyphagia, mental retardation, and hypogonadism suggests a hypothalamic defect, the etiology of the Prader-Willi syndrome is unknown. Several sets of siblings have been described suggesting autosomal recessive inheritance, but the familial cases have been clinically atypical and the great majority of affected individuals are sporadic (<u>72</u>,<u>83</u>).

Achondroplastic Dwarfism

Although Collip *et al.* (<u>9</u>) reported a high prevalence of glucose intolerance in children with achondroplasia and postulated a defect in carbohydrate metabolism as the responsible mechanism for the skeletal dwarfism, these studies were not well controlled and not corrected for obesity. Because of the frequent obesity in achondroplasia, we have studied glucose intolerance and insulin secretion in 26 achondroplastic dwarfs ranging in age from 10 months to 56 years (<u>45</u>). A standard dose per body weight of oral glucose was utilized and the patients were divided into obese and nonobese categories on the basis of Quetelet's index (W/H^2) (Table 3). Abnormal glucose tolerance was found in three of twenty achondroplasts over 18 years of age and one of six children. Three of the ten obese adult achondroplasts had abnormal glucose tolerance; the one child with abnormal glucose tolerance was the only obese child. Moreover, all four of the achondroplastic individuals with abnormal glucose tolerance were obese. Thus, glucose intolerance does not appear to be a major complication of achondroplastic dwarfism and when it is present, it appears to be entirely secondary to the obesity. Furthermore, plasma insulin concentrations following oral glucose in those achondroplasts with abnormal glucose tolerance showed a delayed high peak with delayed return to normal, similar to that of other patients with obesity. Those achondroplastic dwarfs with normal glucose tolerance, had normal insulin secretory responses. Thus, achondroplastic dwarfism does not appear to be associated with a high prevalence of glucose intolerance nor a primary

Table 3. Glucose tolerance in achondroplasia[a]

	Adults (>18 yp)	Children
Abnormal GTT in all achondroplasts	3/20	1/6
Abnormal GTT in obese achondroplasts[b]	3/10	1/1
Obesity in achondroplasts with abnormal GTT	3/3	1/1

[a]Conn and Fajans' criteria.
[b]Quetlet's index.

defect in carbohydrate metabolism and the postulated role of tolbutamide in treating the skeletal disorder probably has no basis at all.

Miscellaneous Syndromes Associated with Glucose Intolerance

The following syndromes include a number of disorders with glucose intolerance, but which do not fit into any of the above pathogenetic categories. A number of the syndromes have been described in only one family and may therefore be "private," secondary to an isolated gene mutation, although further search for these disorders in the general population is certainly warranted.

Steroid-Induced Ocular Hypertension

The increase in ocular pressure following topical dexamethasone has been shown to be a genetically determined trait that appears to be one of the determinants of open angle glaucoma (2). Three genotypes have been identified on the basis of the degree of increase in ocular pressure following dexamethasone; $p^L p^L$ - less than 6 mm Hg; $p^L p^H$ - 6 to 15 mm Hg, and $p^H p^H$ - greater than 15 mm Hg. Armaly (3) studied glucose tolerance in individuals with all three genotypes and found that the frequency on fasting hyperglycemia, abnormal glucose tolerance, mean levels of blood glucose following an oral glucose load, and clinical diabetes were significantly higher in individuals with the $p^H p^H$ phenotype, less in the $p^L p^H$ heterozygotes and least in the $p^L p^L$ homozygotes. They postulated that the p^H gene is one of the genes involved in determining the diabetic genotype, but the relationship of this genetic trait to diabetes mellitus cannot be determined from the data at hand.

Mendenhall's Syndrome

In 1950, Mendenhall (53) described three siblings with an unusual syndrome consisting of severe insulin-resistant diabetes mellitus, an old-appearing face with heavy features, hyperpigmentation of the skin, protruding abdomen, thickened and hardened nails, early dentition, and enlarged genitalia. The genital changes were apparent in infancy. The diabetes had its onset from 3 to 7 years of age and was associated with severe insulin resistance; in one sibling there was little change in blood glucose concentrations following a single injection of 1000 units of insulin. All three children died of infection and were found to have large hyperplastic pineal glands and severe fibrosis of the pancreas at autopsy (64). Although there have been no further reports of this syndrome, it may well represent a distinct entity inherited as an autosomal recessive trait.

Epiphyseal Dysplasia and Infantile-Onset Diabetes Mellitus

Wolcott and Rallinson (93) have described three siblings with an unusual syndrome consisting of severe infantile-onset diabetes mellitus with ketosis, a skeletal disorder compatible with an epiphyseal dysplasia and abnormalities of the feet and skin. The diabetes was severe and had its onset within the first 2 months of life. The skeletal radiographs were interpreted as multiple epiphyseal dysplasia, but in one of the cases, obvious metaphyseal changes were present and a biopsy of the iliac crest showed marked disorganization of the growth plate, unlike the regular growth plate seen in cases of typical multiple epiphyseal dysplasia (67). The teeth were discolored and there was scaliness and pigmentary abnormalities of the skin. Infantile-onset diabetes mellitus with epiphyseal dysplasia may well represent a distinct autosomal recessive syndrome. In view of the rarity of infantile-onset diabetes, all such patients should have radiographs to rule out a skeletal disease.

Diabetes Mellitus, Hyperlipemia, Hypogonadism, and Short Stature

Lynch et al. (49) reported a kindred in which two brothers had severe juvenile-onset, ketoacidotic diabetes mellitus, hyperlipemia, short stature, hypogonadism, and probably hypopituitarism. Juvenile diabetes mellitus was present in three relatives, hyperlipemia in ten, and short stature in ten. None of the other relatives, however, had the complete syndrome. Although they postulated that this may represent a distinct autosomal dominant syndrome, it is quite likely that all of the features can be explained by uncontrolled diabetes mellitus resulting in short stature, hypogonadism, hypopituitarism, and hyperlipidemia (Mauriac's disease), in association with familial hyperlipidemia and familial short stature. It is therefore unlikely that this family has a distinct primary syndrome and cannot be counted among the genetic syndromes associated with diabetes mellitus.

Cytogenetic Disorders Associated with Glucose Intolerance

Several cytogenetic anomalies have been reported to have an increased prevalence of glucose intolerance. These disorders are discussed in detail in Chapter 14, p. 125.

References

1. Alstrom, C.H., Hallgren, B., Nilsson, L.B., Asander, H.: Retinal degeneration combined with obesity diabetes mellitus, and neurogenous deafness. A specific syndrome (not hitherto described) distinct from the Laurence-Moon-Biedl syndrome. A clinical endocrinological and genetic examination based on a large pedigree. Acta Psychiat. Neurol. Scand. 34, 1 (1959)

2. Armaly, M.F.: The heritable nature of dexamethasone-induced ocular hypertension. Arch. Ophthal. 75, 32 (1966)

3. Armaly, M.F.: Dexamethasone ocular hypertension and eosinopenia and glucose tolerance test. Arch. Ophthal. 78, 193 (1967)

4. Balcerzak, S.P., Mintz, D.H., Westerman, M.P.: Diabetes mellitus and idiopathic hemochromatosis. Amer. J. Med. Sci. 255, 53 (1968)

5. Ballard, H.S., Frame, B., Hartsock, R.J.: Familial multiple endocrine adenoma-peptic ulcer complex. Medicine 43, 481 (1964)

6. Bottazzo, G.F., Florin-Christensen, A., Doniach, D.: Islet-cell antibodies in diabetes mellitus with autoimmune polyendocrine deficiencies. Lancet 2, 1279 (1974)

7. Bretz, G.W., Baghdassarin, A., Graher, J.D., Zacherle, B.J., Norum, R.A., Blizzard, R.M.: Coexistence of diabetes mellitus and insipidus and optic atrophy in two male siblings. Amer. J. Med. 48, 398 (1970)

8. Carpenter, C.C.J., Solomon, N., Silverberg, S.G., Bledsoe, T., Northcutt, R.C., Klinenberg, J.R., Bennett, I.L., and Harvey, A.M.: Schmidt's syndrome (thyroid and adrenal insufficiency): A review of the literature and a report of fifteen new cases including ten instances of coexistent diabetes mellitus. Medicine 43, 153 (1964)

9. Collip, P.J., Sharma, R.K., Thomas, J., Maddaiah, V.T., Chen, S.Y.: Abnormal glucose tolerance in children with achondroplasia. Am. J. Dis. Child. 124, 682 (1972)

10. Collis, W.J., Engel, W.K.: Glucose metabolism in five neuromuscular disorders. Neurology 18, 915 (1968)

11. Cooper, I.S., Rynearson, E.H., Bailey, A.A., MacCarty, C.S.: The relation of spinal cord disease to gynecomastia and testicular atrophy.(Proc. staff meet.). Mayo Clin. 25, 320 (1950)

12. Danowski, T.S., Khurana, R.C., Gonzales, A.R., Fisher, E.R.: Capillary basement membrane thickness and the pseudodiabetes of myopathy. Brit. J. Ophthalmol. 51, 757 (1971)

13. Davidson, P., Constanza, D., Swieconek, J.A., Harris, J.B.: Hereditary pancreatitis. A kindred without gross aminoaciduria. Ann. Intern. Med. 68, 88 (1968)

14. Drucker, W.D., Rowland, L.P., Sterling, K., Christy, N.P.: On the function of the endocrine glands in myotonic muscular dystrophy. Amer. J. Med. 31, 941 (1961)

15. Elders, M.J., Garland, J.T., Daughaday, W.A., Fisher, D.A., Whitney, J.E., Hughes, E.R.: Laron Dwarfism: studies on the nature of the defect. J. Pediat. 83, 253 (1973)

16. Epstein, C.J., Mertin, G.M., Schultz, A.L., Motulsky, A.G.: Werner's syndrome. Medicine 45, 117 (1966)

17. Field, J.B., Loube, S.D.: Observations concerning the diabetes mellitus associated with Werner's syndrome. Metabolism 9, 118 (1960)

18. Fraccaro, M., Gastaldi, F.: La patologia della sindrome di Laurence-Moon-Biedl, Folia, Hered. Et Path. 2, 177 (1953)

19. Fraser, G.R.: Heredity in juvenile diabetes. Brit. Med. J. 1, 433 (1964)

20. Frey, H.M.M., Vogt, J.H., Nerup, J.: Familial poly-endocrinopathy. Acta Endocr. 72, 401 (1973)

21. Fujimoto, W.Y., Greene, M.L., Seegmiller, J.E.: Cockayne's syndrome: report of a case with hyperlipoproteinemia, hyperinsulinemia, renal disease and normal growth hormone. J. Pediat. 75, 881 (1969)

22. Furukawa, T., Takagi, A., Nakao, K., Tsukagoshi, H., Tsubaki, T.: Hereditary muscular atrophy with ataxia, retinitis pigmentosa, and diabetes mellitus. Neurology 19, 942 (1968)

23. Gharib, H., Gastineau, C.F.: Coexisting Addison's disease and diabetes mellitus: report of 24 cases with review of literature. Mayo Clin. Proc. 44, 217 (1969)

24. Goldstein, J.L., Fialkow, P.J.: The Alstrom syndrome: report of three cases with further delineation of the clinical, pathophysiological, and genetic aspects of the disorder. Medicine 52, 53 (1973)

25. Gorden, P., Griggs, R.C., Nissley, S.P., Roth, J., Engel, W.K.: Studies of plasma insulin in myotonic dystrophy. J. Clin. Endocr. 29, 684 (1969)

26. Gross, J.B., Gambill, E.E., Ulrich, J.A.: Hereditary pancreatitis. Description of a fifth kindred and summary of clinical features. Amer. J. Med. 33, 358 (1962)

27. Handwerger, S., Roth, J., Gordon, P., di Sant Agnese, P., Carpenter, D.F., Peter, G.: Glucose intolerance in cystic fibrosis. New Eng. J. Med. 281, 451 (1969)

28. Herrmann, C., Jr., Augilar, M.J., Sacks, O.W.: Hereditary photomyoclonus associated with diabetes mellitus, deafness, nephropathy, and cerebral dysfunction. Neurology 14, 212 (1964)

29. Herschberg, A.D., Coirault, R., Giboudeau, J.: Le métabolisme du glucose dans la myopathie progressive de Duchenne. Ann. Endocr. 25, 447 (1964)

30. Hewer, R.L., Robinson, N.: Diabetes mellitus in Friedreich's ataxia. J. Neurol. Neurosurg. Psychiat. 31, 226 (1968)

31. Heycock, J.E., Wilson, J.: Diabetes mellitus in a child showing features of Refsum's syndrome. Arch. Dis. Child. 33, 320 (1958)

32. Holsclaw, D.S., Auruskin, T., Soeldner, S.J., Schwachman, H.: The development of diabetes mellitus in cystic fibrosis. Abstracts of the Annual Meeting, Society for Pediatric Research, 1970

33. Howell, R.R., Ashton, D.M., Wyngaarden, J.B.: Clucose-6-phosphate deficiency glycogen storage disease. Pediatrics 29, 553 (1962)

34. Huff, T.A., Horton, E.S., Lebovitz, H.E.: Abnormal insulin secretion in myotonic dystrophy. New Eng. J. Med. 277, 837 (1967)

35. Huff, T.A., Lebovitz, H.E.: Dynamics of insulin secretion in myotonic dystrophy. J. Clin. Endocr. 28, 992 (1968)

36. Ikkos, D.G., Fraser, G.R., Matsouki-Gavra, Petrochilos, M.: Association of juvenile diabetes mellitus, primary optic atrophy and perceptive hearing loss in three sibs, with additional idiopathic diabetes mellitus insipidus in one case. Acta Endocrinologia 65, 95 (1970)

37. Ionasecu, V., and Luca, N.: Investigations on carbohydrate metabolism in progressive muscular dystrophy. Psychiat. Neurol. 146, 309 (1963)

38. Jarnerot, G.: Diabetes mellitus with optic atrophy-thalassemia-like sideroblastic anemia and weak isoagglutinins – a new genetic syndrome. Acta Med. Scand. 193, 359 (1973)

39. Klein, D., Ammann, F.: The syndrome of Laurence-Moon-Bardet-Biedl and allied diseases in Switzerland. J. Neurol. Sci. 9, 479 (1969)

40. Kolodny, E.H., Hass, W.K., Lane, B., Drucker, W.D.: Refsum's syndrome. Arch. Neurol. 12, 583 (1965)

41. Lancet Editorial: Autoimmune diabetes mellitus. Lancet II, 1549 (1974)

42. Landwirth, J., Schwartz, H., Grunt, J.A.: Prader-Willi syndrome. Amer. J. Dis. Child. 116, 211 (1968)

43. Laron, E., Karp, M., Pertzelan, A., Kauli, R., Keret, R., Doron, M.: The syndrome of familial dwarfism and high plasma immunoreactive human growth hormone (IR-HGH). In: Growth and Growth Hormone. Pecile, A., Muller, E. (eds.). Amsterdam: Excerpta Medica, 1972, p. 458

44. Lee, F.I., Hughes, D.T.D.: Systemic effects in dystrophia myotonica. Brain 87, 521 (1964)

45. Levine, M., Rimoin, D.L., Bray, G.A.: Glucose tolerance in achondroplasia. In preparation

46. Lippe, B., Sperling, M.A., Dooley, R.: Pancreatic alpha and beta cell function in children with cystic fibrosis. Pediat. Res. 8, 435 (1974)

47. Lockwood, D.H., Merimee, T.J., Edgar, P.J., Greene, M.D., Fujimoto, W.Y., Seegmiller, J.E., Howell, R.R.: Insulin secretion in type I glycogen storage disease. Diabetes 18, 755 (1969)

48. Loridan, L., Sadeghi-Nejad, A., Senior, B.: Hypersecretion of insulin after the administration of L-leucine to obese children. J. Pediat. 78, 53 (1971)

49. Lynch, H.T., Kaplan, A.R., Henn, J.J., Krush, A.J.: Familial coexistence of diabetes mellitus, hyperlipemia, short stature, and hypogonadism. Amer. J. Med. Sci. 252, 323 (1966)

50. MacCuish, A.C., Barnes, E.W., Irvine, W.J., Duncan, L.J.P.: Antibodies to pancreatic islet cells in insulin-dependent diabetics with coexistent autoimmune disease. Lancet 2, 1529 (1974)

51. MacDonald, W.B., Fitch, K.D., Lewis, I.C.: Cockayne's syndrome, a heredo-familial disorder of growth and development. Pediatrics 25, 996 (1960)

52. McFarlin, D.E., Strober, W., Waldmann, T.A.: Ataxia telangiectasia. Medicine 51, 281 (1972)

53. Mendenhall, E.N.: Tumor of the pineal body with high insulin resistance. J. Indiana Med. Assoc. 43, 22 (1950)

54. Merimee, T.J., Fineberg, S.E., McKusick, V.A., Hall, J.: Diabetes mellitus and sexual ateliotic dwarfism: a comparative study. J. Clin. Invest. 49, 1096 (1970)

55. Merimee, T.J., Siperstein, M.D., Hall, J.D., Fineberg, S.E.: Capillary basement membrane structure: a comparative study of diabetics and sexual ateliotic dwarfs. J. Clin. Invest. 49, 2161 (1970)

56. Milner, A.D.: Blood glucose and serum insulin levels in children with cystic fibrosis. Arch. Dis. Child. 44, 351 (1969)

57. Najjar, S.S., Mahmud, J.: Diabetes insipidus and diabetes mellitus in a six-year-old girl. J. Pediat. 73, 251 (1968)

58. Nakano, K.K., Dawson, D.M., Spence, A.: Machado disease. A hereditary ataxia in Portuguese emigrants to Massachusetts. Neurology 22, 49 (1972)

59. Neill, C.A., Dingwall, M.M.: A syndrome resembling progeria: a review of two cases. Arch. Dis. Child. 25, 213 (1950)

60. Niemeyer, G., Marquardt, J.L.: Retinal function in an unique syndrome of optic atrophy, juvenile diabetes mellitus, diabetes insipidus, neurosensory hearing loss, autonomic dysfunction, and hyperalanineuria. Invest. Ophthal. 11, 617 (1972)

61. Podolsky, S., Leopold, N.A., Sax, D.S.: Increased frequency of diabetes mellitus in patients with Huntington's chorea. Lancet I, 1356 (1972)

62. Podolsky, S., Sheremata, W.A.: Insulin dependent diabetes mellitus and Friedreich's ataxia. Metabolism 19, 555 (1970)

63. Prader, A., Labhart, A., Willi, H.: Ein Syndrom von Adipositas, Kleinwuchs, Kryptorchidismus und Oligophrenia nach myotonieartigem Zustand im Neugeborenenalter. Schweiz. Med. Wschr. 86, 1260 (1956)

64. Rabson, S.M., Mendenhall, E.N.: Familial hypertrophy of pineal body, hyperplasia of adrenal cortex and diabetes mellitus. Amer. J. Clin. Path. 26, 283 (1956)

65. Raiti, S., Plotkin, S., Newns, G.H.: Diabetes mellitus and insipidus in two sisters. Brit. Med. J. 2, 1625 (1963)

66. Rimoin, D.L.: Genetics of Diabetes Mellitus. Diabetes 16, 346 (1967)

67. Rimoin, D.L.: The Chondrodystrophies. Advances in Human Genetics 5, 1 (1975)

68. Rimoin, D.L., Schechter, J.E.: Histological and ultrastructural studies in isolated growth hormone deficiency. J. Clin. Endocrinol. Metab. 37, 725 (1973)

69. Rimoin, D.L., Schimke, R.N.: Genetic Disorders of the Endocrine Glands. St Louis: C.V. Mosby, 1971

70. Rorsman, G., Soderstrom, N.: Optic atrophy and juvenile diabetes mellitus with familial occurrence. Acta Med. Scand. 182, 419 (1967)

71. Rose, F.C., Fraser, G.R., Friedmann, A.I., Kohner, E.M.: The association of juvenile diabetes mellitus and optic atrophy. Quart. J. Med. 35, 385 (1966)

72. Royer, P.: Le diabète sucré dans le syndrome de Willi-Prader. Journées Ann. Diabet. Hôtel Dieu 4, 91 (1963)

73. Saddi, R., Peingold, J.: Idiopathic haemochromatosis and diabetes mellitus. Clin. Gen. 5, 242 (1974)

74. Savir, A., Dickerman, Z., Karp, M., Laron, Z.: Diabetic retinopathy in an adolescent with Prader-Labhart-Willi syndrome. Arch. Dis. Child. 49, 963 (1974)

75. Schalch, D.S., McFarlin, D.E., Barlow, M.H.: An unusual form of diabetes mellitus in ataxia telangiectasia. New Eng. J. Med. 282, 1396 (1970)

76. Solis-Cohen, S., Weiss, E.: Dystrophia adiposogenitalis, with atypical retinitis pigmentosa and mental deficiency - the Laurence-Biedl syndrome. Amer. J Med. Sci. 169, 489 (1925)

77. Spark, H.: Cachectic dwarfism resembling the Cockayne-Neill type. J. Pediat. 66, 41 (1965)

78. Spergel, G., Bleicher, S.J., Ertel, N.H.: Carbohydrate and fat metabolism in patients with pheochromocytoma. New Eng. J. Med. 278, 803 (1968)

79. Stahl, M., Girard, J., Rutishauser, M., Nars, P.W., Zuppinger, K.: Endocrine function of the pancreas in cystic fibrosis: evidence for an impaired glucagon and insulin response following arginine infusion. J. Pediat. 84, 821 (1974)

80. Stimmler, L., Jensen, N., Toseland, P.: Alaninuria, associated with microcephaly, dwarfism, enamel hypoplasia, and diabetes mellitus in two sisters. Arch. Dis. Child. 45, 682 (1970)

81. Swash, M., van den Noort, S., Craig, J.W.: Late-onset proximal myopathy with diabetes mellitus in four sisters. Neurology 20, 694 (1970)

82. Thoren, C.: Diabetes mellitus in Friedreich's ataxia. Acta Paediatrica 51, 239 (1962)

83. De Fraites, E.B., Thurmon, T.F. and Farbadian, H.: Familial Prader-Willi syndrome. In: Genetic Forms of Hypogonadism, Birth Defects Original Article Series. XI (4): 123, 1975

84. Tunbridge, R.E., Paley, R.G.: Primary optic atrophy in diabetes mellitus. Diabetes 5, 295 (1956)

85. Vance, J.E., Buchanan, K.D., O'Hara, D., Williams, R.H., Porte, D.: Insulin and glucagon responses in subjects with pheochromocytoma: effects of alpha adrenergic blockade. J. Clin. Endocr. 29, 911 (1969)

86. Wang, C.I.: Intertwining genetics of cystic fibrosis and diabetes mellitus. Abstracts of the Eighth Annual Meeting of Cystic Fibrosis Club, National Cystic Fibrosis Research Foundation, New York, 1967

87. Waxman, A.D., Schalch, D.S., Odell, W.D., Tschudy, D.P.: Abnormalities of carbohydrate metabolism in acute intermittent porphyria. J. Clin. Invest. 46, 1129 (1967)

88. Waxman, A.D., Berk, P., Schalch, D., Tschudy, D.: Isolated adrenocorticotrophic hormone deficiency in acute intermittent porphyria. Ann. Intern. Med. 70, 317 (1969)

89. Weinstein, R.L., Kliman, B., Scully, R.E.: Familial syndrome of primary testicular insufficiency with normal virilization, blindness, deafness, and metabolic abnormalities. New Eng. J. Med. 281, 969 (1969)

90. Welsh, D.: Study of a family with a new progeroid syndrome. In: New Chromosomal and Malformation Syndromes, Birth Defects Original Article Series. XI (5): 25, 1975

91. Whitten, D.M., Feingold, M., Eisenklam, E.J.: Hereditary pancreatitis. Amer. J. Dis. Child. 116, 426 (1968)

92. Wilber, J.F., Turtle, J.R., Crane, N.A.: Inhibition of insulin secretion by a pheochromocytoma. Lancet 2, 733 (1966)

93. Wolcott, C.D., Rallison, M.L.: Infancy-onset diabetes mellitus and multiple epiphyseal dysplasia. J. Pediat. 80, 292 (1972)

94. Wolfram, D.J.: Diabetes mellitus and simple optic atrophy among siblings: report of four cases. (Proc. staff meet. Mayo Clin.) 13, 715 (1938)

95. Zellweger, H., Schneider, H.J.: Syndrome of hypotonia-hypomentia-hypogonadism-obesity (HHHO) or Prader-Willi syndrome. Arch. Dis. Child. 115, 588 (1968)

96. Zucker-Franklin, D., Rifkin, H., Jacobson, H.G.: Werner's syndrome. An analysis of ten cases. Geriatrics 23, 123 (1968)

8. The Natural History of Idiopathic Diabetes Mellitus. Heterogeneity of Insulin Responses in Latent Diabetes

S. S. FAJANS

Idiopathic diabetes mellitus is a disorder of metabolism which in its fully developed clinical expression is characterized by fasting hyperglycemia, atherosclerotic and microangiopathic vascular disease, and neuropathy. Diabetes may present clinically also in a mild or asymptomatic form with relatively mild carbohydrate intolerance, and with normal fasting blood glucose levels.

There is common agreement that idiopathic diabetes is a disease in which an inherited susceptibility plays an important part. This susceptibility has its origin at conception and may exist for prolonged periods before additional pathogenetic factors cause the emergence of a recognizable abnormality of carbohydrate metabolism. The genetic defect may remain without clinical expression indefinitely. Thus, a definition of genetic or idiopathic diabetes mellitus should include stages in the natural history of the disease which presently cannot be recognized since we lack a marker for "genetic diabetes."

Before discussing further arbitrary definitions of the stages in the natural history of idiopathic diabetes, it is important to recognize several recent findings and concepts which are discussed in detail elsewhere in this volume. These findings suggest a revision in interpretation of a previously proposed scheme of the natural history of diabetes (13,15,17).

The biochemical and clinical manifestations of the disease encompass a spectrum from the recognizable but asymptomatic form of the disease to symptomatic diabetes with acute metabolic decompensation (ketoacidosis, hyperosmolar coma) or with chronic complications or associations (cataracts, complications of pregnancy, neuropathy, atherosclerosis, microangiopathy). Hyperglycemia and these complications are found in both maturity-onset type and juvenile-onset type diabetes. These two types of diabetes usually have been thought to represent only a quantitative difference in the defect in insulin secretion or action, and attendent sequelae. However, a growing body of evidence suggests the existence of heterogeneity of idiopathic diabetes mellitus in terms of (1) inheritance, (2) insulin responses to glucose in maturity-onset type diabetes, and (3) prevalence of vascular disease.

A difference in the inheritance of diabetes has been shown between the families of maturity-onset type diabetes in young people and families of patients with classical juvenile-onset type diabetes (48), as is discussed in Chapter 10. The genetic heterogeneity found among sets of identical twins of which at least one had diabetes mellitus is discussed in Chapter 21. Concordance of diabetes among the pairs of identical twins was very high (92%) among those in whom the age of onset of diabetes in the index twin was 40 years or more (mostly maturity-onset type), while concordance was found with a frequency of only 53% in those in whom diabetes was diagnosed under 40 years of age in one twin (mostly juvenile-onset type) (47). This suggests that there is a difference in genetic as well as in environmental factors in the etiology and pathogenesis of diabetes between those two groups of identical twins (47).

A difference in the inheritance between juvenile-onset and maturity-onset type diabetes may be associated with a difference in the frequency of occurrence of certain histocompatibility types or HL-A antigens (HL-A8 and/or W15) (9,30), and a difference in the frequency with which viral and autoimmune processes may be involved, as is discussed in Chapter 12. At least in a proportion of patients with juvenile-onset type diabetes an increased susceptibility to beta cell damage by viral agents may be due to a defective immune response influenced by genes in the HL-A chromosomal region and leading to an autoimmune process (9, 30). The presence of cell-mediated immunity to pancreas antigen was reported to be more frequent in patients with insulin-dependent diabetes than in patients with insulin-independent diabetes (28,30). These findings also support the concept that these two types of diabetes differ from each other and have been cited to indicate that they are two different disease entities in etiology and pathogenesis (30).

Let us now return to a consideration of the stages in the natural history of diabetes mellitus which have been based on the absence or presence, and on the degree, of abnormality of glucose metabolism (13,15, 17).

Table 1 depicts the natural history of diabetes divided into four stages. The terminology employed in this table draws on the definitions used by our group (13,15,17) and by the British Diabetic Association and the World Health Organization (17).

Overt (or clinical) diabetes is the most advanced of these stages. Classical symptoms may be present; there is gross fasting hyperglycemia; there is no insulin secretory response to administered glucose. This stage can be divided further into the ketotic and nonketotic forms of the disease which, at least in part, may differ in etiology and pathogenesis (30,47,48).

The preceding stage is latent (or asymptomatic, chemical) but clinically detectable diabetes. A latent diabetic is an individual who has no symptoms, signs, or complications referable to the disease (except for reactive hypoglycemia in some patients) but in whom a diagnosis of diabetes can be established by presently accepted laboratory procedures. This stage may also be characterized by an elevated fasting blood glucose level but of lesser severity than in overt diabetes. When the fasting level of blood glucose is below diagnostic levels this stage can be recognized by a definitely abnormal glucose tolerance test. The heterogeneous nature of the plasma insulin response to administered glucose in this stage will be discussed subsequently.

An earlier stage is subclinical diabetes or latent diabetes by the WHO definition. In this stage, not only the fasting blood glucose level but also the glucose tolerance test is normal under usual circumstances. However, diabetes may be suspected because of evidence of insufficient functional reserve of the islet cells under stress. An example would be a woman who has a normal glucose tolerance test but who has a history of abnormality of glucose tolerance during pregnancy. The latter has been termed pregnancy or gestational diabetes. A high proportion of such women develop latent or overt diabetes in the years that follow. A delayed and subnormal insulin secretory response to glucose has been demonstrated in some patients with gestation diabetes (29). Another

Table 1. Stages in the natural history of diabetes mellitus

Terminology by: University of Michigan	Prediabetes →	Subclinical diabetes	Latent Diabetes	Overt diabetes
World Health Organization	Potential diabetes	Latent diabetes	Asymptomatic diabetes (subclinical or chemical)	Clinical diabetes
FBS	Normal	Normal	Normal or	←
GTT	Normal	Normal Abnormal during pregnancy, stress	Abnormal	Not necessary for diagnosis
Cortisone-GTT	Normal	Abnormal	Not necessary	-----
Delayed and/or decreased insulin response to glucose	None or +	++	+++	++++

example of subclinical diabetes may be an individual with a normal glucose tolerance test but an abnormal cortisone-glucose tolerance test in the nonpregnant state. The plasma insulin response in groups of subjects with abnormal steroid-glucose tolerance tests is delayed and lower as compared to those found in subjects with normal steroid-glucose tolerance tests (27,44).

The earliest stage is prediabetes or potential diabetes (WHO). This stage exists prior to the onset of identifiable diabetes mellitus whether it be overt, latent, or subclinical. It identifies the interval time from conception until the demonstration of impaired glucose tolerance in an individual predisposed to diabetes on genetic grounds. This period can be identified only retrospectively. Prediabetes or potential diabetes can be suspected to be present in individuals who have an increased probability of developing diabetes on genetic grounds, such as some nondiabetic identical twins of diabetic patients or some offspring of two diabetic parents. During the prediabetic period, glucose tolerance and cortisone-glucose tolerance tests are normal.

Recent evidence would suggest that there is more than one form of "genetic prediabetes." A normal insulin secretory response to glucose has been found in young nondiabetic monozygotic twins of diabetic patients (20,46,47). Also, as reviewed earlier, concordance of diabetes in monozygotic twins has been found to be relatively low in those pairs where the index twin developed diabetes under the age of 40 years (47). This may suggest that the nondiabetic twin is not "prediabetic," or more likely, that in these twins diabetes evolves from "prediabetes" only with the superimposition of a specific environmental factor such as a viral infection and/or development of autoimmunity.

Another form of genetic prediabetes may be found in offspring of two diabetic parents who may have a reduced insulin secretory response to glucose (20). This defect is similar in nature to that demonstrated in the majority of patients with latent and subclinical diabetes (19, 44). In these offspring of two diabetic parents and in the older nondiabetic monozygotic twins representing a different type of genetic predisposition from the prediabetic who will develop juvenile-onset diabetes, and in maturity-onset type diabetics in general, more common environmental factors such as overnutrition and resulting obesity, or pregnancy may lead to hyperglycemia.

In the natural history of diabetes progression or regression from one stage to the next stage may never occur, may occur very slowly over many years, or may be rapid or even explosive (13,15,17) depending on the type of genetic predisposition (type of "prediabetes") and the type of environmental factor involved. For example, a patient with a genetic susceptibility to juvenile-onset type, ketosis-prone diabetes may remain a "prediabetic" for life if the necessary viral and/or autoimmune, or other factors do not supervene. When clinical diabetes does occur it usually is manifested by an abrupt onset of insulin insufficiency without previously known abnormality of carbohydrate intolerance. Thus, there is rapid progression from prediabetes to overt diabetes without recognition of subclinical or latent diabetes (Table 2). Occasionally by prospective testing, in siblings of patients with juvenile-onset type diabetes, carbohydrate intolerance can be recognized before decompensation to insulin-requiring, ketotic diabetes, which occurs usually within 2 years of diagnosis (Fig. 1). On the other hand, in young maturity-onset type diabetic patients, with a different genetic susceptibility, intervals of time from 2-18 years have been recorded, before progression to hyperglycemia or to insulin-requiring but nonketotic diabetes (17) (Table 3). Among young people (under 25 years at diagnosis) with asymptomatic maturity-onset type diabetes, glucose intolerance does not pro-

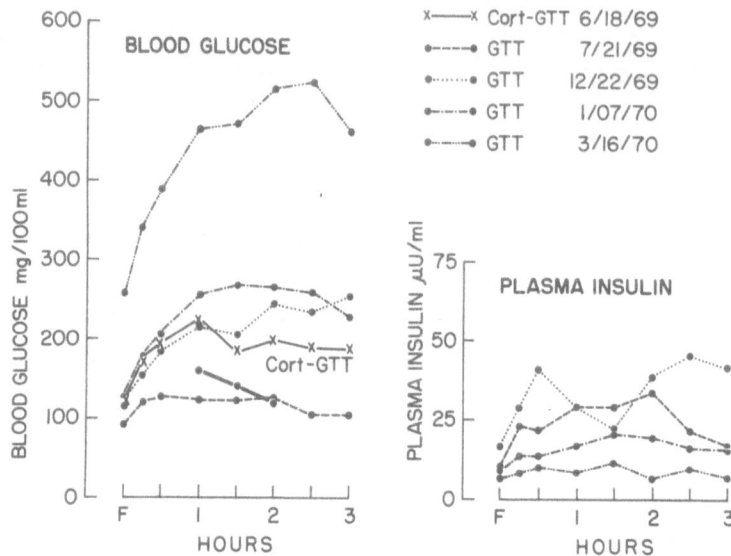

S.N., Male, Age 11 1/2 ; F.H.D.M.: Father, Sister

BLOOD GLUCOSE

x———x Cort-GTT 6/18/69
•-----• GTT   7/21/69
•·······• GTT   12/22/69
•-·-·-• GTT   1/07/70
•-----• GTT   3/16/70

BLOOD GLUCOSE mg/100ml

Cort-GTT

PLASMA INSULIN µU/ml

PLASMA INSULIN

HOURS

HOURS

Fig. 1. Decompensation from subclinical diabetes to latent diabetes and to overt, insulin-requiring, ketotic diabetes within 9 months in an 11-1/2-year-old brother of a juvenile-onset type, ketotic diabetic sister

Table 2. Glucose tolerance test
Rapid progression from "prediabetes" to overt diabetes
K.G.: Male
F.H.: Father, mother, 2 siblings with D.M.

Date	Age	Test	F	1/2	1	1-1/2	2	2-1/2	3
						mg/100 ml			
12/2/54	16	GTT	82	106	88	85	74	85	79
12/3/54	16	Cort-GTT	81	121	91	84	90	98	67
11/55	17		350 - 7 weeks of polyuria, polydipsia, 30-lb. weight loss, fatigue						

gress in severity in approximately 80% of patients followed for as long as 20 years (17). This can be observed in nonobese patients with extremely low insulin responses to glucose. Some of these studies will be reviewed in greater detail below.

The concept that there may be fluctuations in the expression of the carbohydrate aspects of the disease in either direction is an important one in any study of the natural history of the disease or in genetic studies. Such fluctuations are particularly common when carbohydrate intolerance is mild (26,31) as in maturity-onset type diabetes. However, even the overt stage of the disease may regress. Extreme examples such as regression from overt ketotic diabetes to prediabetes have been reported in individuals who have been in diabetic coma and who subsequently exhibited normal standard and normal cortisone-glucose tolerance tests (32). Remission of overt (clinical) diabetes with ketoacidosis to latent (chemical, asymptomatic) diabetes after a period of therapy with

68

Table 3. Maturity-onset type diabetes in childhood

A.P.S., Female; F.H. diabetes:

(1) Father: died of vascular disease
(2) Mother: died of vascular disease
(3) Two brothers (one died of vascular disease) and one sister

Date	Age	Glucose tolerance test							Ht	Wt (lb)
		F	1/2	1	1-1/2 mg/100 ml	2	2-1/2	3		
1/12/54	10	94	146	214	207	161	160	135	4'9"' 1400 calorie diet	118
11/29/54	10	85	–	129	146	100	118	104		110
5/8/58	14	82	105	136	142	150	105	–	5'2-1/2"	177
5/19/59	15	92	144	185	157	156	164	133	5'2-1/4" 1400 calorie diet	178
11/23/59	15	91	125	132	⬧106	136	120	102		160
1/16/61	17	Delivery: M, 8 lb, 6 oz								
3/6/62	18	Delivery: F, 11 lb, 8 oz								
3/4/63	19	88	–	224	–	207	162	–	5'3"	205
7/4/66	22	Delivery: M, 10 lb, 8 oz								
1/11/68	24	87	169	–	182	168			5'3"	185
11/12/69	26	85	149	207	222	212	161	131		170
11/30/70	27	101	210	269	238	246	227	165		199
5/11/72	28	134		258	274	288	288	248		208
7/5/72	29	118								198
1/4/73	29	191								204
7/27/73	30	117								189
8/12/74	31	274								205
9/6/74	31	109							Chlorpropamide 500 mg q.d.	

insulin has been documented more frequently (reviewed by Pirart and Lauvaux, ref. 35). Recently this has been shown to be associated with improvement of B-cell secretory activity (2); this paper contains references to previous relevant reports). However, as we have reported before, in individual patients there may be no consistent relationship between glucose tolerance and the· insulin response to glucose as measured by plasma levels of insulin in peripheral blood by conventional radioimmunoassay (14,16). These findings suggest that factors in addition to the abnormal pancreatic insulin response to glucose may determine normality or abnormality of glucose tolerance.

Earlier I reviewed evidence which has been presented to suggest that there are differences in genetic and environmental factors between insulin-dependent and insulin-independent diabetes. Now I would like to present our evidence for heterogeneity of insulin responses in latent diabetes (18).

There is disagreement among investigators as to the magnitude and patterns of plasma insulin responses to glucose in nonobese patients with latent or chemical or asymptomatic diabetes. When comparing the insulin response to a glucose load of nonobese mildly diabetic patients with that of control subjects, investigators have considered (a) the early, and (b) the later increases in plasma insulin above fasting levels. All patterns of insulin responses possible have been reported (Table 4).

Table 4. Insulin responses to administration of glucose in latent diabetic patients

Type	Early insulin response[a]	Later insulin response[a]	References
1	Delayed	Subnormal	1,4,8,12,14,16,17,22,23, 25,34,40,45,46
2	Delayed	Normal	5,7,25,43,49
3	Delayed	Supernormal	11,12,33,45,50,51
4	Normal	Normal	8,21,24,39,40,41
5	Normal	Supernormal	6,14,16,17,24,36,37,43, 45,50
6	.Supernormal	Supernormal	3,10,21,34,36,40,41,43

[a]Increases above basal levels.

Since our patients with latent diabetes showed a variety of insulin responses to oral glucose (14,16,17), we have examined the pattern of distribution of insulin responses of 59 nonobese latent diabetic patients. Their insulin responses were compared to those of 67 nonobese control subjects who did not have a family history of diabetes or large newborn. The 59 diabetic patients were 9-45 years old at diagnosis (mean age 22.3 years). Forty-three were less than 25 years old at diagnosis; most had a strong family history of diabetes.

On the initial diagnostic tests of the 59 patients all blood glucose levels were significantly higher than those of control subjects (Fig.2). The mean increase in plasma insulin of the diabetic group was significantly lower at 1/2 and 1 hour of the tests (Fig. 2, Table 5).

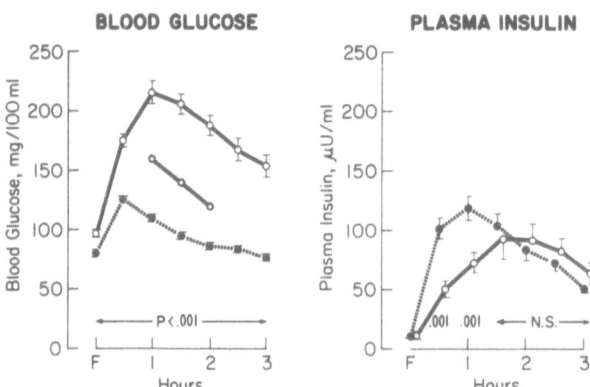

Fig. 2. Glucose tolerance tests in 59 latent diabetic patients and in 67 healthy control subjects. In diabetic patients, blood glucose levels represent mean values of tests on which initial diagnosis of diabetes was made. Plasma levels of insulin represent mean of insulin levels obtained at time of the diagnostic glucose tolerance test or during first glucose tolerance tests after 1961. Oral glucose load was 1.75 g/kg of ideal body weight

Table 5. Increments and distribution of increments in plasma insulin 30 minutes after ingestion of glucose in latent diabetic patients as compared to the mean of control subjects

		Increments of plasma insulin, µU/ml, at 30 min			
	N	Mean	S.D.	S.E.M.	P
Control subjects	67	90	60	8	<.001
Diabetic patients	59	36	38	5	

Distribution of 59 diabetic patients around				
-S.D.		Mean of control subjects	+S.D.	
32	24		2	1
54.2%	40.7%		3.4%	1.7%
95%			5%	

The distribution of the patients' increments in plasma insulin 30 min after ingestion of glucose around the mean increment of the control subjects is given in Table 5. Although 95% of the 30-min values of the diabetic patients are less than the mean of the control subjects, the distribution is wide, with a few values exceeding the mean of the control subjects (Table 5).

In Table 6 the magnitude and distribution of the total insulin response (sum of increments = sum of increases above fasting levels of all half-hourly intervals during the 3-hour glucose tolerance test) is shown in a similar way. The values of the control subjects vary considerably as reflected by the large standard deviation (S.D.) of the mean, 321 µU/ml. Among the diabetic patients the magnitude of individual total insulin responses is even more variable (Table 6). The distribution of the individual sums of increments of the diabetic patients is skewed to the left as compared to the control subjects. We have examined the responses of patients with the lowest and those with the highest insulin responses. Sixteen patients had sum of increments more than 1 S.D. below the mean of the control subjects. Eight patients had sum of increments in plasma insulin greater than 1 S.D. above the mean of the increments of the control subjects (Table 6); four were greater than 2 S.D. above the mean of the controls.

The initial insulin responses to glucose in the latent diabetic patients classified as having "low" and "high" insulin responses, respectively, are contrasted in Figure 3. The difference in plasma levels of insulin are striking. In those with "low" insulin responses mean blood glucose levels were higher than in those with "high" insulin responses, particularly during the glucose tolerance tests from which diabetes was first diagnosed (Fig. 4). In this analysis 3 of the "low" responders who progressed to insulin-requiring diabetes (inability to maintain blood glucose below 120 mg/dl consistently with diet and sulfonylureas) are excluded as is one of the "high" responders lost to follow-up. Mean blood glucose levels of the initial diagnostic glucose tolerance tests in the two groups (solid line, left vs. right panel) were significantly different at the 2-1/2- and 3-hour intervals (p < 0.025).

During follow-up, glucose intolerance of the 13 patients with the "low" insulin responses initially improved with therapy (3 on diet, 10 on diet plus sulfonylurea), as did that of the 7 patients with "high" insulin responses initially who were being treated (3 with diet, 4 with diet plus sulfonylurea) (Fig. 4). Eleven of the 16 patients with "low"

responses, but none of the 8 patients with "high" insulin responses,
had occasional fasting hyperglycemia.

Table 6. Sum of increments and distribution of sum of increments in plasma insulin
above fasting levels during 3-hour glucose tolerance tests of latent diabetic patients as compared to mean of control subjects

	N	Sum of increments in plasma insulin, µU/ml			P
		Mean	S.D.	S.E.M.	
Control subjects	67	464	321	39	<.08
Diabetic patients	59	372	415	54	

Distribution of 59 diabetic patients around				
−S.D.		Mean of control subjects	+S.D.	
16	30		5	8
27.1%	50.8%		8.5%	13.6%
78%			22%	

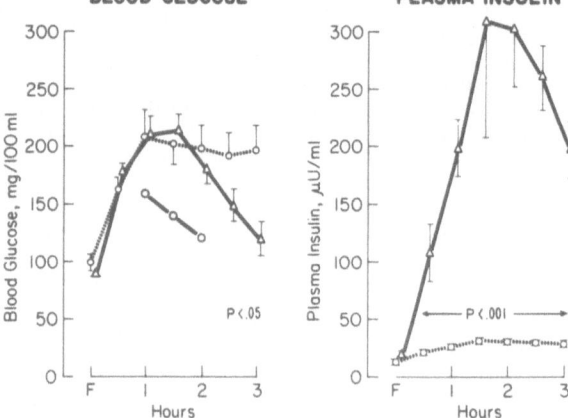

o————o "Low" Insulin Responses   N = 16   Mean Age 21.6 ± 2.1 years
△————△ "High" Insulin Responses   N = 8   Mean Age 31.0 ± 4.0 years

Fig. 3. Blood levels of glucose and plasma levels of insulin during glucose tolerance tests on which first insulin determinations were made in latent diabetic patients
with "low" and "high" insulin responses to glucose (see text)

The initial insulin response to glucose of the 13 "low insulin responders" who did not progress to insulin-requiring diabetes, and their
current response after 2.9-11.4 years of therapy are shown in Figure
5. Mean plasma insulin currently is significantly higher at 1/2 and 1
hour of the test. For the "high" insulin responders current tests show
a significant reduction in the high insulin levels that characterize
this group (Fig. 6). These data are summarized in Figure 7 as the means
± S.E.M. of the sum of increments in plasma insulin.

Factors in addition to severity of carbohydrate intolerance and age
(Figs. 3 and 4) distinguish patients with "low" from patients with "high"

72

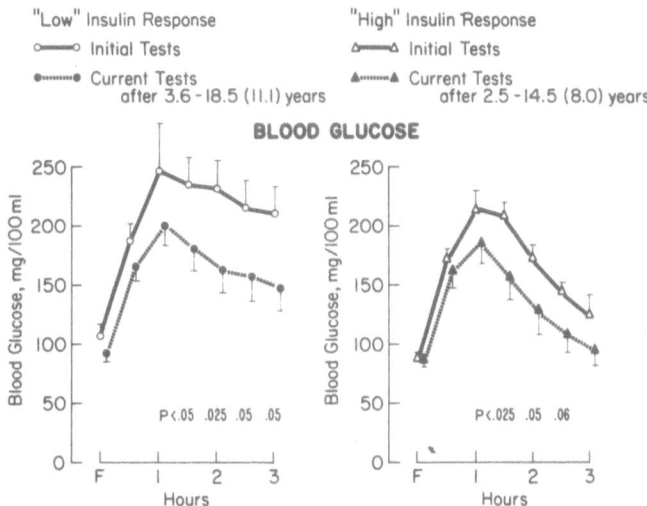

Fig. 4. Initial diagnostic glucose tolerance tests and current glucose tolerance tests in patients with latent diabetes (13 patients with "low" insulin responses and 7 patients with "high" insulin responses; see text)

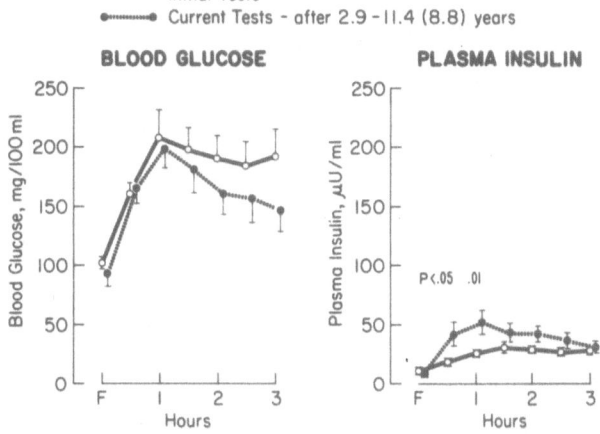

Fig. 5. Blood levels of glucose and plasma levels of insulin in response to glucose in 13 latent diabetic patients with "low" insulin responses to glucose. Initial tests are glucose tolerance tests on which the first insulin determinations were made. Current tests are mean of last glucose tolerance tests on follow-up with therapy (see text)

insulin responses. Several patients in each group had degrees of glucose intolerance and ages similar to that of individuals in the other group. Yet, the insulin levels of these individuals were comparable to the mean levels of their corresponding groups.

Subsequent to the above analysis of data a fourth patient with a "low" insulin response to glucose progressed to insulin-requiring diabetes.

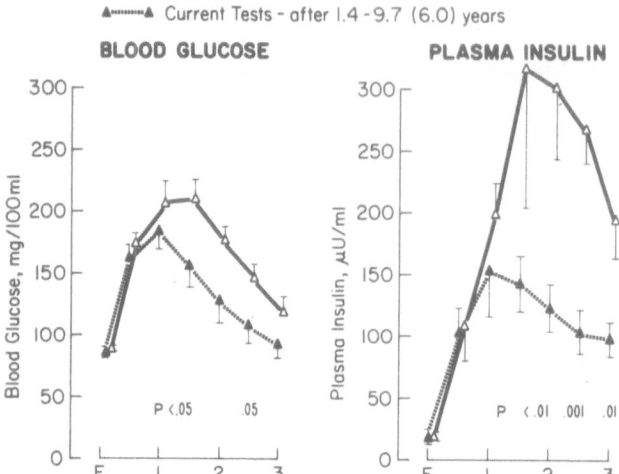

Fig. 6. Blood levels of glucose and plasma levels of insulin in response to glucose in 7 latent diabetic patients with "high" insulin responses to glucose. Initial tests are glucose tolerance tests on which first insulin determinations were made. Current tests are mean of last glucose tolerance tests on follow-up with therapy (see text)

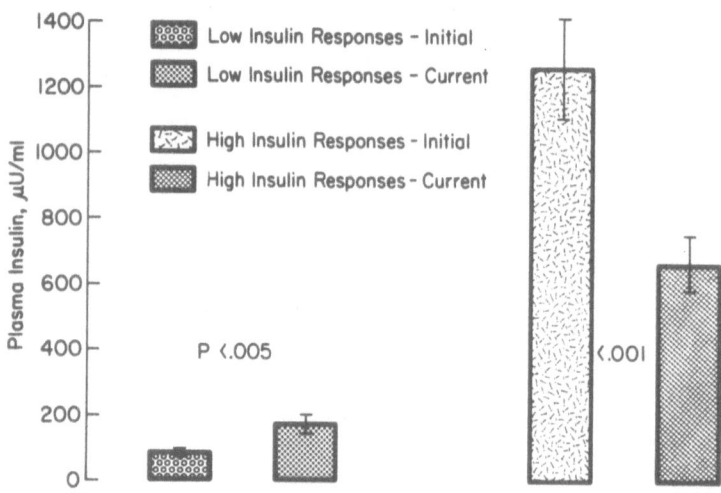

Fig. 7. Mean sum of increments in plasma insulin above fasting levels during three hours of glucose tolerance tests in latent diabetic patients. Bars represent 13 patients with "low" insulin responses and 7 patients with "high" insulin responses

The interval between diagnosis and requirement of insulin was 0.3, 2.0, 3.2, and 8.8 years for the 4 patients. Initially, they had very low 1/2-hour increments in plasma insulin (24, 15, 0 and 2 µU/ml, respectively) and sums of increments in plasma insulin of 114, 125, 11 and 36 µU/ml, respectively. Of the 59 patients, 4 additional patients progressed to insulin-requiring diabetes. Their respective sums of increments in plasma insulin, 193, 181, 185, and 258 µU/ml, fell between the mean (464 µU/ml) and mean −1 S.D. (143 µU/ml) of the controls. Their 1/2-hour increments in plasma insulin were 7, 38, 23, and 31 µU/ml, respectively. The interval between initial diagnosis and progression to insulin-requiring diabetes was 1.5, 4.9, 8.4, and 15.2 years, respectively. In contrast, none of the patients with "high" insulin responses, or with responses exceeding the mean of the control cubjects, have progressed to insulin-requiring diabetes.

The results of these studies have led us to the following conclusions: (1) Most of our latent diabetic patients have a significantly delayed increment in plasma insulin in response to glucose but the magnitude of the individual insulin responses to glucose encompasses a wide spectrum. At one extreme, greatly decreased insulin responses appear to be determinant, at least in part, of abnormal carbohydrate tolerance. On follow-up with therapy, the insulin responses were greater and glucose levels were lower. At the other extreme were the patients with glucose intolerance who had insulin responses which were supernormal. On follow-up with therapy their insulin responses decreased toward or to normal and carbohydrate tolerance improved. This suggests that in these latter patients hyperinsulinemia is secondary or compensatory to factors which cause glucose intolerance. Studies of variations in insulin moieties in plasma and of the activity of target cell receptors for insulin, which have been initiated, may help to clarify the cause and nature of the hyperinsulinemia. (2) The demonstration of heterogencity of insulin responses to glucose among nonobese patients with latent diabetes supports the view that so-called idiopathic diabetes mellitus includes more than one disorder associated with hyperglycemia. (3) Progression to insulin-requiring diabetes (some to ketosis-prone type) occurred only in individuals who had insulin responses which were delayed and lower than the mean response of the control subjects. Such an insulin response appears to be a more reliable prognostic indicator of decompensation to insulin-requiring diabetes at a later date than the degree of abnormality of carbohydrate intolerance or the fasting level of glucose at presentation. The data of Johansen indicate also that young latent diabetics who progressed to insulin-requiring diabetes had had delayed and subnormal insulin responses to oral glucose (23,25). Among young patients reported by various investigators at the Workshop on Chemical Diabetes Mellitus in Childhood (42), only those patients with "low insulin responses" progressed to insulin-requiring diabetes. None of the children with elevated insulin responses, comprising the majority of those reported, were said to have progressed to insulin-requiring diabetes. The interval between recognition of diabetes and the last examination was relatively short in most. Nevertheless, these findings would support our interpretations that in the young the pattern of insulin responses associated with carbohydrate intolerance has prognostic implications.

References

1. Bagdade, J.D., Bierman, E.L., Porte, D.J.: The significance of basal insulin levels in the evaluation of the insulin response to glucose in diabetic and nondiabetic subjects. J. Clin. Invest. 46, 1549 (1967)

2. Block, N.B., Rosenfield, R.L., Mako, M.E., Steiner, D.F., Rubenstein, A.H.: Sequential changes in beta-cell function in insulin-treated diabetic patients assessed by C-peptide immunoreactivity. N. Eng. J. Med. 288, 1144 (1973)

3. Burrows, S.: Insulin response in glucose tolerance tests. Amer. J. Clin. Path. 47, 709 (1967)

4. Cerasi, E., Luft, F.: Plasma insulin responses to glucose infusions in healthy subjects and in diabetes mellitus. Acta Endocrin. 55, 278 (1967)

5. Cerasi, E., Effendic, S., Luft, R.: Dose-response relation between plasma-insulin and blood-glucose levels during oral glucose loads in prediabetic and diabetic subjects. Lancet 1, 794 (1973)

6. Chiles, R., Tzagournis, M.: Excessive serum insulin response to oral glucose in obesity and mild diabetes. Diabetes 19, 458 (1970)

7. Chiumello, G., DelGurcio, M., Carnelutti, M., Bidone, G.: Relationship between obesity, chemical diabetes, and beta pancreatic function in children. Diabetes 18, 238 (1969)

8. Colle, E., Belmonte, M.M.: Chemical diabetes in the juvenile patient. Metabolism 22, 345 (1973)

9. Cudworth, A.G., Woodrow, J.C.: HL-A antigens and diabetes mellitus. Lancet 2, 1153 (1974)

10. Danowski, T.S., Lombardo, Y.B., Mendelsohn, L.B., Corredor, D.G., Morgan, C.R., Sabeh, G.: Insulin patterns prior to and after onset of diabetes. Metabolism 18, 731 (1969)

11. Danowski, T.S., Khurana, R.R., Nolan, S., Stephan, T., Gegick, C., Chae, S., Vidalon, C.: Insulin patterns in equivocal glucose tolerance tests (chemical diabetes). Diabetes 22, 808 (1973)

12. Ehrlich, R.M., Martin, J.M.: Early diabetes mellitus in children. Metabolism 22, 391 (1973)

13. Fajans, S.S., Conn, J.W.: Prediabetes, subclinical diabetes, and latent clinical diabetes: interpretation, diagnosis, and treatment. In: On the Nature and Treatment of Diabetes. Excerpta Medica Int'l. Cong. Series No. 84. Leibel, B.S., Wrenshall, G.A. (eds.). New York, 1965, p. 641

14. Fajans, S.S., Floyd, J.C., Jr., Pek, S., Conn, J.W.: The course of asymptomatic diabetes in young people, as determined by levels of blood glucose and plasma insulin. Trans. Assoc. Amer. Phys. 82, 211 (1969)

15. Fajans, S.S.: What is diabetes? Definition, diagnosis and course. Med. Clin. N. Amer. 55, 793 (1971)

16. Fajans, S.S., Floyd, J.C., Jr., Pek, S., Conn, J.W.: Studies on the natural history of asymptomatic diabetes in young people. Metabolism 22, 327 (1973)

17. Fajans, S.S., Taylor, C.I., Floyd, J.C., Jr., Conn, J.W.: Some aspects of the natural history of diabetes mellitus. Excerpty Medica Int'l. Cong. Series No. 312. Malaisse, W.J., Pirart, J. (eds.). Amsterdam 1974, p. 329

18. Fajans, S.S., Floyd, J.C., Jr., Taylor, C.I., Pek, S.: Heterogeneity of insulin responses in latent diabetes. Trans. Assoc. Amer. Phys. 87, 83 (1974)

19. Floyd, J.C., Jr., Fajans, S.S., Conn, J.W., Thiffault, C., Knopf, R.F.: Secretion of insulin induced by amino acids and glucose in diabetes mellitus. J. Clin. Endocrin. 28, 266 (1968)

20. Johansen, K., Soeldner, J.S., Gleason, R.E.: Insulin, growth hormone, and glucagon in prediabetes mellitus - a review. Metabolism 23, 1185 (1974)

21. Jackson, W.P.O., VanMiegham, W., Keller, P.: Insulin excess as the initial lesion in diabetes. Lancet 1, 1040 (1972)

22. Johansen, K., Lundbaek, K.: Plasma insulin in mild juvenile diabetes. Lancet 1, 1257 (1967)

23. Johansen, K.: Mild carbohydrate intolerance developing into classic juvenile diabetes. Acta Medica Scand. 189, 337 (1971)

24. Johansen, K.: Normal initial plasma insulin response in mild diabetes. Metabolism 21, 1177 (1972)

25. Johansen, K.: Mild diabetes in young subjects. Clinical aspects and plasma insulin response pattern. Acta Medica Scand. 193, 23 (1973)

26. Kahn, C.B., Soeldner, J.S., Gleason, R.E., Rojas, L., Camerini-Davalos, R.A., Marble, A.: Clinical and chemical diabetes in offspring of diabetic couples. N. Eng. J. Med. 281, 343 (1969)

27. Kalkhoff, R.K., Richardson, B.L., Stoddard, F.J.: Defective plasma insulin response during prednisolone glucose tolerance tests in subclinical diabetic mothers of heavy infants. Diabetes 17, 37 (1968)

28. MacCuish, A.C., Jordan, J., Campbell, C.J., Duncan, L.J.P., Irvin, W.J.: Cell-mediated immunity to human pancreas in diabetes mellitus. Diabetes 23, 293 (1974)

29. Metzger, B.E., Nitzan, M., Freinkel, N.: The beta cell in gestational diabetes: Victim or culprit? Clin. Res, 22, 651A (1974)

30. Nerup, J., Platz, P., Andersen, O.: HL-A antigens and diabetes mellitus. Lancet 2, 864 (1974)

31. O'Sullivan, J.B., Hurwitz, D.: Spontaneous remissions in early diabetes mellitus. Arch. Intern. Med. 117, 769 (1966)

32. Peck, F.B., Jr., Kirtley, W.R., Peck, F.B., Sr.: Complete remission of severe diabetes. Diabetes 7, 93 (1958)

33. Perley, M., Kipnis, D.M.: Plasma insulin responses to glucose and tolbutamide of normal weight and obese diabetic and nondiabetic subjects. Diabetes 15, 867 (1966)

34. Pildes, R.: Adult onset diabetes mellitus in childhood. Metabolism 22, 307 (1973)

35. Pirart, J., Lauveaux, J.P.: Remission in diabetes, In: Handbook of Diabetes, Vol. II. Munich: Lehmanns, 1971

36. Reaven, G., Miller, R.: Study of the relationship between glucose and insulin responses to an oral glucose load in man. Diabetes 17, 560 (1968)

37. Reaven, G.M., Shen, S.W., Silvers, A., Farquhar, J.W.: Is there a delay in plasma insulin response of patients with chemical diabetes mellitus. Diabetes 20, 416 (1971)

38. Reaven, G.M., Olefsky, J., Farquhar, J.W.: Does hyperglycemia or hyperinsulinemia characterize the patient with chemical diabetes? Lancet 1, 1247 (1972)

39. Rimoin, D.L., Saiki, J.H.: Diabetes mellitus among the Navajo: plasma glucose and insulin responses. Arch. Int. Med. 122, 6 (1968)

40. Rimoin, D.S.: Ethnic variability in glucose tolerance and insulin secretion. Arch. Int. Med. 124, 695 (1969)

41. Rosenbloom, A.: Insulin responses of children with chemical diabetes mellitus. N. Eng. J. Med. 282, 1228 (1970)

42. Rosenbloom, A.L., Drash, A., Guthrie, R.A. (eds.): Workshop on Chemical Diabetes in Childhood, Metabolism 22, 211 (1973)

43. Rosenbloom, A.: Criteria for interpretation of the oral glucose tolerance tests in children and insulin responses with normal and abnormal tolerance. Metabolism 22, 301 (1973)

44. Rull, J.A., Conn, J.W., Floyd, J.C., Jr., Fajans, S.S.: Levels of plasma insulin during cortisone glucose tolerance tests in nondiabetic relatives of diabetic patients. Implications of diminished insulin secretory reserve in subclinical diabetes. Diabetes 19, 1 (1970)

45. Seltzer, H., Allen, E., Herron, A., Brennan, M.: Insulin secretion in response to glycemic stimulus: Relation of delayed initial release to carbohydrate intolerance in mild diabetes. J. Clin. Invest. 46, 323 (1967)

46. Soeldner, J.S., Johansen, K., Gleason, R.E., Smith, T.M.: Serum insulin and growth hormone responses to four types of tests in young monozygotic twins of a juvenile diabetic twin-mate. Diabetes 23, 350 (1974)

47. Tattersall, R.B., Pyke, D.A.: Diabetes in identical twins. Lancet 2, 1120 (1972)

48. Tattersall, R.B., Fajans, S.S.: A difference between the inheritance of classical juvenile-onset and maturity-onset type diabetes of young people. Diabetes 24, 44 (1975)

49. Varsano-Ahron, N., Echemendia, E., Yalow, R., Berson, S.: Early insulin responses to glucose and to tolbutamide in maturity-onset diabetes. Metabolism 19, 409 (1970)

50. Yalow, R.S., Berson, S.A.: Immunoassay of endogenous plasma insulin in man. J. Clin. Invest. 39, 1157 (1960)

51. Yalow, R.S., Berson, S.A.: Plasma insulin concentrations in nondiabetic and early diabetic subjects. Diabetes 9, 254 (1960)

Supported in part by USPHS Grants AM-00888, AM-02244, and TI-AM-5001 from the National Institute of Arthritis, Metabolism, and Digestive Diseases and by grants from the Upjohn Company, Kalamazoo, Michigan, and Charles Pfizer, Inc., New York.

9. Genetic Heterogeneities within Idiopathic Diabetes

J. KÖBBERLING

One of the main purposes in studying the genetics of diabetes mellitus is to determine heterogeneities. Many special types of diabetes, with various types of etiology and pathogenesis and sometimes distinct clinical pictures, have been described. After separation of these special types all remaining diabetics are summarized as idiopathic diabetics. There is conclusive evidence that heredity plays a major role in the eiology in this group of idiopathic diabetics. It is very unlikely that it represents a homogeneous disease. Most probably it consists of various types of diseases with different etiologies, both exogenous and genetic, and even the genetic diabetes is most probably heterogenous. As long as we are not able to subdivide the idiopathic diabetes according to etiology, pathogenesis, or clinical type, we have to confine ourselves to genetic differences between groups of patients which may be classified according to sex, age at onset, weight, or other measurable parameters.

A. Genetic Heterogeneities between Juvenile and Adult-Onset Diabetes

The age at onset is highly correlated with the clinical types of so-called juvenile-onset and adult-onset diabetes. Most authors have preferred to subdivide by age at onset or age at diagnosis and not according to the clinical diagnosis, which is prone to arbitrary classification in some borderline cases. Various approaches have been used to determine whether the genetic control of juvenile diabetes is different from that of adult-onset-diabetes.

I. Method of Heritability of Liability to Diabetes

This method, which was introduced by Falconer (2), is based on the following idea: All the causes, both genetic and environmental, that make an individual more or less likely to develop the disease can be combined into a single measure called the individual's "liability." The liabilities of individuals in a population form a continuous variable and the apparent discontinuity between affected and normals arises from a "threshold" at a certain level of liability. Individuals with a liability above the threshold are affected and individuals below it are not. The liability of an individual cannot be measured, but the mean liability of the population or of subpopulations or groups can be evaled from the incidence of the disease in that population or group.

The heritability is a mathematical expression giving the proportion of the phenotypic variance that is due to additive genetic variance. The analysis provides an estimate of the correlation between relatives in respect of liability and this leads to an estimate of the heritability of liability to a given group of subjects.

Two groups of investigators have applied this method in an attempt to answer the question as to whether the genetic control of juvenile diabetes is the same as that in adult-onset diabetes. They came to essentially opposite conclusions.

Simpson (20) has calculated the heritability of liability to diabetes for the first-degree relatives of 6600 Canadian diabetics. The estimates of heritability in parents, siblings and children of diabetics were related to the age-at-onset of the proband cases. It declined from 55% in the youngest group (0-19 years) to 36% in the middle (20-39 years) and to 27% in the late-onset group ($\geq$ 40 years). Genetic correlations showed that the early and late groups had only a moderate number of genes in common. It was concluded, therefore, that early and late age-at-onset are different genetically. Falconer (3) has also observed a drop of the heritability with increasing age (from 70-80% to about 30-40%) but Smith *et al.* (21) concluded that the two disorders have the same or a very similar causation.

Several objections to the application of heritability in studying the genetics of diabetes have to be made. An increase of liability may be due to an increase of the mean liability with equal variance or due to an increased variance with equal mean (3). Consideration of the changes of liability that individuals may undergo as they grow older shows that an increase of variance with increasing age is to be expected. Since the additional variance is likely to be mainly environmental, a reduction of heritability is to be expected. There are other, more general objections to the method. The main objection is that it is based on the assumption that diabetes is a multifactorially inherited disease with additive gene action. If diabetes is, in part, controlled by a major gene or genes, heritability will underestimate the total degree of genetic determination of the disease. Extensive evidence has been presented that diabetes is a heterogenous group of disorders and not primarily a single disease which is multifactorially inherited. This method seems not to be valid when applied to diabetes.

II. The Method of the So-called "K-ratio"

This method was suggested by Penrose (14): The ratio of frequency of diabetes in relatives of special classes of diabetics to relatives of corresponding controls has to be calculated. This ratio is usually called the K-ratio. Thus the study requires the investigation of normal controls from the general population, or a sample of it, which have to be matched at least for age and sex. There have been several studies which used this approach to investigate the question of heterogeneity between juvenile- and adult-onset diabetes (5,7,17,19). Again, the results are conflicting. Most authors have found that the relative risk of diabetes among relatives of diabetics who were young at the age of onset was greater than that for relatives of diabetics who were older at age of onset. It has been concluded, that the genetic control of juvenile diabetes may be different from that for adult-onset diabetes (18,19). In the study by Keen and Track (7) the values for the K-ratio for the relatives of diabetics of younger onset are also higher than those for the relatives of older-onset cases, when estimates are based upon the analysis of verbal family histories. However, when glucose tolerance status is more fully ascertained by submitting "normal" relatives to examination and including abnormal response to glucose in the calculation of the ratios, this difference between older-onset cases is found to be much less marked.
There are several reasons for the conflict between results from different authors who have used the K-ratio. These more or less serious ob-

jections have been pointed out by Keen and Track (7) and by Köbberling (8).

To consider the extreme cases: If general population frequencies are
extremely low or nil in youth, then a very few affected relatives of
diabetic probands will give a very high value for the K-ratio. At the
other extreme, the general population frequency may be so high that it
is not possible to exceed it significantly. A hypothetical model is
given by Keen and Track (Fig. 1) in which diabetes frequency in a population composed of siblings of diabetics is compared with that in a
population composed of siblings of controls. Two assumptions are made:
(1) The frequency of diabetes in the general population rises with age
from zero to a total of 2%. (2) A genetic factor, operating equally at
all ages, causes diabetes in an extra 4% among the siblings of diabetics.
The values of the K-ratio calculated on these assumptions are much higher
at younger than older ages. Thus a result which postulates different
modes of inheritance can arise from a population which is, by definition,
genetically homogeneous. Considering this and some further difficulties in using the K-ratio, the results obtained by this method may not
be regarded as a support of the hypothesis that there are different
modes of inheritance of the two clinical types of diabetes, especially
not as evidence for the higher genetic influence in juvenile-onset diabetes compared to adult-onset diabetes.

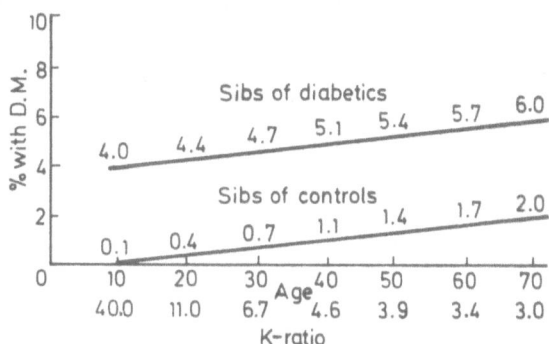

Fig. 1. A hypothetical model showing that, even assuming a constant genetic factor
causing a fixed increase of 4% in the rate of affected siblings of diabetics at all
ages, there is considerable fall with age in calculated K-ratios.[From Keen, H.,
Track, N.S.: Diabetologia 4, 317 (1968)]

III. Prevalence of Adult-Onset Diabetes in Relatives of Juvenile-Onset
Diabetics Compared to Normal Controls

This method is rather close to the calculation of the K-ratio. It also
requires incidence estimation in a control group but it restricts itself to the question as to whether the genetic control of juvenile diabetes is the same as that of adult-onset diabetes.

Three studies have been reported using this method: Joslin et al. (6)
reported that the incidence of diabetes among parents and grandparents
of 841 diabetic children was twice the incidence of diabetes in general
population. However, their data on the incidence of diabetes in the

81

general population was derived from previous mortality statistics. For several reasons this might not be regarded as conclusive.

Lestradet *et al.* (10) published the results of a survey of diabetes among the relatives of 300 nondiabetic children who were selected identically to a group of 926 diabetic children. Their data show that the incidence of non insulin-dependent diabetics was equal to that among the parents and grandparents of nondiabetics. The incidence of insulin-dependent diabetes, however, was significantly higher among the families of nondiabetics. They concluded from these data that inheritance of juvenile diabetes is completely independent from the inheritance of adult-onset diabetes.

Very similar results were yielded in a study performed by MacDonald (11). The incidence of individuals diagnosed as diabetic after age 45 among 423 grandparents of diabetic children was not significantly differnt from that among 395 grandparents of control children who were very thoroughly matched. This is also interpreted as evidence that juvenile and adult onset diabetes are under different genetic control. In this study the families of diabetic children reported twice the incidence of adult-onset diabetics among nonrelatives than did families of nondiabetic children. Thus the "awareness" of diabetes is quite different between diabetics and controls, a factor which might influence all studies based on control groups.

IV. Age Corrections by the Modified Strömgren-Method

The method, derived by Strömgren (22) for studies in schizophrenia and modified by Köbberling (8), is useful for incidence calculation of diseases with a variable age of onset. No control groups are necessary. The calculations do not give figures of actual incidence but the hypothetical incidence if all persons reach an assumed maximal age. This maximal age was classified as 25 years for juvenile-onset diabetes and 85 years for adult-onset diabetes (8). For the calculation the age at onset of diabetes in a representative group of patients is required. The diabetic probands themselves may serve as this group (Fig. 2). The

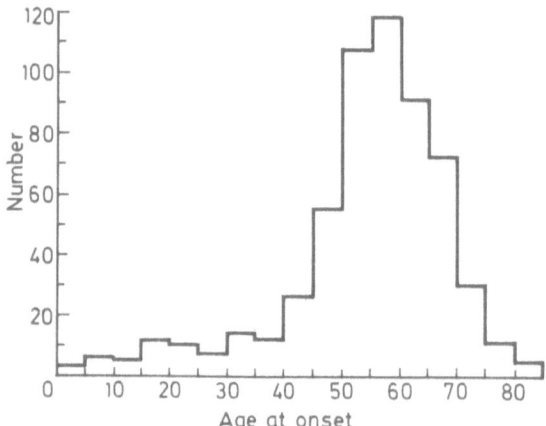

Fig. 2. Diabetic probands, assorted in groups of 5 years according to age at onset. (From Köbberling, J.: Diabetologia 5, 392 (1969)

number of diagnoses made within classes of 5 years is divided by the
number of persons of this age group in the general population, derived
from statistical year-books. These figures are then given as a percent
of the overall number, thus giving the proportional chance to become
diabetic within this age group for all those who become diabetic at
any age. If these figures are summed it will give, by definition,
a 100% chance to become diabetic at the previously defined maximal age
(Fig. 3). For example: a person who would develop diabetes between the
age of 25 and 85 years has a 60% chance to be diagnosed as diabetic
by the age of 63 years or younger. The chance of being diagnosed as
juvenile onset diabetic is 100%, by definition, for all those older
than 25 years. All living family members and those who have died are
calculated not as "one" but as the value derived from the calculation
for proportional chance. This calculation renders the method independent of the incidental age of the probands and their relatives.

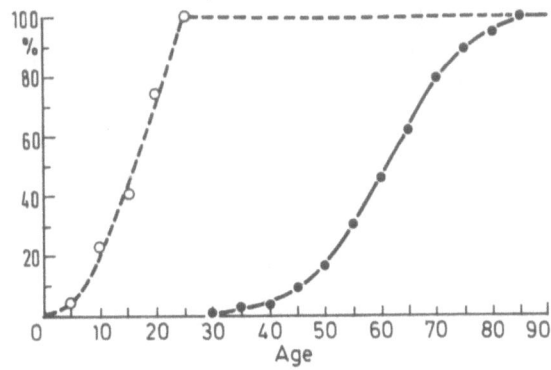

Fig. 3. Chance to be diagnosed as diabetic at a special age for all those who will
become diabetic at any age. Dotted line: juvenile diabetes. Solid line: adult-onset
diabetes. (From Köbberling, J.: Diabetologia 5, 392 (1969))

There are certainly many objections to this method, e.g., the age of
onset in the diabetic population may not be representative for the age
at onset of all diabetics. The proportional risk figures on which the
calculations are based, especially those for adult-onset diabetes, may
have been previously quite different. The absolute values should be
regarded with caution, but there is a striking difference in the pattern
of familiar occurrence of diabetes between juvenile-onset and adult-
onset probands. Juvenile diabetes is rare among siblings and children
of adult-onset diabetics (Table 1). Adult-onset diabetes among the parents of juvenile diabetics is also rare (Table 2). The incidence of
adult-onset diabetes among parents of juvenile diabetics may well be
within the incidence in the general population.

Thus the results are in accordance with some of the results from other
authors derived with different methods, suggesting that juvenile-onset
and adult-onset diabetes are genetically heterogeneous. The question
as to whether genetic factors play a more important role in juvenile-
or in adult-onset diabetes may be answered, if at all, only in that
adult-onset diabetes seems to be under greater genetic control than
juvenile-onset diabetes. In this respect there is a discordance to the
previous studies.

Table 1. Juvenile diabetes (after age correction) among relatives of diabetics of different types

Proband cases	Parents	Siblings	Children
Juvenile diabetics	1.6 ± 1.3%	10.9 ± 3.9%	no calculation
Adult-onset diabetics	no calculation	0.4 ± 0.1%	0.3 ± 0.2%

Table 2. Adult-onset diabetes (after age correction) among relatives of diabetics of different types

Proband cases	Parents	Siblings	Children
Juvenile diabetics	8.5 ± 5.6%	no calculation	no calculation
Adult-onset diabetics	no calculation	25.8 ± 1.5%	33.4 ± 6.4%

B. Genetic Heterogeneities within the Adult-Onset Diabetes

The same method for evaluation of familial incidence has been applied to investigate whether heterogeneities exist within the group of adult-onset diabetics, defined as age at onset after 25 years (9). Subgroups were classified according to need of therapy, degree of overweight, and number of pregnancies. The incidence of diabetes among the siblings was estimated using the modified Strömgren method of age correction (8).

The degree of overweight was calculated as follows: The percentage of deviation from the normal weight at the time of diagnosis of diabetes was multiplied by the time in years in which it had existed before onset of diabetes. These are certainly rather rough estimates based on the patients' reports. The patients were grouped into three classes:

   I. Product of overweight and time under 400
  II. Product between 400 and 1000
 III. Product over 1000 e.g., 50% overweight for 20 years or more

The incidence of diabetes among the siblings is given in Figure 4, which shows that the frequency of diabetes among siblings is reduced with increasing overweight of the probands.
This observation can be interpreted by the model of additive gene function, known as "multifactorial" inheritance. Since overweight is an additional pathogenetic factor, persons with a high degree of overweight require only a smaller "dose of genes" to become diabetic. This explanation is analogous to what geneticists call the "Carter effect" (1) in multifactorial inheritance, but one can certainly imagine various types of heterogeneity that could lead to this observation. There might exist types of diabetes with high penetrance not depending on overweight and others with a low or zero genetic background and overweight as the main pathogenetic factor.

This relationship, as shown in Figure 4, has only been observed in non-insulin-treated diabetics. A similar calculation in insulin-treated diabetics has revealed that no such relationship between overweight and incidence of diabetes among siblings existed (Fig. 5). Thus the factor overweight seems not to be relevant in the pathogenesis of insulin-dependent diabetes. One can, therefore, assume heterogeneity between insulin-dependent and non insulin-dependent diabetes.
A similar observation has been made with respect to the number of pregnancies. Multiparity is regarded as an additional pathogenetic factor in diabetes since the incidence of diabetes in women increases steadily

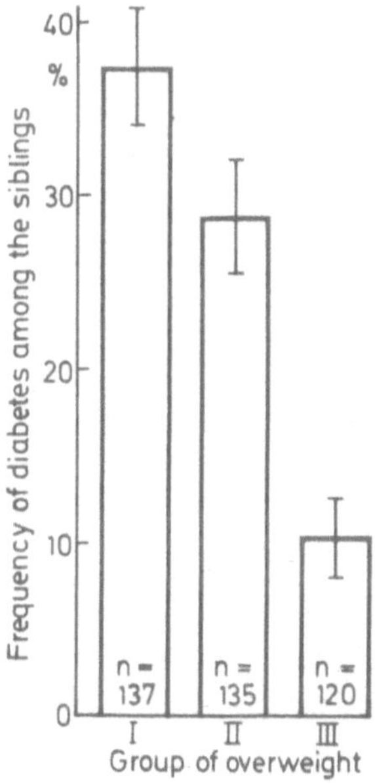

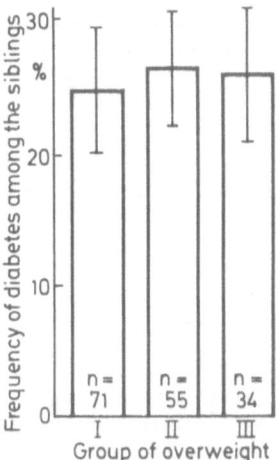

Fig. 4. Frequency of diabetes among siblings in relation to degree of overweight. Probands: adult-onset
diabetics with oral or dietetic therapy in three groups
of different overweight. n = number of probands. (From
Köbberling, J.: Diabetologia 7, 46 (1971))

Fig. 5. Frequency of diabetes among siblings in relation to degree of overweight. Probands: adult-onset
diabetics with insulin therapy in three groups of different overweight. n = number of probands. (From Köbberling, J.: Diabetologia 7, 46 (1971))

with increasing parity (4,13,15). Female patients with a high number
of pregnancies before the onset of diabetes have a lower incidence of
diabetes among the siblings (Fig. 6). Again, this only applies to non-
insulin-treated diabetics. No such relationship has been observed in
insulin-treated diabetics.

A relationship between the number of pregnancies and the frequency of
diabetes among family members has also been described by Pyke (16).
Middleton and Caird (12), on the other hand, found no such relationship. Perhaps a different proportion of insulin-dependent and nonde-
pendent individuals among the proband cases can be responsible for this
discrepancy. Information about types of treatment are not given by
Middleton and Caird.

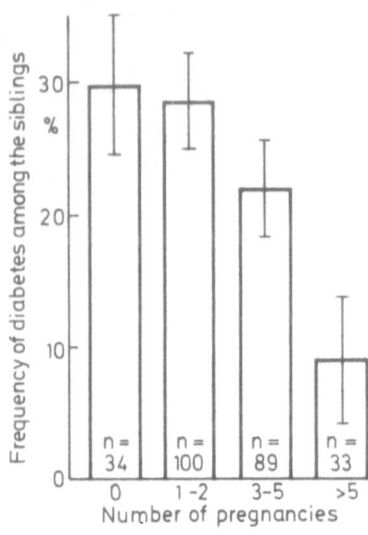

Fig. 6. Frequency of diabetes among siblings in relation to parity. Probands: female adult-onset diabetics with oral or dietetic therapy in four groups with different number of pregnancies. n = number of probands. (From Köbberling, J.: Diabetologia $\underline{7}$, 46 (1971))

The above data and the review of the literature do not help to separate special types of diabetes among those classified as idiopathic. However, the studies show that idiopathic diabetes cannot be regarded as one group with a similar genetic background. Various heterogeneities exist, at least according to age at onset, weight before onset of diabetes, insulin dependence, and number of pregnancies. Further investigations are needed to separate genetically homogeneous groups, but it seems likely that there will always remain a group of diabetics who cannot at the moment be further subdivided but still comprise a heterogeneous group of disorders.

References

1. Carter, C.D.: The inheritance of common congenital malformations. In: Progress in Medical Genetics, Steinberg, A.G., Bearn, A.G. New York, London: Grune and Stratton, 1965, Vol. IV

2. Falconer, D.S.: The inheritance of liability to certain diseases, estimated from the incidence among relatives. Ann. Hum. Genet. (Lond.). $\underline{29}$, 51 (1965)

3. Falconer, D.S.: The inheritance of liability to diseases with variable age of onset, with particular reference to diabetes mellitus. Ann. Hum. Genet. (Lond.) $\underline{31}$, 1-20 (1967)

4. Fitzgerald, M.G., Malins, J.M., O'Sullivan, D.J., Wall, M.: The effect of sex and parity on the incidence of diabetes mellitus. Quart. J. Med. $\underline{30}$, 57 (1961)

5. General practitioners: The family history of diabetes. Report of a working party appointed by the college of general practitioners. Brit. Med. J. $\underline{1}$ (1960/1965)

6. Joslin, E.P., Dublin, L.I., Marks, H.H.: Studies in diabetes mellitus. Amer. J. Med. Sci. $\underline{193}$, 8 (1937)

7. Keen, H., Track, N.S.: Age of onset and inheritance of diabetes: The importance of examining relatives. Diabetologia $\underline{4}$, 317 (1968)

8. Köbberling, J.: Untersuchungen zur Genetik des Diabetes mellitus. Eine geeignete Methode zur Durchführung von Alterskorrekturen. Diabetologia $\underline{5}$, 392 (1969)

9. Köbberling, J.: Studies on the genetic heterogeneity of diabetes mellitus. Diabetologia $\underline{7}$, 46 (1971)

10. Lestradet, H., Battistelli, J., Ledoux, M.: L'hérédité dans le diabète infantile. Le Diabète 20, 17 (1972)

11. MacDonald, M.J.: Equal incidence of adult-onset diabetes among ancestors of juvenile diabetics and nondiabetics. Diabetologia 10, 767 (1974)

12. Middleton, G.D., Caird, F.I.: Parity and diabetes mellitus. Brit. J. Prev. Soc. Med. 22, 100 (1968)

13. Munro, N.H., Eaton, J.C., Glen, A.: Survey of a Scottish diabetic clinic; a study of the etiology of diabetes mellitus. J. Clin. Endocr. 9, 48 (1949)

14. Penrose, L.S.: The genetical background of common diseases. Acta Genet. (Basel) 4, 257 (1953)

15. Pyke, D.A.: Parity and the incidence of diabetes. Lancet 1, 818 (1956)

16. Pyke, D.A.: The incidence of diabetes and its preponderance among women. Acta Genet. (Basel) 7, 91 (1957)

17. Simpson, N.E.: The genetics of diabetes: A study of 233 families of juvenile diabetics. Ann. Hum. Genet. (Lond.) 26, 1 (1962)

18. Simpson, N.E.: Multifactorial inheritance. A possible hypothesis for diabetes. Diabetes 13, 462 (1964)

19. Simpson, N.E.: Diabetes in the families of diabetics. Can. Med. Ass. J. 98, 427 (1968)

20. Simpson, N.E.: Heritability of liability to diabetes when sex and age at onset are considered. Ann. Hum. Genet. (Lond.) 32, 283 (1969)

21. Smith, C., Falconer, D.S., Duncan, L.J.P.: A statistical and genetical study of diabetes. Ann. Hum. Genet. (Lond.) 35, 282 (1972)

22. Strömgren, E.: Zum Ersatz des Weinberg'schen "abgekürzten Verfahrens." Zugleich ein Beitrag zur Frage von der Erblichkeit des Erkrankungsalters bei der Schizophrenie. Zbl. ges. Neurol. Psychiat. 153, 784 (1935)

10. The Inheritance of Maturity-Onset Type Diabetes in Young People

R. TATTERSALL

In children, adolescents, and young adults two phenotypically distinct forms of diabetes can be recognized (Table 1). The classical and commoner form is characterized by an abrupt clinical onset, severe symptoms, lack of stimulated insulin output and a tendency to ketoacidosis (classical Juvenile-Onset Diabetes or JOD). The other form resembles typical maturity-onset diabetes of middle age in that symptoms at diagnosis are either mild or absent, stimulated insulin output is retained although delayed and diminished, there is no ketonuria and hyperglycemia can be controlled without insulin (Maturity-Onset type Diabetes of Young people or MODY). In practice there is inevitably some overlapping between these two arbitrary categories and the classification can only be made with certainty in retrospect (27).

Table 1. Phenotypic features of classical juvenile-onset (JOD) and maturity-onset type diabetes of young people (MODY)

	Onset	Symptoms	Keto-nuria	Stimulated in-sulin response	Course
JOD	Abrupt	Severe weight loss ++	Present	None	Exogenous insulin necessary to prevent symptoms and ketosis
MODY	Insidious	Mild or absent weight loss 0	Absent	Present but reduced and late	Can be treated without insulin indefinitely

Historically the first reference to MODY may have been in Rollo's *An Account of two Cases of Diabetes Mellitus* (1798) (22) wherein are described a father, two children, and a grandchild with diabetes of a mild type. Reservations must be expressed about this and other reports antedating 1916 since, without blood sugar measurements, mild diabetes cannot definitely be distinguished from renal glycosuria which may be inherited, usually as a dominant condition (5,10). Joslin (13) and Graham (8) described patients diagnosed at 9, 11, and 20 years of age with unequivocal biochemical evidence of diabetes who could be satisfactorily controlled for at least 5 years by dietary measures alone. The discovery of insulin with its near miraculous effect in restoring the strength and vitality of children with diabetes tended to obscure the existence of MODY until its rediscovery in 1960 by Fajans and Conn (6). At first MODY was thought to be an early stage of classical juvenile diabetes which had been detected by chance (18). However, although some cases do progress to classical insulin-deficient juvenile diabetes (9,11) it has now been established by long-term prospective follow-up in several centers that this is uncommon and that most patients with MODY show little or no progression in severity over 20 years or more

(7,23). This lack of progression suggested that MODY and JOD might be
different diseases rather than different stages in the evolution of
a single disease.

Evidence suggesting a specific mode of inheritance for MODY was obtained
from the study of three unusual families at King's College Hospital,
London (26). The propositi of these families (Table 2) were striking
because, although diagnosed at young ages and having had diabetes for
a mean of 40 years, all were treated with oral hypoglycemic agents.
In each case there was a strong family history of diabetes with at least
10 affected relatives. The phenotypic manifestations of diabetes in
the 20 relatives who were still alive (deceased relatives also had a
phenotypically similar form of diabetes) were similar to those in the
propositi (Table 3). Diabetes had been diagnosed under the age of 20
years in half the cases (mean age at diagnosis 22 years). The classical
onset of juvenile diabetes was never seen and significant weight loss
was never a feature. The diagnosis of diabetes had often been made by
chance; eleven patients had been diagnosed as a result of urine testing
carried out for reasons other than their known family history of diabetes (e.g., at insurance or school medical examinations). In spite of
the young ages at diagnosis and the long duration of diabetes (mean
22 years) none had ever been ketoacidotic and only one was still on
insulin (this patient was not insulin-dependent since she only took 4
units of insulin daily and had omitted this for periods of 3 weeks
without any deterioration in diabetic control).

Table 2. Propositi of three families with MODY (13)

Propositus of:	Age at diagnosis	Duration of diabetes	Present treatment	Complications	Number of diabetic relatives
Family M	12	30	Sulphonylurea	none	13
Family H	14	46	Sulphonylurea	1 microaneurysm	10
Family R	22	45	Sulphonylurea	none	15

Table 3. Clinical features in 20 living diabetics in 3 MODY families (13)

Age at diagnosis	22 years (9-42)
Presentation	
Routine urine test	11
Symptoms	9
Duration of diabetes	22 years (2-54)
Ketoacidosis	0
Still on insulin	1
Retinopathy	Present: 2, Absent: 18
Proteinuria	0
Neuropathy	0

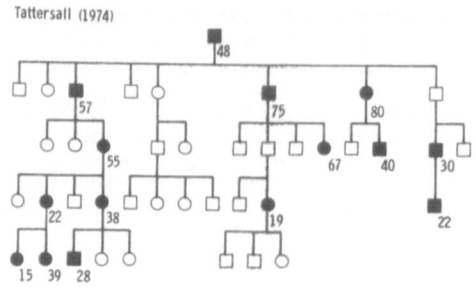

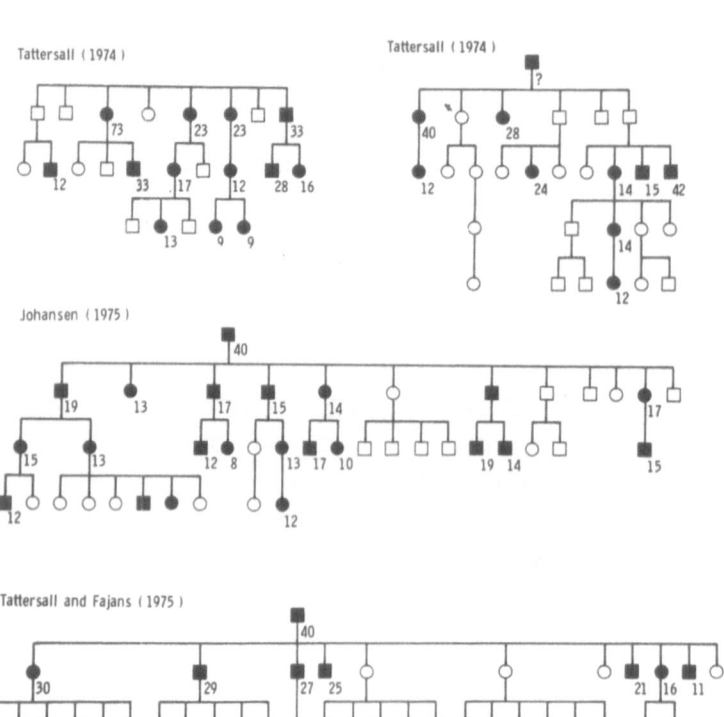

Fig. 1. Pedigrees of maturity-onset type diabetes of young people illustrating the features of dominant inheritance. Subscripts indicate age at diagnosis of diabetes

Representative pedigrees of the three families described above with two additional ones (12,28) are shown in Figure 1. In all three families diabetes appeared to be inherited as a dominant character because:

1. In each family there was direct transmission through at least three generations.
2. Almost every diabetic had a diabetic parent.
3. Diabetics had diabetic and nondiabetic offspring in a ratio of 1:1.

In a further study on the inheritance of MODY carried out in Ann Arbor, Michigan (27), a maturity-onset diabetic of young age (MODY) was defined as a patient developing diabetes under the age of 25 years in whom fasting hyperglycemia, if present, could be normalized without insulin for more than 2 years. A classical juvenile-onset diabetic (JOD) was a diabetic patient who required insulin within 2 years of diagnosis to prevent fasting hyperglycemia.

Two groups of first-degree relatives were investigated (Table 4): (1) the families of 26 MODY propositi diagnosed at a mean age of 19 and controlled without insulin for a mean of 9.3 years, and (2) the families of 35 classical JOD propositi who had been diagnosed at a mean age of 12 years. All presented with classical symptoms of diabetes, 47 of 61 (77%) siblings of MODY propositi, had glucose tolerance tests at a mean age of 19 years and 68 of 99 (69%) siblings of JOD propositi at a mean age of 16 years.

Table 4. Ages at diagnosis and testing of propositi with MODY and JOD and their siblings (1)

| | Propositi | | | Siblings | |
	No.	Age at diagnosis	Total No.	No. tested	Age at testing
MODY	26	19 yr	61	47	19 yr
JOD	35	12 yr	99	68	16 yr

This comparison (Table 5) showed that in the families of MODY: (1) 22 of 26 (85%) propositi had a diabetic parent; (2) 4 siblings were already known to have a maturity-onset type of diabetes (mean age at diagnosis 30 years) and a further 21 were found to have latent diabetes - a total of 53% of siblings with diabetes; (3) nearly half the families showed direct vertical transmission of diabetes through three generations (no glucose tolerance tests were carried out on grandparents so this may be an underestimate); and (4) the diabetic phenotype was consistent with most individuals having noninsulin-requiring disease. These findings are compatible with autosomal dominant inheritance of MODY although they do not conclusively exclude multifactorial inheritance.

Table 5. Comparison of close family history of diabetes in MODY and JOD (1)

| | Diabetic siblings | | | Diabetic parent | Diabetic grandparent |
	already known	discovered	% diabetic		
MODY	4	21	53	22 (85%)	12 (46%)
JOD	6	2	11	4 (11%)	2 (6%)

In contrast to MODY, in the families of JOD (1) only 4 propositi (11%) had a diabetic parent; (2) although 6 siblings were already known to have typical JOD, only 2 latent diabetics were found among 68 tested siblings (3%); and (3) three-generation inheritance was found in only 2 of JOD families (6%).

The results of other studies support the concept of autosomal dominant inheritance of MODY. Joslin (13) emphasized that all his and Naunyn's (10) cases of young-onset diabetes surviving for more than 10 years in

the preinsulin era had strong family histories of diabetes. Both Naunyn (19) and Cammidge (1) emphasized that cases in which diabetes could
be traced through two or three generations tended to be comparatively
mild even if they were young at onset. Pedigrees showing three-generation inheritance of MODY have also been reported by Colle (2), Paulsen
(20), and Johansen (11).

A maturity-onset type of diabetes in young people may be relatively
more common in South Africa, India and the Middle East and was reported
in India as long ago as 1907 (4). In Caucasians the frequency of MODY
is difficult to extimate because: (1) the condition is often asymptomatic, even in the presence of marked glucose intolerance, and may remain unsuspected until diagnosed either accidentally at an insurance
or school examination or alternatively as a result of systematic testing
of families of diabetics. (2) The terms "insulin-dependent" and "insulin taking" are often used loosely and synonymously. Cases of Mody may
be treated with insulin because of their age and the assumption that
it will be necessary sooner or later rather than because their clinical
condition warrants it. Thereafter their need for insulin is rarely
reviewed (26). Since the description of the original three families
at King's College Hospital, the author has seen several other probable
examples in three separate clinics suggesting that the condition may
be more common than was originally thought.

Carbohydrate intolerance in maturity-onset diabetes of middle age is
often asymptomatic and it has been shown that young patients can have
asymptomatic diabetes for as long as two decades. Dominant inheritance
of typical maturity-onset diabetes in middle age has been postulated
(14) and it is possible that MODY may be "typical" maturity-onset diabetes detected at an unusually early age. On the other hand maturity-
onset diabetes may itself be a heterogeneous condition of which MODY
is a distinct variety. The remarkable freedom from clinically significant complications in MODY even after long durations of diabetes is
not entirely explicable in terms of the mildness of carbohydrate intolerance and may be a manifestation of the specific type of diabetes (26).

Heterogeneity between classical juvenile diabetes and typical maturity-
onset diabetes of middle age has been postulated by Rimoin (21), Köbberling (15), and Simpson (24). The work reported here supports the
suggestion from twin studies that diabetes in the young is itself a
heterogeneous condition (25).

Although the findings in this small series of relatives of JOD do not
lead to any new conclusions about the inheritance of JOD, they do confirm (1) the infrequency of latent diabetes among the siblings of Jod
(26); and (2) that the frequency of adult-onset diabetes is no greater
among the parents and grandparents of classical juvenile-onset diabetics
than the controls (16,17).

It is suggested from these studies that populations, in which the genetics of diabetes is analized, should be as clearly defined as possible
in terms of phenotype rather than amalgamated under the umbrella of
"diabetes." Furthermore, more attention should be given to clear definition of the term "insulin-dependent."

In conclusion: The clinical course of Maturity-Onset Diabetes of Young
People (MODY), with a majority of cases showing insulin independence
and little or no progression in severity for twenty or more years, suggests that it may be a different disease from the insulin-dependent,
classical Juvenile-Onset Type Diabetes (JOD).
Studies of the inheritance of MODY suggest that it is inherited as an

autosomal dominant because: (1) 85% of propositi have a diabetic parent; (2) 53% of tested siblings had diabetes; (3) 46% of families showed direct vertical transmission of diabetes through three generations; and (4) the diabetic phenotype in three families was consistent, most affected individuals having a noninsulin-requiring type of disease.

In contrast, in the families of JOD: (1) only 11% of propositi had a diabetic parent; (2) three generation inheritance was found in only 6% of families; and (3) of 74 tested siblings 8 had diabetes, 6 classical JOD and 2 latent.

The history of MODY is reviewed. The difference between the inheritance of JOD and MODY provides further evidence of the genetic heterogeneity of diabetes mellitus and indicates the need for careful definition of the phenotype in populations in which the genetics of diabetes is to be analysed.

References

1. Cammidge, P.J.: Diabetes mellitus and heredity. Brit. Med. J. 2, 738 (1928)

2. Colle, R., Belmonte, M.M.: Chemical diabetes in the juvenile patient. Metabolism 22, 345 (1973)

3. Deschamps, I., Lestradet, H.: L'Epreuve d'hyperglycémie provoquée par voie buccale chez les frères et soeurs d'enfants diabétiques. Arch. Franc. Ped. 25, 761 (1968)

4. Discussion on diabetes in the tropics. Brit. Med. J. 2, 1051 (1907)

5. Elsas, L.J., Rosenberg, L.E.: Familial renal glycosuria: a genetic reappraisal of hexose transport by kidney and intestine. J. Clin. Invest. 48, 1845 (1969)

6. Fajans, S.S., Conn, J.W.: Tolbutamide-induced improvement in carbohydrate tolerance of young people with mild diabetes mellitus. Diabetes 9, 83 (1960)

7. Fajans, S.S., Taylor, C.I., Floyd, J.C., Jr., Conn, J.W.: Some aspects of the natural history of diabetes mellitus. Excerpta Medica, Int'l. Cong. Series 312, 329 (1974)

8. Graham, G.: Two cases of diabetes mellitus of an unusual type. Proc. R. Soc. Med. 14, 18 (1921)

9. Hales, C.N.: Plasma levels of glucose, non-esterified fatty acid, glycerol and insulin, four years before the onset of diabetic ketosis. Lancet 2, 389 (1967)

10. Hjarne, V.: A study of orthoglycemic glycosuria with particular reference to its hereditability. Acta Med. Scand. 67, 423 (1927)

11. Johansen, K.: Mild carbohydrate intolerance developing into classic juvenile diabetes. Acta Med. Scand. 189, 337 (1971)

12. Johansen, K.: Personal communication, 1975

13. Joslin, E.P.: The treatment of diabetes mellitus with observations based on three thousand cases. London: H. Kimpton, 1924

14. Köbberling, J., Appels, A., Köbberling, G., Creutzfeldt, W.: Glucose tolerance tests in 727 first-degree relatives of maturity-onset diabetics. Germ. Med. Monthly 14, 290 (1969)

15. Köbberling, J.: Untersuchungen zur Genetik des Diabetes Mellitus. Diabetologia 5, 392 (1969)

16. Lestradet, H., Battiselli, J., Ledoux, M.: L'hérédité dans le diabète infantile. Le Diabète 20, 17 (1972)

17. MacDonald, M.J.: Equal incidence of adult-onset diabetes among ancestors of juvenile diabetics and nondiabetics. Diabetologia 10, 767 (1974)

18. Murthy, D.Y.N., Guthrie, R.A., Womack, W.N.: Progressive decrease in insulin reserve in children with chemical diabetes. J. Pediatrics 72, 567 (1968)

19. Naunyn, B.: Der Diabetes Mellitus. Vienna: Hokler, 1906

20. Paulsen, E.P.: Experiences in Sulphonylurea therapy. Metabolism 22, 381 (1973)

21. Rimoin, D.L.: Inheritance in diabetes mellitus. Med. Clin. N. Amer. 55, 807 (1971)

22. Rollo, J.: An account of two cases of the diabetes mellitus. London: C. Dilly, 1797

23. Rosenbloom, A.L., Drash, A., Guthrie, R.: Chemical diabetes mellitus in childhood - report of a conference. Diabetes 21, 45 (1972)

24. Simpson. N.E.: Heritabilities of liability to diabetes when sex and age at onset are considered. Ann. Hum. Genet. 32, 283 (1969)

25. Tattersall, R.B., Pyke, D.A.: Diabetes in identical twins. Lancet 2, 1120 (1972)

26. Tattersall, R.B.: Mild familial diabetes with dominant inheritance. Quart. J. Med. 43, 339 (1974)

27. Tattersall, R.B., Fajans, S.S.: A difference between the inheritance of classical juvenile-onset and maturity-onset type diabetes in young people. Diabetes 24, 44 (1975).

11. A Possible Virus Etiology for Juvenile Diabetes

D. R. GAMBLE

A number of animal models of virus-induced diabetes have now been described; Encephalomyocarditis (EMC) virus (4), foot-and-mouth virus (2), and Coxsackie B4 virus (3) have all been found to be diabetogenic in animals. The diabetes described in these reports has usually been mild and transient, and although of great interest, it may not be relevant to the problem of diabetes in man.

The investigation of the possibility of a virus etiology in human diabetes is beset with difficulties (5). Virus-induced diabetes would probably be a late manifestation of infection, too late for the conventional techniques of virus isolation or the demonstration of rising antibody titers. The only approach may be to seek an excess of virus antibodies in groups of diabetics over levels found in matched groups of controls. If, as seems likely, a number of viruses are involved, patients with antibody to a particular etiological virus may be heavily outnumbered by patients with diabetes due to other viruses. The sucessful use of this procedure may therefore only be possible if very large numbers of patients are tested, unless patients with diabetes due to a particular virus can be identified in some other way - by an outbreak for example.

Virological studies on patients have not yet produced convincing evidence of a virus etiology, although there are some indications that Coysackie B4 virus may be involved in some cases (10,11). Much of our current effort is concentrated on epidemiologic studies of which one object is the identification of groups of similar patients in whom a common etiology is probable. At the same time serum specimens are being collected for the estimation of antibodies to any viruses that the epidemiologic results may suggest are potential candidates. In the present paper some preliminary results of these epidemiologic studies are discussed.

Methods

In 1972 the British Diabetic Association invited physicians and pediatricians in the United Kingdom and Eire to notify new cases of diabetes in children for inclusion on a register, to be used as a basis for suitable research projects. An epidemiologic investigation was started in 1973 based on information obtained by questionnaire from the physicians notifying cases to the register (12). Most of the data included here form part of this investigation which will be reported in full in due course.

Secular Trends

Seasonal Incidence

The seasonal incidence by month of onset for the first 1 1/2 years of
the survey (Fig. 1) showed a winter peak about December and an autumn
peak in September. This confirms the results of earlier surveys (1,10,
12). More recent results not included in the figure show a repetition
of this pattern in 1974 but the autumn peak was smaller and occurred
somewhat later, in October. The seasonal pattern, therefore, although
consistent in its main features, may vary in detail from year to year.
The shape of the winter peaks also supports this impression in that
the peak in the winter of 1972-1973 was broader and flatter than that
of the second winter.

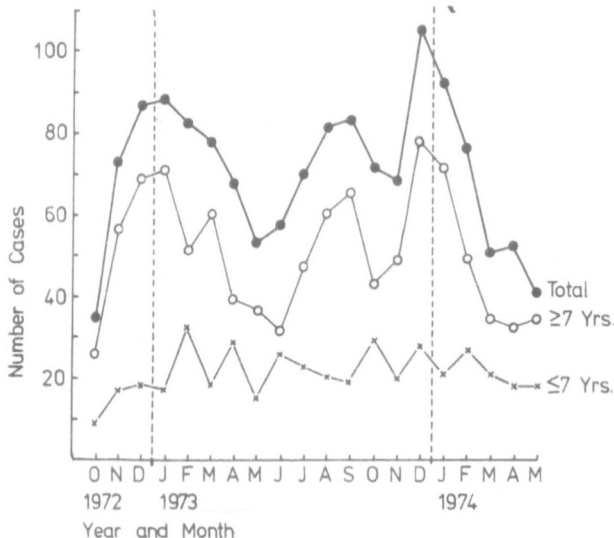

Fig. 1. Seasonal incidence of diabetes in children aged less than 16 years by month
of onset (● = all cases; ○ = patients aged 7 years or over; x = patients aged less
than 7 years)

The seasonal variation described was·most marked in children aged 7
years or over. Children aged less than 7 years showed little seasonal
variation in 1973, but in 1974 there was a marked decline in the summer
months. The different patterns in the two groups may imply different
etiologies.

The classical incidence of diabetes may arise in a number of different
ways, and some possibilities that affect its interpretation are as
follow:

1. It may reflect the simultaneous seasonal variation of an environmental etiological factor - viral or nonviral.
2. There may be a latent period between the etiological event and the
   onset of diabetes. The seasonal incidence of diabetes would then
   reflect the variation of the etiological factor with a lag equal to
   the latent period. It seems unlikely, however, that the latent period would be longer than a few months without the seasonal pattern
   becoming blurred or lost.

3. It may reflect a nonviral seasonal factor which precipitates or
   reveals latent diabetes in patients who have previously sustained
   islet cell damage.

Climatic Variables

The high incidence of diabetes in winter suggests the possibility that
it is due to cold weather, but a comparison of the number if new cases
reported per week with the mean recorded temperatures at Kew (22) fails
to support this suggestion (Fig. 2). The peak incidence at the end of
December occurred before the cold weather of January to March, during
which the incidence fell. Several individual weeks (e.g., week 8, 1974)
had an unusually high incidence but these weeks appeared to precede
rather than follow a temperature drop. The winter of 1974-1975 was the
warmest winter· for 50 years, but the December peak was as high as in
either of the preceding winters.

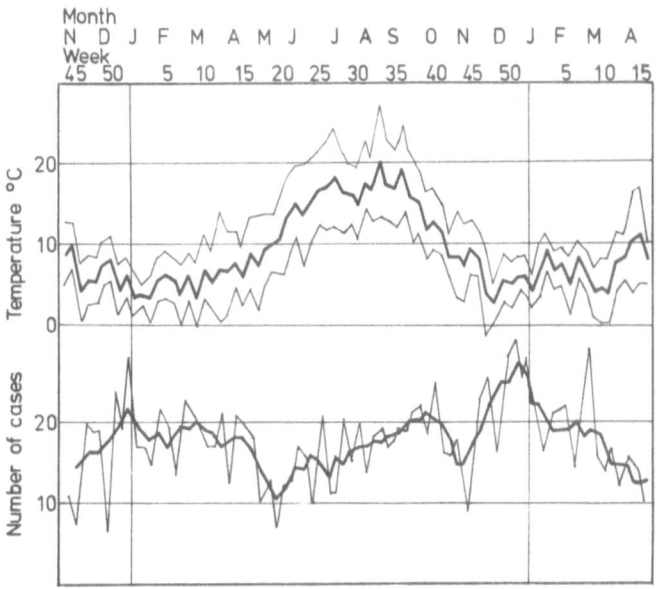

Fig. 2. Above: Average weekly temperatures at Kew (London) from November 1972 to
April 1974. Mean (heavy line) minimum and maximum temperatures (faint line). Below:
Number of cases of juvenile diabetes by week of onset (faint line) and 4-week moving
average (heavy line) from November 1972 to April 1974. Only patients for whom a
completed questionnaire was received are included

The autumn peak showed even less correlation with temperature; the
rise occurred during the summer, reaching its peak incidence when the
temperature was already declining.

It would seem unlikely therefore that the onset of diabetes is related
to temperature and although details of rainfall are not shown these
seem even less likely to be implicated.

Other Seasonal Variables

Many seasonal events like holidays, school attendance, feasts, and festivals occur at fixed times in the calendar but the incidence of diabetes lacks this regularity. Other factors such as type of clothing or calorie intake are probably related to temperature and might follow its general trends. Although nonifective factors cannot be definitely excluded, the majority of seasonal illnesses are due to infection which seems to be the most likely explanation of the seasonal pattern of diabetes.

Seasonal Variation of Virus Infection

In the UK the total incidence of all infectious illnesses has a high incidence from December to March, the peak most commonly occurring in the first quarter of the year, and the lowest incidence in summer – usually August (Kendall, unpublished data). A similar pattern has been reported in the USA (7). Respiratory infections, which make up more than three-quarters of all infections, follow the same pattern. The agents mainly responsible for these infections appear therefore to arrive too late to be associated with diabetes with its peaks in autumn and December.

We have been unable to find a virus which regularly has its peak in December to match the peak of diabetes and it therefore seemed more likely that if these cases are associated with virus infection there is a latent period before the onset of diabetes. Since the latent period would probably not exceed a few months, these viruses which are most prevalent in the autumn seem the most likely candidates.

The picorna group of viruses which includes the Coxsackie and ECHO viruses are most prevalent in the second half of the year. The highest incidence usually occurs in the autumn, the peak month varying from year to year, and this variability would be consistent with our limited observations of the seasonal pattern of diabetes. The picorna viruses, like most viruses, have an epidemic pattern with isolated years of high prevalence intersporsed by a varying number of years of low prevalence. Diabetes does not display this epidemicity. Although there are seasonal fluctuations, the annual incidence appears to vary little from year to year. If, therefore, a substantial proportion of juvenile diabetes is induced by viruses, the involvement of a number of different viruses is likely to account for the more or less steady flow of cases.

Even if the apparent absence of epidemicity of diabetes is largely explained in this way, a regular incidence pattern accords poorly with the usual pattern of virus infection. There is, however, some evidence to suggest some irregularity in the incidence of diabetes. Gunderson (13) reported considerable variation in the annual mortality among 10–20-year-old diabetics in Norway prior to the introduction of insulin, and in our current survey in the UK, a number of diabetic clinics have reported striking increases in the numbers of new cases seen in some of the last few years. Clearly more data are required for the objective assessment of long-term secular trends. If there is an infectious element in diabetes it is perhaps surprising that most cases occur singly, even in families, among whom infections normally spread readily. It is interesting, therefore, that in the past 2 years diabetes occurring almost simultaneously in siblings of different ages has been reported to us on four occasions. Two siblings were affected within a week in two instances, and in a third family two siblings acquired diabetes within a month. The fourth incident involved three siblings who developed diabetes within 3 months.

A fifth instance has been reported in the UK during the same period by Cudworth and Woodrow (6). Simultaneous diabetes in siblings might be expected to occur on rare occasions by chance but it is surprising that there should be five instances within 2 years, particularly when three siblings are affected in one family, and the influence of the environmental factor must be suspected. On the other hand, if virus infection is responsible it is perhaps more surprising that it does not occur more often. It may be, therefore, that the conditions necessary for the induction of diabetes are in some way critical, involving a particular combination of host and environmental factors, or that an event occurs at some stage in the etiological chain which involves an element of chance.

Age Incidence

Age Incidence in Juvenile Diabetics

It appears from the age incidence of childhood diabetes found in the present survey (Fig. 3) and from previous investigations (12) that the pattern is bimodal with peaks at about 5 and 11 years. These may represent two groups of different etiology.

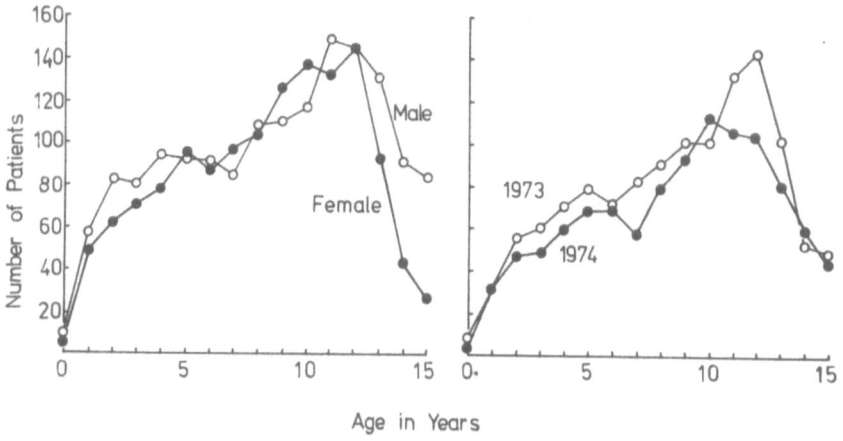

Fig. 3. Age at diagnosis of diabetes by sex and year of onset

The sex ratio shows a male excess from 0-4 years, a female excess from 5-9 years, and a male excess from 10-15 years, overall there is a slight male excess. These differences may be due to hormonal factors or to differnces in behavior between boys and girls, but sex differences also occur in infection rates of some viruses (23).

Comparing the incidence in the first 2 years of the survey there were slightly fewer cases in 1974 (Fig. 3b). There may have been a fall in the ascertainment rate, but the decrease was confined to the autumn peak from July to mid-November and it mainly affected 10- and 11-year-old children. It is perhaps more likely, therefore, to be due to a changing environmental factor.

The results for the 2 years also suggest taht the ages at which the peak incidence occurs may change from year to year. Thus the peak incidence occurred in 12-year-old children in 1973 and in 10-year-old children in 1974.

Puberty and Growth Rates

The pattern of age incidence in juvenile diabetes has been attributed to puberty or spurts in the growth rate (25). Figure 4 shows the age incidence by sex and the percentage growth rate by year of age, based on figures quoted by Stewart and Stevens (24). The fastest growth occurs in the first 2 years of life when diabetes has its lowest incidence. Both sexes have a peak in diabetes incidence at the age of about 5 years although boys have a growth spurt at 5 but girls do not. From age 6-10 years diabetes incidence increases but growth rate decreases. The second diabetes peak occurs at about the age of 11 years but the "peak height velocity" (20,21) occurs at 14 in boys and at 12 in girls. Menarche at the age of about 13 years in girls is later still. Moreover the seasonal onset of diabetes in 11-year-olds makes it unlikely that it is the result of pubertal changes.

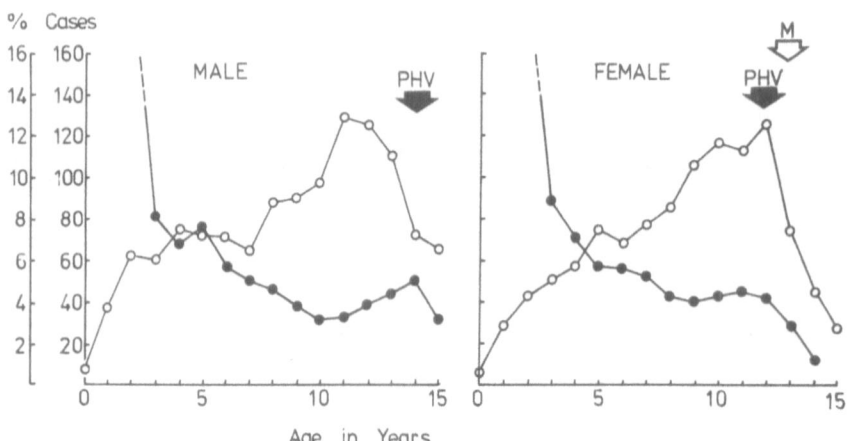

Fig. 4. Number of male and female cases of diabetes by age at onset (•) and percentage growth rate by year (o) (see text)

Another weakness of the "puberty theory" is that pubertal changes show a remarkable regularity in the ages at which they occur. Marshall and Tanner (20,21) have found that the ages at which the various pubertal changes take place have a normal distribution with a standard deviation of about 1 year. This means that observations in 1000 children should then establish the mean age at which, say, menarche or the "peak height velocity" occurs, with a standard error of about two weeks ($\frac{S.D.}{\sqrt{1000}}$).

Replicate estimations should not, therefore, vary by more than about a month either way. By contrast, the age peaks in the incidence of diabetes, which are based on data from more than 1000 cases for each of the 2 years, appear to vary by as much as 2 years. The factor responsible for these peaks must therefore be subject to a lot more variation than pubertal changes or growth spurts, which are unlikely to be major determinants of the onset of diabetes although their effects cannot be discounted completely.

School Attendance

The major environmental changes in childhood are associated with school attendance. In the UK children start school at the age of about 4 or 5 years, and transfer from primary to secondary school at about 11 years. At these times cohorts of susceptible pupils are introduced into school communities and waves of infection occur, and it has been suggested that this may be related to the peaks in age incidence of diabetes in childhood (12). If diabetes is associated with starting school, children who attend nursery schools before the usual starting age may develop diabetes earlier than those who start at the conventional age of 5 years.

A preliminary analysis suggested that this was so (12) but we have subsequently found that a great increase has occurred in recent years in the number of places available in nursery schools in the UK (14) and that the results at least in part reflect this fact. Since information about the ages of children in nursery schools is unobtainable we are now investigating this problem in another way. Cohorts of children born in particular years are being followed to see at what age they develop diabetes in relation to the age at which they start school. Figure 5 shows the results to date for children born in 1966-1967. They are now 8-9 years old and of these who started school at five 76 have developed diabetes, and of those who started school at less than five 155 are diabetic. Figure 5 shows a tendency for those who started school first to develop diabetes at an earlier age but we need to collect data for several more years to confirm this finding and to assess how important this factor is.

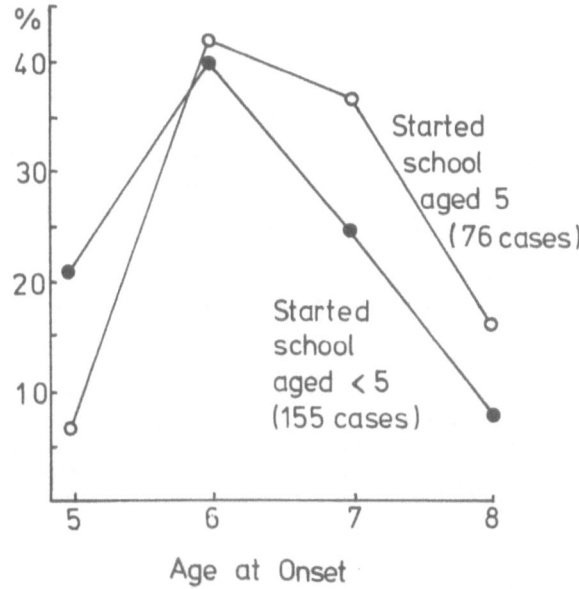

Fig. 5. Age of onset of diabetes in children born in 1966-1967 in relation to age of starting school

Age Incidence of Virus Infection

Most viruses have their highest incidence at the age of 5 or 6 years in
children who have just started school. Some viruses like the common
cold attack preschool children because adults have no immunity to these
infections and parents carry infection into the home. A few viruses
attack older people because their infectivity is lower, or because they
are transmitted in an unusual way such as serum hepatitis, arthropod-
borne viruses, or infectious mononucleosis.

How can the age incidence of diabetes with its peak at 11 years be reconciled with that of viral infection which is likely to occur at an
earlier age? There are a number of possibilities.

1. Diabetes may be due to a virus of low infectivity that has its peak
   incidence of infection at about 11 years.
2. There may be a long latent period between infection and the development of overt diabetes. If this were of the order of 5 years it
   would then be difficult to account for the seasonal variation in
   diabetes.
3. There may be an increasing susceptibility to diabetes with age, just
   as the likelihood of paralysis from poliovirus infection increases
   with the age at which infection occurs.
4. A single pancreatropic infection may produce subdiabetogenic damage
   and several such infections may be required to produce overt diabetes. This would postpone the age at which diabetes occurs.
5. Some viruses may cause reinfection when antibodies provoked by the
   primary infection have waned - probably after several years. Such
   reinfection in the presence of a low level of residual antibody
   might provoke a damaging hypersensitivity reaction.

Congenital Infections and Diabetes in Infancy

Forrest *et al.* (8) have recently reported a high incidence of diabetes
in patients with congenital rubella. Of 87 cases, 8 have developed diabetes and this is far more than would be expected in patients of this
age - they are all under 30 years of age. They have also found 10 more
patients whose glucose tolerance curves indicate that they have latent
diabetes; if these are included 21% of the 87 patients might be considered diabetic. This certainly suggests that rubella virus infestion
can produce pancreatic damage that may lead to diabetes.

An interesting aspect of this report is the age incidence. The onset
of diabetes in the 15 cases quoted occurred at the age 1 (4 cases), 3
(1 case), 12 (2 cases), 17 (1 case), 19 (1 case) and between 20 and
30 in the remainder. Patients with onset at age of 12 or less had insulin-dependent diabetes. If pancreatic damage occurred in these patients
before birth, why should it have taken between 1 and 30 years before
diabetes developed? A persistent latent infection of the islet cells
with rubella virus might shorten their lifespan, or the initial damage
might trigger an immunologic reaction which eventually destroys the
cells, but in neither case does it seem likely that the duration of
the destructive process would vary by as much as 30 years. It is perhaps more likely, at least in those cases where diabetes took many years
to develop, that the disease was precipitated by a second event nearer
to the time of onset.

It is surprising that although virus infections are common in young
infants diabetes is rare. Is the pancreas resistant at this age? It
would appear not because diabetes is not uncommon in the first year of
life, and the pancreas may be involved in generalized virus infections

of the newborn (15,16). Does the pancreas in young animals have greater powers of recovery? The diabetes induced in mice by EMC or Coxsackie virus infection is usually mild, and full recovery generally occurs within a few weeks. Similarly the few recorded cases of diabetes in the newborn unsually recover normal glucose tolerance. Since the B-cells are capable of hyperplasia in mice (17), sand rats (18) and monkeys (19), some regeneration may also occur in man, and if the regenerative capacity enables the pancreas to withstand a degree of damage one might expect this capacity to be greatest in the young. This suggestion would be consistent with the idea that diabetes may occur as a result of repeated and cummulative pancreatic damage when the capacity of regeneration is exhausted.

A Hypothetical Model

I would like to conclude with a hypothetical model of the age and secular trands in juvenile diabetes. The age incidence of childhood diabetes ascertained in our current survey may comprise three separate groups.

Group A (Fig. 6) represents cases associated with congenital infection. It appears that congenital rubella infection may lead to diabetes and if this is so other viruses may act in the same way.

Group B comprises children of whom the majority would be under the age of 7 years with a modal age of about 5 years. There is some evidence that the onset of diabetes in this group may be related to starting school.

Group C comprises children of whom the majority would be aged 7 years or over, with a modal age of about 11 years. This group has a pronounced seasonal incidence suggesting a viral etiology.

The seasonal incidence patterns suggest further subdivisions of these groups. Thus Group B had a variable seasonal incidence pattern which may have a summer and a winter component (Fig. 6, Groups B1 and B2). If both occur together in the same year the incidence would show little seasonal pattern, but in years in which one or other was absent, either a summer or winter prevalence would result. This changing seasonal pattern would be very much in line with the secular trends of virus infection.

Group C includes the older children who fall into two subgroups constituting the autumn and winter peaks (Fig. 6, Groups C1 and C2) for which different viral etiologies seem likely.

This model allows us to divide cases of juvenile diabetes into subgroups and tissue typing may permit further subdivision which should facilitate virologic studies. But although there is now a great deal of evidence that infection would be a plausible explanation, there is as yet little direct evidence for the viral hypothesis in man.

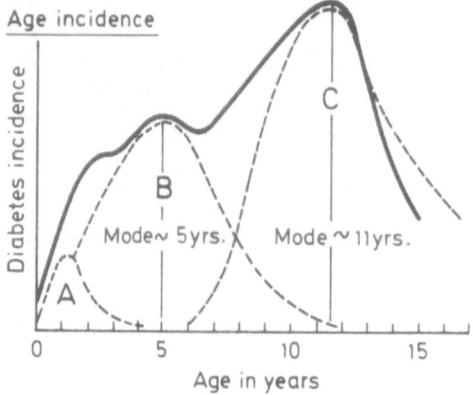

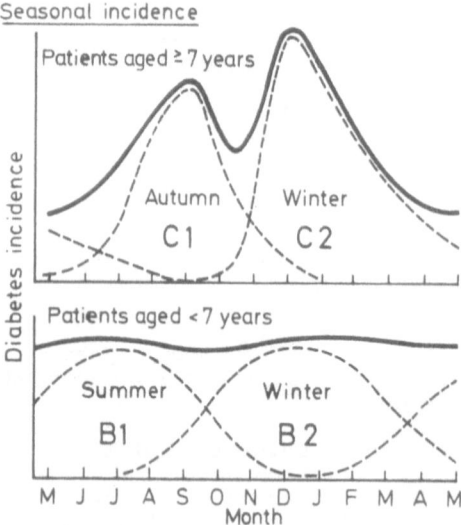

Fig. 6. Hypothetic model of the age and seasonal incidence of diabetes in children (see text)

References

1. Adams, S.F.: The seasonal variation in the incidence of acute diabetes. Arch. Int. Med. 17, 861 (1926)

2. Barboni, E., Manocchio, I.: Alterazioni pancreatiche in bovini con diabete mellito post-aftoso. Arch. Vet. Ital. 13, 477 (1962)

3. Coleman, T.J., Gamble, D.R., Taylor, K.W.: Diabetes in mice after Coxsackie B4 virus infection. Brit. Med. J. III, 25 (1973)

4. Craighead, J.E., McLane, M.F.: Diabetes Mellitus: induction in mice by encephalo-mycarditis virus. Science 162, 913 (1968)

5. Craighead, J.E.: Workshop on viral infection and diabetes mellitus in man. J. Infect. Dis. 125, 568 (1972)

6. Cudworth, A.G., Woodrow, J.C.: HL-A antigens and diabetes mellitus. Lancet 2, 1153 (1974)

7. Dingle, J.H., Badger, G.F., Jordan, W.S.: Illness in the Home. A study of 25,000 illnesses in a group of Cleveland families. Cleveland: 1964, Western Reserve Univ. Press

8. Forrest, J.M., Menser, M.A., Burgess, J.A.: High frequency of diabetes mellitus in young adults with congenital rubella. Lancet 2, 332 (1971)

9. Gamble, D.R., Kinsley, M.L., Fitzgerald, M.G., Bolton, R., Taylor, K.W.: Viral antibodies in diabetes mellitus. Brit. Med. J. 3, 627 (1969)

10. Gamble, D.R., Taylor, K.W.: Seasonal incidence of diabetes mellitus. Brit. Med. J. 3, 631 (1969)

11. Gamble, D.R., Taylor, K.W., Cumming, H.: Coxsackie viruses and diabetes mellitus. Brit. Med. J. 4, 260 (1973)

12. Gamble, D.R.: Epidemiological and virological observations on juvenile diabetes. Postgrad., ed. J., 50, 538 (1974)

13. Gunderson, E.: Is diabetes of infectious origin? J. Infect. Dis. 41, 197 (1927)

14. Health and Personal Social Service Statistics for England. London: Her Majesty's Stationary Office, 1973

15. Kibrick, S., Benirschke, K.: Acute aseptic myocarditis and meningoencephalitis in the newborn child infected with Coxsackie virus group B, type 3. New. Eng. J. Med. 255, 883 (1956)

16. Kibrick, S., Benirschke, K.: Severe generalized disease (encephalohepatomyocarditis) occurring in the newborn period and due to infection with Coxsackie virus group B - evidence of intra-uterine infection with this agent. Pediatrics 22, 857 (1958)

17. Like, A.A., Jones, E.E.: Studies on experimental diabetes in the Wellesley hybrid mouse. IV morphological changes in islet tissue. Diabetologia 3, 179 (1967)

18. Like, A.A., Miki, E.: Diabetic syndrome in sand rats. IV morphological changes in islet tissue. Diabetologia 3, 143 (1967)

19. Like, A.A., Chick, W.L.: Pancreatic beta cell replication induced by glucocorticoids in subhuman primates. Am. J. Path. 75, 329 (1974)

20. Marshall, W.A., Tanner, J.M.: Variations in the pattern of pubertal changes in girls. Arch. Dis. Childh. 44, 291 (1969)

21. Marshall, W.A., Tanner, J.M.: Variations in the pattern of pubertal changes in boys. Arch. Dis. Childh. 45, 13 (1970)

22. The Register General's Statistical Review for England and Wales. (weekly returns for England and Wales). 1972-1974

23. Spicer, C.C.: The incidence of poliomyelitis virus in normal children aged 0-5 years. J. Hyg. (Camb.) 59, 143 (1961)

24. Stewart, H.C., Stevenson, S.S.: Textbook of Pediatrics, 7th ed. Nelson, W.E. (ed.). Philadelphia: Saunders 1959, p. 50

26. White, P.: Diabetes in Childhood & Adolescence, Philadelphia: Lea and Febiger, 1932, p. 47

12. HLA, Autoimmunity and Insulin-Dependent Diabetes Mellitus

J. NERUP, P. PLATZ, O. ORTVED ANDERSEN, M. CHRISTY, J. EGEBERG, J. LYNGSØE, J. E. POULSEN, L. P. RYDER, M. THOMSEN, and A. SVEJGAARD

The etiology and pathogenesis of juvenile diabetes mellitus (JDM), i.e., insulin-dependent diabetes in nonobese individuals, are still poorly understood.

None of the many hypotheses as yet proposed has been able to explain the essential pathologic finding in this disease: The functioning B-cell mass is reduced due to reduction of the total amount of islet tissue as well as a striking reduction of the number of B-cells (15, 19).

The purpose of this presentation is to propose a hypothesis concerning the etiology and pathogenesis of insulin-dependent diabetes based on a review of observations reported during recent years:

1. There is a well-known tendency to aggregation of diabetes in families, but no pattern of inheritance has been established (16,21). In mono-zygous twins a surprisingly low concordance rate, of about 50% of JDM, suggests that exogenous factors play an important part in the development of the disease (47).

Thus, what is inherited is not the disease JDM as such but rather a susceptibility to develop JDM under the influence of certain environmental factors.

2. Evidence that viral infections might be of importance has been reported. High titers of virus-neutralizing antibodies against Coxsackie B4 and other viruses have been demonstrated with unexpected high prevalences in JDM patients (10,17,18). In mice a diabetic state can be induced by Coxsackie B4 and EMC virus (3,4,8,10,12,26). Interestingly enough this susceptibility to diabetogenic viruses in mice is observed only in certain strains and might therefore be genetically determined (11).

3. Indirect evidence that autoimmunity is involved in the pathogenesis of JDM stems from the observation that clinical and chemical diabetes occurs in combination with organ-specific autoimmune endocrine disorders (Graves' disease, myxedema, Hashimoto's disease, idiopathic Addison's disease, hypergonadotropic hypogonadism and idiopathic hypoparathyroidism) more often than expected by chance alone (1,22,35,36). Furthermore, lymphocytic infiltration in and around the islets of Langerhans - insulitis - is a characteristic finding in JDM of short duration (19,24,27).

4. Direct experimental evidence that organ-specific autoimmune phenomena play a part in patients suffering from JDM has also been reported. Nerup et al. (38,40) found antipancreatic cell-mediated immunity (APCI) directed against antigenic determinants in the endocrine pancreas in patients with JDM of short duration. Other workers have confirmed this finding (30,43). Recently Botazzo et al., Irvine et al., and Lendrum et al. (2,28,29) have reported the occurrence of an IgG antibody di-

rected against the pancreatic islet cells in patients with JDM. This islet cell antibody (ICA) was found with the highest frequency in patients with JDM of recent onset. By immunization of experimental animals with homogenates of isolated islets of Langerhans, a transient diabetes-like syndrome can be induced, that is characterized by reduced glucose tolerance, cell-mediated immunity against the endocrine pancreas, discrete lymphocytic inflammation in the islets of Langerhans, and B-cell degeneration and destruction (37).

The exact biochemical nature and characteristics of the antigenic determinant in the endocrine pancreas against which these autoimmune phenomena were directed is still unknown, but the antigen(s) is organ-specific, species nonspecific, and different from insulin. During the past few years several investigations have shown that different antigens of the major human histocompatibility system, the HLA-system, are found with increased frequency in patients suffering from different diseases showing aggregation in families and in which virus and autoimmunity seem to be involved (31,46).

It was of interest, therefore, to investigate the prevalence of different HLA antigens in diabetic patients (41). A total of 146 patients with diabetes mellitus were HLA-typed. In 85 patients diabetes was diagnosed before the age of 40 (juvenile diabetes) and in the remaining 61 patients age at onset was 41 years or more (maturity onset diabetes). All patients were unrelated Danish Caucasian out-patients. The number of obese (i.e. > 125% of normal weight) and of insulin-dependent patients is shown in Table 3.

For the HLA-typing the microlymphocytotoxicity test was used (25). In all patients and in 1967 unrelated Danish Caucasian controls the presence or absence of 23 different HLA antigens of the A and B series were determined (see Table 1 for details about the antigens in question and the new and old nomenclature of HLA antigens. In this presentation the new nomenclature will be used).

Table 1. HLA nomenclature – new and old (only antigens tested for in this study are included)

A-series	(LA)	B-series	(Four)	D-series	(MLC)
New	Old	New	Old	New	Old
HLA-A1	HL-A1	HLA-B5	HL-A5	HLA-Dw2	7a
HLA-A2	HL-A2	HLA-B7	HL-A7	HLA-Dw3	8a
HLA-A3	HL-A3	HLA-B8	HL-A8	HLA-Dw4	W15a
HLA-A9	HL-A9	HLA-B12	HL-A12		
HLA-A10	HL-A10	HLA-B13	HL-A13		
HLA-A11	HL-A11	HLA-B14	W 14		
HLA-A28	W28	HLA-B18	W 18		
HLA-Aw19	W19	HLA-B27	W 27		
		HLA-Bw15	W 15		
		HLA-Bw16	W 16		
		HLA-Bw17	W 17		
		HLA-Bw21	W 21		
		HLA-Bw22	W 22		
		HLA-Bw35	W 5		

Ref: IUIS Nomenclature Report. In: Kissmeyer-Nielsen (ed.) Histocompatibility Testing. Copenhagen: Munksgaard, 1975.

The relative risk was calculated as described by Svejgaard *et al.* (45). The only antigens appearing with increased frequencies were HLA-B 8 and HLA-Bw15. As shown in Table 2 the increased frequency of B 8 was restricted to the group of juvenile diabetics, whereas Bw15 was found with increased frequency in juvenile diabetics as well·as in maturity onset diabetics, although not significantly so in the latter. Table 3 shows that the group of insulin-dependent, nonobese diabetics (i.e., juvenile diabetics irrespective of age) was responsible for the increase in HLA-B 8. The so-called relative risk indicates the calculated risk of healthy carriers of a certain HLA antigen for developing the disease in question.

Table 2. Some HLA frequencies in patients with diabetes mellitus and in normal individuals

	Control	Diabetics total	Juvenile diabetics	Maturity onset diabetics
	N = 1967	N = 146	N = 85	N = 61
HLA-B 8	23.7%	37.7%[a]	44.7%[b]	27.9%
HLA-Bw15	17.9%	31.5%[b]	32.9%[b]	29.5%
HLA-B 7	26.8%	15.8%	10.6%[c]	23.0%

Statistics: Fisher's exact test. P-values corrected for one-sidedness of the test ($x2$) and for the number of antigens investigated ($x23$).
[a] $p < 0.01$.
[b] $p < 0.001$.
[c] $p < 0.05$.

Table 3. HLA-B 8 and Bw15 in diabetes mellitus: correlation with obesity and insulin dependency

	Obesity		Insulin dependency		Controls
	No (N = 112)	Yes (N = 31)	Yes (N = 109)	No (N = 37)	(N = 1967)
HLA-B 8	46 (41.1%)	8 (25.5%)	46 (42.4%)	9 (24.3%)	(23.7%)
HLA-Bw15	36 (32.1%)	9 (29.0%)	38 (34.9%)	8 (21.6%)	(17.9%)
HLA-B 8 and/or Bw15	70 (62.5%)	14 (45.2%)	70 (64.2%)	16 (43.2%)	(39.2%)

In Table 4 it is shown that HLA-B 8- or Bw15-positive individuals carry a risk of about 2.5 times that of HLA-B 8- or Bw15-negative individuals of developing juvenile diabetes (i.e., insulin-dependent diabetes in the nonobese patient). In contrast they carry no increased risk as far as maturity onset diabetes was concerned. It is noteworthing, (1) that persons positive for HLA-B 8 and Bw15 carry a risk that is the sum of the calculated relative risk of each of the individual, (2) that hetero- and homozygous carriers of HLA-B 8 or Bw15 have identical relative risks (46).

Table 4. Relative risk of insulin-dependent and non insulin-dependent diabetes in HLA-B 8- and Bw15-positive subjects

	Insulin-dependent diabetes mellitus	Non insulin-dependent diabetes mellitus
	Relative risk	Relative risk
HLA-B 8	2.4 $(p = 1.9 \times 10^{-5})$	1.0 (N.S.)
HLA-Bw15	2.5 $(p = 3.2 \times 10^{-5})$	1.3 (N.S.)

Statistics: Fisher's exact test.

These findings have to be interpreted in the following way: (1) HLA-B 8 and Bw15 seem to predispose to different diabetes-provoking factors. (2) No gene-dose effect of HLA-B 8 and Bw15 exists. Thus, the highest prevalence of diabetes mellitus should be expected amongst siblings of JDM patients positive for both HLA-B 8 Bw15. The results shown in Table 5 confirm this expectation. The significantly increased frequency of HLA-B 8 and Bw15 in patients with JDM has now been confirmed by others (5,13,23).

Table 5. Prevalence of diabetes in siblings of juvenile diabetics with different HLA types

Patient HLA type	Diabetic siblings	
	No.	%
HLA-B 8	10/99	10.1
HLA-Bw15	9/79	11.4
HLA-B 8 and Bw15	7/34	20.6
Other HLA types	7/127	5.5

HLA-B 8 and Bw15 thus seem to be genetic markers of insulin-dependent diabetes mellitus. This type of diabetes is further characterized by an early age of onset, normal weight, lymphocytic infiltration in and around the islets of Langerhans, reduction of the functioning B-cell mass, antipancreatic cellular immunity (APCI), and high titers of islet cell antibodies (ICA). Therefore these findings support the concept that juvenile, insulin-dependent diabetes in nonobese patients is a disease entity of its own different from non insulin-dependent diabetes with respect to etiology and pathogenesis (41).

Figure 1 demonstrates a family including several cases of insulin-dependent diabetes. It is seen that the phenotype diabetes follows the HLA-haplotype. The significance of the occurrence of this HLA-haplotype in the nondiabetic family members is discussed briefly below. Cudworth and Woodrow also found that aggregation of diabetes in families is closely connected to the HLA region on chromosome No. 6 and especially to the HLA types B 8 and Bw15 (14). HLA-B 8 and/or Bw15 can be demonstrated in 65% of patients suffering from JDM as compared to only 39%

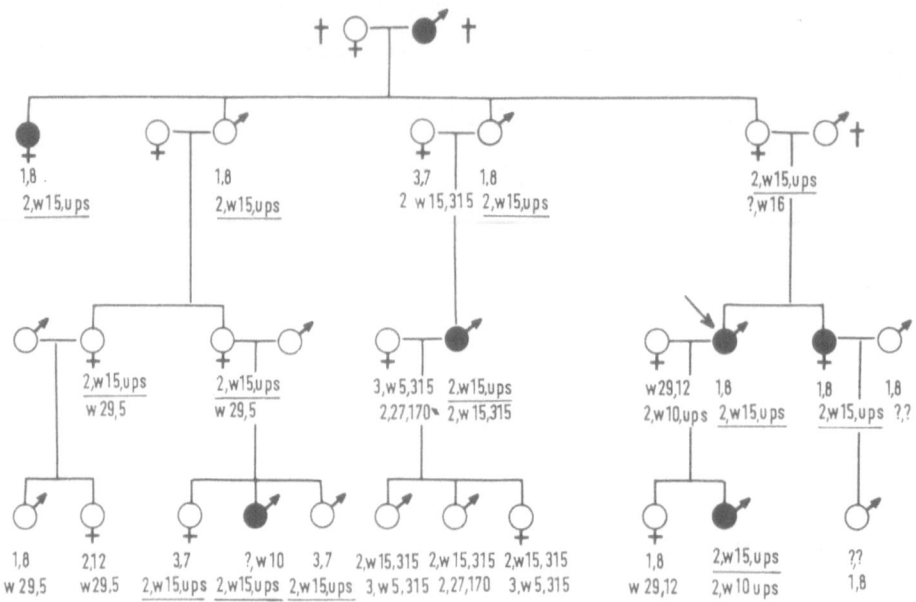

Fig. 1. HLA genotypes in a family including 7 cases of diabetes (black). Propositus is marked by an arrow. The HLA-A2, Bw15, CW3 haplotype shared by all diabetic members of the family (and some nondiabetics) is underlined
? = haplotypes that could not be definitely established

Table 6. D-Types (MLC types) in insulin-dependent (juvenile) diabetes mellitus

	Diabetics	Controls N = 35	Relative risk
Dw3	29/50 (58%)	16%	6.4
Dw4	33/75 (42%)	16%	3.7

in the background population. An even stronger association was demonstrated between insulin-dependent diabetes mellitus and the HLA-Dw3 and Dw4 antigens of the D-series of the HLA system (previously known as LD or MLC types) (Table 6).
The antigens of this fourth locus of the major human histocompatibility region on chromosome No. 6 can at present only be typed by means of unidirectional mixed lymphocyte cultures and thus, they differ from other histocompatibility antigens (for further details see Thomsen *et al.* (<u>48</u>)).
Dw3 and/or Dw4 was found to occur in 80% of patients compared to 24% of the control population. In other words: a genetic marker for insulin-dependent diabetes mellitus could be demonstrated in 80% of the juvenile diabetics.

It is still unknown how the HLA factors confer the susceptibility to develop insulin-dependent diabetes. As mentioned above, diabetes is often seen together with other endocrine disorders. For this reason it is worth noting that HLA-B 8 and Dw3 also occur with increased frequency in patients suffering from Addison's disease (20), Graves' disease (20,33), and certain cases of hypergonadotropic hypogonadism (7). Thus Dw3 or possibly one or more immune response gene(s) linked to Dw3 could be involved as a common denominator of organ-specific auto-immune endocrinopathy. Some preliminary observations suggest future lines of research in this field. It has been demonstrated (Table 7) that islet cell antibodies (ICA) in juvenile diabetics were found predominantly in the sera of the HLA-B 8-positive patients in small series (6).

Table 7. Islet cell antibody (ICA) and juvenile diabetes mellitus

	HLA-B 8	Other HLA types	Total
ICA	13/18 .	8/20	21/38
	(72%)[a]	(40%)[a]	(55%)

[a]P = 0.05 (Fisher's exact test).
Mean duration of diabetes: 3.2 years, range (1-20 years).

No correlation was found between the occurrence of ICA and APCI. This is, however, in accordance with the findings in other autoimmune endocrinopathies, e.g., idiopathic Addison's disease (34). Autoimmunity (ICA and/or APCI) was present in 73% of the juvenile diabetics (Table 8) and it is worth noting that autoimmunity against the endocrine pancreas was found to be statistically significant more often in the HLA-B 8-positive patients (89%), when compared to HLA-B 8-negative diabetics. However, the mean duration of disease in this small series was 3.2 years. Since ICA as well as APCI seems to fade away with increased duration of disease, we anticipate autoimmunity to be present with an even higher prevalence in juvenile diabetics when examined at time of diagnosis or, perhaps, of even greater significance in the months preceding clinical manifestation.

Table 8. Autoimmunity (ICA and/or APCI) in juvenile diabetes mellitus

	HLA-8 positive	Other HLA types	Total (N = 37)
ICA and/or APCI	16/18	11/19	27/37
	(89%)[a]	(58%)[a]	(73%)

[a]P = 0.04 (Fisher's exact test).

Similarly, a tendency toward a correlation between HLA-B 8 and high titers of neutralizing antibodies against Coxsackie B4 virus was demonstrated, but the correlation was not statistically significant in this small retrospective study. Further evidence in support of an association between HLA and viral infections was provided by the observation that more than 70% of the children with congenital rubella who developed diabetes were HLA-B 8-positive (22). Furthermore, the seasonal variation in the incidence of JDM was reported to be accounted for by the HLA-B 8-positive cases (44). Thus evidence is accumulating to suggest that immune response genes associated with HLA-B 8 predispose to the development of JDM through the susceptibility to isletotrophic viruses leading to B-cell destruction directly or through the triggering of autoimmune reactions.

As previously mentioned, B 8 and Bw15 seem to predispose to the development of JDM through different mechanisms. Data to elucidate the possible action of Bw15 are sparse. However, studies of the early insulin response as estimated by the method of Thorell (49) suggest that in the Bw15-positive nondiabetic members of the family shown in Figure 1 the insulin response to intravenous glucose is lower than in the non-Bw15 nondiabetic members. This might implicate the presence of an inherited insensitivity to glucose, an inherited reduced B-cell mass, or an impaired regeneration capacity to subclinical islet damage.

In conclusion: A statistically significant correlation between HLA-B 8 and Bw15 and insulin-dependent diabetes mellitus (juvenile diabetes) has been found. In addition, some preliminary - as yet incomclusive - findings suggest the existence of more specific connections between HLA-B 8 and viral infections, between HLA-Bw15 and low insulin response, and between both these HLA factors and antipancreatic autoimmune reactions. With this background the following hypothesis for the etiology and pathogenesis of insulin-dependent diabetes mellitus is proposed:

1. The inherited susceptibility in certain individuals to develop juvenile diabetes mellitus when exposed to some environmental factors (virus? chemical agents?) is at least in part conferred by HLA-Dw3- and Dw4-associated immune response genes (Ir-genes).

2. In susceptible individuals these Ir-genes cause a defective T cell response (T-B lymphocyte cooperation) against environmental factors, leading to B-cell destruction directly or through autoimmune mechanisms.

References

1. Bastonie, P.A.: Immunity, autoimmunity and diabetes. In: Diabetes. VIIIth Congress Internat. Diabetes Federation. Malaisse, W.J.. Pirart, J. (eds.) Amsterdam: Excerpta Medica, 1974, p. 3

2. Botazzo, G.F., Florin-Christensen, A., Doniach, D.: Islet-cell antibodies in diabetes mellitus with autoimmune polyendocrine deficiencies. Lancet II, 1279 (1974)

3. Burch, G.E., Tsui, C.Y., Harb, J.M.: Pancreatic islets cell-damage in mice produced by Coxsackie B 1 and encephalomyocarditis virus. Experentia 28/3, 310 (1972)

4. Burch, G.E., Tsui, C.Y., Harb, J.M., Colcolough, H.L.: Pathologic findings in the pancreas of mice infected with Coxsackie virus B4. Arch. Int. Med. 128, 40 (1971)

5. Cathelineau, G., Cathelineau, L., Hors, J., Schmid, M., Dausset, J.: HL-A and juvenile diabetes. Diabetologia 11, 335 (1975)

6. Christy, M., Botazzo, G.F., Doniach, D., Nerup, J., Platz, P., Thomsen, M., Ryder, L.P., Svejgaard, A.: Association between HLA-B 8 and autoimmunity in juvenile diabetes mellitus.(In preparation)

7. Christy, M., Thomsen, M., Platz, P., Ryder, L., Staub Nielsen, L., Starup, J., Svejgaard, A., Nerup, J.: HL-A antigens and hypergonadotropic hypogonadism. (In preparation)

8. Coleman, T.J., Gamble, D.R., Taylor, K.W.: Diabetes in mice after Coxsackie B4 virus infection. Brit. Med. J. 3, 25 (1973)

9. Coleman, T.J., Taylor, K.W., Gamble, D.R.: The development of diabetes following Coxsackie B virus infection in mice. Diabetologia 10, 755 (1974)

10. Craighead, J.E.: The role of viruses in the pathogenesis of pancreatic disease and diabetes mellitus. Prog. Med. Virol. 19, 161 (1975)

11. Craighead, J.E., Higgins, D.A.: Genetic influences affecting the occurrence of diabetes mellitus-like disease in mice infected with the encephalomyocarditis virus. J. Exp. Med. _139_, 414 (1974)

12. Crainghead, J.E., McLane, M.F.: Diabetes mellitus induction in mice by encephalo-myocarditis virus. Science _162_, 913 (1968)

13. Cudworth, A.G., Woodrow, J.C.: HL-A antigens and diabetes mellitus. Lancet _II_, 1153 (1974)

14. Cudworth, A.G., Woodrow, J.G.: Evidence for HL-A-linked genes in "juvenile" diabetes mellitus. Brit. Med. J. _3_, 133 (1975)

15. Doniach, I., Morgan, A.G.: Islets of Langerhans in juvenile diabetes mellitus. Clin. Endocrinology _2_, 233 (1973)

16. Frias, J.L., Rosenbloom, A.L.: The genetics of diabetes. Metabolism _22_, 355 (1973)

17. Gamble, D.R., Kinsley, M.L., Fitzgerald, M.G., Bolton, R., Taylor, K.W.: Viral antibodies in diabetes mellitus. Brit. Med. J. _3_, 627 (1969)

18. Gamble, D.R., Taylor, K.W., Cumming, H.: Coxsackie viruses and diabetes mellitus. Brit. Med. J. _4_, 260 (1973)

19. Gepts, W.: Pathologic anatomy of the pancreas in juvenile diabetes mellitus. Diabetes _14_, 619 (1965)

20. Grumet, C., Konishi, J., Payne, R., Kriss, J.P.: Association of Graves' disease with HL-A 8. Clin. Res. _21_, 493 (1973)

21. Harvald, B.: Genetic perspectives in diabetes mellitus. Acta Med. Scand. Suppl. _476_, 17 (1967)

22. Irvine, W.J., Clarke, B.F., Scarth, L., Cullin, L.J.P.: Thyroid and gastric auto-immunity in patients with diabetes mellitus. Lancet _II_, 163 (1970)

23. Jansen, F.K., Bertrams, J., Grünekke, D., Drost, H., Reis, H.S., Bever, J., Kuwert, E., Gries, F.A., Actrock, E.: Genetic association of insulin antibody production with histocompatibility (HL-A)-antigens in diabetics. Diabetologia _11_, 352 (1975)

24. Junker, K., Egeberg, J.C., Kromann, H., Nerup, J.: The pathology of the islets of Langerhans in early juvenile diabetes mellitus. Diabetologia _11_, 354 (1975)

25. Kissmeyer-Nielsen, F., Kjerbye, K.E.: Lymphocytotoxic microtechnique. Purification of lymphocytes by flotation. In: Histocompatibility Testing. Copenhagen. Munksgaard, 1967, p. 381

26. Kromann, H., Faber Vestergaard, B., Nerup, J.: Glucose intolerance in mice infected with encephalomyocarditis virus. Acta. Endocrinol. (Copenhagen) _76_, 670 (1974)

27. LeCompte, P.M.: "Insulitis" in early juvenile diabetes. Arch. Path. _66_, 450 (1958)

28. Lendrum, R., Walker, G., Gamble, D.R.: Islet-cell antibodies in juvenile diabetes mellitus of recent onset. Lancet _I_, 880 (1975)

29. MacCuish, A.C., Barnes, E.W., Irvine, W.J.: Antibodies to pancreatic islet-cells in insulin-dependent diabetics with coexistant autoimmune disease. Lancet _II_, 1529 (1974)

30. MacCuish, A.C., Jordan, J., Campbell, C.J., Duncan, L.J.P., Irvine, W.J.: Cell-mediated immunity to human pancreas in diabetes mellitus. Diabetes _23_, 693 (1974)

31. McDevitt, H.O., Bodmer, W.F.: HL-A, immune-response genes, and disease. Lancet _I_, 1269 (1974)

32. Menser, M., Forrest, J.M., Honeyman, M.C.: Diabetes, HL-A antigens and congenital rubella. Lancet _II_, 1509 (1974)

33. Nerup, J., Bech, K., Melholm Hansen, J.E., Ortved Andersen, O., Friis, T., Thomsen, M., Platz, P., Ryder, L., Staub Nielsen, L., Svejgaard, A.: HL-A antigens and Graves' disease. (In preparation)

34. Nerup, J., Bendixen, G.: Antiadrenal cellular hypersensitivity in Addison's disease. II correlation with clinical and genological findings. Clin. Exp. Immunol. 5, 341 (1969)

35. Nerup, J., Bendixen, G., Binder, C.: Autoimmunity in diabetes mellitus. Lancet II, 610 (1970)

36. Nerup, J., Binder, C.: Thyroid, gastric and adrenal autoimmunity in diabetes mellitus. Acta Endocrinol. (Copenhagen) 72, 279 (1973)

37. Nerup, J., Ortved Andersen, O., Bendiyen, G., Egeberg, J., Gunnarsson, R., Kromann, H., Poulsen, J.E.: Glucose intolerance and islet damage in mice immunized with homologous endocrine pancreas – a preliminary communication. Horm. Metab. Res. 6, 173 (1974)

38. Nerup, J., Ortved Andersen, O., Bendixen, G., Egeberg, J., Poulsen, J.E.: Antipancreatic cellular hypersensitivity in diabetes mellitus. Diabetes 20, 424 (1971)

39. Nerup, J., Ortved Andersen, O., Bendixen, G., Egeberg, J., Poulsen, J.E.: Antipancreatic hypersensitivity in diabetes mellitus. Antigenic activity of fetal calf pancreas and correlation with clinical type of diabetes. Acta Alberg. (Copenhagen) 28, 223 (1973)

40. Nerup, J., Ortved Andersen, O., Bendixen, G., Egeberg, J., Poulsen, J.E: Cellular hypersensitivity to islets antigen(s) different from insulin in diabetes mellitus. In: Immunity and Autoimmunity in Diabetes Mellitus, Bastenie, P.A., Gepts, W. (eds.). Amsterdam: Excerpta Med., 1974, p. 107

41. Nerup, J., Platz, P., Ortved Andersen, O., Christy, M., Lyngsøe, J., Poulsen, J.E., Ryder, L.P., Staub Nielsen, L., Thomsen, M., Svejgaard, A.: HL-A antigens and diabetes mellitus. Lancet II, 864 (1974)

42. Platz, P., Ryder, L., Staub Nielsen, L., Svejgaard, A., Thomsen, M., Christy, M.: HL-A and idiopathic Addison's disease. Lancet II, 289 (1974)

43. Richens, E.: Personal communication (1974)

44. Rolles, C.J., Rayner, P.H.W., Mackintosh, P.: Etiology of juvenile diabetes. Lancet II, 230 (1975)

45. Svejgaard, A., Jersild, C., Staub Nielsen, L., Bodmer, W.F.: HL-A antigens and disease. Statistical and genetical considerations. Tissue Antigens 4, 95 (1974)

46. Svejgaard, A., Platz, P., Ryder, L.P., Staub Nielsen, L., Thomsen, M.: HL-A and disease associations. A sruvey. Transplant. Rev. 22, 3 (1975)

47. Tattersall, R.B., Pyke, D.A.: Diabetes in identical twins. Lancet II, 1120 (1972)

48. Thomsen, M., Nerup, J., Platz, P., Christy, M., Ortved Andersen, O., Ryder, L.P., Staub Nielsen, L., Rasmussen, K., Svejgaard, A.: MLC typing in juvenile diabetes mellitus and idiopathic Addison's disease. Transplant. Res. (In press)

49. Thorell, J., Nosslin, B., Sterky, G.: Estimation of the early insulin response to intravenous glucose injection. J. Lab. Clin. Med. 82, 101 (1973)

13. Environmental Factors and Genetic Interactions

H. KEEN and R. J. JARRETT

Diabetes mellitus has long been regarded as a disease, the expression of which depends upon an interaction between hereditary susceptibility and environmental determinants. The relative strength of these two components and the precise nature of their interaction in the individual case has not yet been fully documented, but both genetic susceptibility and the environmental determinants are assumed to be multifactorial and to contribute in varying proportion to the "diabetogenic mix." Thus, at one extreme there would be almost entirely genetically determined diabetic, presumably with an acute onset early in life. At the other would be the environmental diabetic, exhibiting, in increasing abundance as the years passed by, the cumulation of life's diabetogenic insults.

In this general theoretical framework, juvenile onset, insulin-dependent diabetes has usually been regarded as a prime example of the genetically mediated form of the disease (one of its many synonyms is genetic diabetes), and the maturity onset variety as the form owing most to influences in the environment. The newer information on the etiology of diabetes of the last few years, however, is compelling us to rethink this rather simple schema. The identical-twin studies from the King's College Hospital group suggest that genetic factors play at least as large a role in the maturity onset type of diabetes as in the juvenile onset, perhaps a larger one (45); infection and autoimmunity may provide at least a partial explanation for diabetes in the young (27,33, 43). Some of the conundrums that have disturbed the sleep of geneticists attempting to explain the inheritance of diabetes have been brought measurably closer to solution by the demonstration of the association of certain histocompatibility antigens with the susceptibility to juvenile diabetes (10). We begin to discern the components of the genetic/environmental mix. This paper will deal with a consideration of some of the environmental influences, especially those which have been studied in the more common, maturity-onset form of diabetes.

Problems of Criteria and Ascertainment

In order to isolate or define factors in the environment which play a role in inducing or repressing diabetes it is necessary to make reasonably standardized estimates of prevalence and incidence of diabetes mellitus in different populations. In so doing, the investigator is confronted with the problems of ascertainment and of "diagnostic criteria". Two classes of information can be used (a) frequency of clinically recognized diabetics under observation or treatment within a defined group or area; (b) evidence from defined population samples subjected to standardized diagnostic procedures, such as the glucose tolerance test in one or other of its forms. The former approach (a) will certainly underestimate diabetes prevalence, sometimes quite markedly so, and will carry the taint of unknown selective influences which determine whose diabetes is diagnosed and whose is not. It may be influenced by systematic differences in diagnostic criteria for diabetes used by different observers (49). The latter method of ascertainment (b) will largely obviate sampling problems, but will emphasize the problem of diagnostic demarcation, for in all populations submitted to tests of glucose tolerance, the range of responses is a continuum. Expressed as a frequency distribution, there is no natural dividing line which separates the clearly normal from the clearly abnormal response. Estimated frequencies can vary severalfold in the same population depending on the criteria of abnormality applied and, by the same token, differing criteria may suggest similar diabetes frequencies though the actual rates of glucose intolerance are very different. There is also the unsolved question of compositional heterogeneity between segments of the very wide range of glucose intolerance. It seems highly unlikely, for example, that the same (or even similar) factors are responsible for a blood glucose concentration of 121mg/dl, which just exceeds a diagnostic cutoff set at say, 120mg/dl, as for a spontaneously occurring blood glucose level of 400mg/dl in a person with severe symptoms. Yet both will be called diabetes. The problem is most acute for the asymptomatic class of diabetic who provides difficulties of both ascertainment and diagnostic criteria; for the grossly hyperglycemic, juvenile-onset diabetic diagnostic criteria are self-evident; but even so, in most populations, ascertainment is far from simple or complete.

Epidemiologic Considerations

There is very little valid evidence regarding the influence of nongenetic factors upon the classical, insulin-dependent form of the disease. Nutrition may play a small part. In Japan, during the years of privation of World War 2 and after, fewer insulin-dependent diabetics first presented themselves for treatment at the Diabetic Clinics compared with the years before and after the period of nutritional inadequacy (16). Over the same period, however, the decline in incidence was much greater for the noninsulin-dependent diabetics. Infection may also play a role in determining the incidence of juvenile diabetes. Gamble and Taylor (15) reported a seasonal variation in the incidence of new cases of insulin-dependent diabetes in patients under 30 years of age attending two British Diabetic Clinics. They postulated a directly deleterious effect upon the pancreas of infections with the Coxsackie B4 virus. Congenital rubella is also clearly linked with increased risk of development of diabetes in early life (30). The relative frequency of the insulin-dependent variety of diabetes seems often to be dissociated from that of maturity-onset type. However, information about the relative prevalence of the two types is incomplete and even sound epidemiologic data concerning diabetes with onset in childhood is itself scarce. One of the best studies is that of Cohen *et al.* (8) in Israel. They estimated the prevalence of known diabetes mellitus in the population aged 2-16 at about 1:1600. This is lower than the estimated prevalence in Northampton, England (4) which is 1:1200 in children aged 5-16 years, and in Erie County, New York (44) where it was 1:1750 in those under the age of 16. In the Israel study, diabetes prevalence was considerably higher among offspring of fathers born in Europe, America, or Israel (0.24 per 1000) compared with offspring of fathers born in Asia and Africa (0.09 per 1000).

Several epidemiologic studies have reported population groups showing very low prevalence of juvenile diabetes mellitus. These include the Eskimos in Alaska (32) and Greenland (40), Indians, Malays, and Negros in Cape Town (29), Indians and Negros in Trinidad (34), Cook Island Maoris (36), in Malta (51), amongst Japanese (46), in Ceylon (11), amongst the Pima American Indians (31), and Navajo American Indians (37).

However, comparative prevalence studies have limited value when the duration of the condition may vary widely from group to group, depending largely upon the quality and quantity of medical care available for diagnosis and treatment. True incidence studies would be more rewarding and informative.

In view of the likelihood that viral infection in genetically susceptible subjects may underlie the appearance of juvenile-onset diabetes, month by month, annual or even longer-term fluctuations in incidence might well relate to waves of infection affecting the population at large. The failure of the epidemic of Coxsackie B4 infection to trigger a wave of new diabetes in the Pribolov Islands (12) may well have been due to the lack of genetic susceptibility of this racial group. Among them, the histocompatibility antigens HL-A8 and W15, clearly associated in other populations with increased risk of diabetes, are rarely found (19). Variation with time in incidence of diabetes of juvenile-onset has been noted by Cohen (8) who recorded a progressive rise in incidence in cohorts of children born in Israel in 1947-51, 1952-56, and in 1957-61. In the British Diabetic Association Register of newly diagnosed diabetic children (6) there are substantial differences in the numbers reported for 1973 and for 1974, unlikely to have arisen simply from variations in reporting. Wadsworth and Jarrett (47) presented evidence suggesting a lower incidence of diabetes before the age of 16 in a cohort of children born in 1946 compared with the cohort born in 1958. These authors also draw attention to the apparent excess incidence in children from nonmanual class homes, further suggesting the operation of environmental determinants. In their study, 14 of the 16 cases of diabetes detected under the age of 26 probably came to light from screening or at a routine medical examination. This suggests that milder (or earlier) forms of diabetes in young people are much commoner than we now suppose and accounts for the fact that only 8 of their 16 cases were taking insulin injections.

Transpositions of Populations

The importance of the environment may be inferred from the wide differences in diabetes prevalence between indigenous and geographically transposed populations. Cohen and his colleagues (7) found diabetes mellitus in only 3 of 5000 (0.06%) Yemenite Jews recently arrived in Israel. In Yemenite Jews who had lived in Israel for 25 years or more, due allowance being made for age and sex composition, diabetes frequency was 2,4%. A 25-year exposure to the new environment had induced this approximately forty-fold increase in the frequency of the disease. It is interesting to speculate on the genetic conclusions that would be drawn under conditions of low prevalence in the Yemen and how they might differ from those in the high prevalence situation of the comparatively long-term Israeli resident. Estimates of gene frequency would certainly have differed widely and so probably would the postulated genetic mechanism.

Similar "transposition gradients" have been described in other population groups. The Indians of South Africa have a reported frequency of diabetes some ten times higher than that in the Punjab population from whom their ancestors were recruited 150 or so years ago to work the sugar plantations (1,20). Transposition gradients, fourfold (1.6% vs. 6.9%) for women and over twentyfold (0.4% vs. 8.7%) for men have been described by Prior (35) for Polynesian peoples in the Pacific living under contrasting environmental conditions as island dwellers or on the New Zealand mainland. Prior and his colleagues, drawing attention to the frequent coexistence of hyperuricemia and gout which preceded the discovery of diabetes, questioned the possibility that hyperuricemia may itself contribute causally to diabetes. Their further studies with inhabitants of the Tokelau Islands and Mainland Maoris showed a high diabetes prevalence in both groups, but with a highly significant two-fold gradient between them.

Some Diabetogenic Factors within Populations

Sex and Age

There are a number of defined factors which are associated with and may directly influence diabetes frequency. Differences in prevalence between sexes and the increase in rates with advancing age were among the earliest etiologic factors recognized, though there is variation in the extent and uncertainty about the mechanisms of their effects. In the carefully recorded experience of the Birmingham (England) Diabetes Clinic, the sex ratio of newly diagnosed diabetics has changed from a probable excess of males at the beginning of the 20th century to a highly significant excess for women and, over the last 20 years, back to a small but probably significant excess in men, a change in ratio with time which has been recorded by others (17,28). In some populations the female excess has probably never occurred. There must be changing environmental factors within these populations which, over a comparatively short time, differentially influence the relative susceptibility to diabetes in the two sexes. The changing fashions in adiposity and the very large reduction in family size may have contributed partially to the changed sex ratio (see below) though the relative timing of these cultural changes and the trends in sex ratio suggest that this is not the complete explanation.

Age

It is in the interpretation of the effects of age on glucose tolerance that the selection of diagnostic cutoff points assumes special importance. In a study of glucose tolerance in an age/sex random sample of the general population of the town of Bedford, England (41), with increasing age there was a progressive mean "loss" of oral glucose tolerance, a phenomenon familiar to all workers who have examined populations in a similar way. Since the same age effect is seen in fasting and postabsorptive blood glucose levels and with intravenous glucose tolerance, it is not ascribable to changing glucose absorption with age. The deterioration in tolerance is such that the *mean* curve for the oldest age group of Bedford women satisfied the British Diabetic Association criteria for a diabetic response (14). When the average behavior of a randomly selected "normal" population group is itself "diabetic", one is compelled to question the applicability of the diagnostic term. If, within each age and sex group, the areas under the glucose tolerance curve are plotted as a frequency distribution histogram, with increasing age there is progressive spread of individual results toward and into the diabetic extreme of the response range. A few individuals separate out, breaking well away from the main distribution; but, using conventional criteria, the division between the normal and the diabetic falls well within the descending limb of the distribution. These findings are compatible with those of the much larger collection of data from the US National Health Survey which recorded blood glucose measured one hour after a glucose challenge in 7710 ostentibly normal subjects (5).

A conspicuously different picture of the influence of the age on the appearance of glucose intolerance was demonstrated in the Pima Indians of Arizona by Miller and his colleagues (31). With increasing age, the progressive emergence of a large, separate subpopulation of "hyperglycemics" or diabetics is evident. It has been argued (42) that similar "bimodality" of blood glucose responses is present in other Western populations, the separation being blurred into "positive skewing" by imperfections of testing methods and the small numbers in the upper reaches of the frequency distribution curve. However, further independent evidence of a more direct and convincing nature is required before the hypothesis of a single distribution, varying only quantitatively, is rejected. Lauvaux and Staquet (26) tackled the question by restricting their study of glucose tolerance to older people, plotting the distributions of blood glucose by decade in subjects aged 50 or more. In both sexes they found apparently unimodal, positively skewed, frequency distributions; the modes, the dispersion of observations, and the upper extreme rose progressively through the three decades studied. The 95th percentile point of the distributions rose faster with age than the 50th and the 5th, and on the basis of this special behavior of the upper extreme, the authors suggested the emergence late in life of a distinct and discrete diabetic subpopulation. However, it seems equally valid to suggest that there is a correlation between level of blood glucose and rate of rise with age without invoking a qualitative difference at the upper extreme. In any case there are serious objections to extrapolating arguments from cross-sectional studies of this sort to the behavior with time of a cohort followed longitudinally.

Kaufman *et al.* (23) claimed that the tendency to accelerated glucose intolerance with age was, at least in part, genetically determined on the basis of a raised frequency of family history of diabetes reported by older individuals in the hyperglycemic tail of the frequency distribution. In a recent collaborative study of a large population of male Civil Servants aged 40 or more in London (39), a systematic enquiry for a family history of diabetes was combined with a screening test of glucose tolerance, consisting of a single measurement of blood glucose made two hours after a 50g oral glucose load taken in the morning after an overnight fast. Those screening above 120 mg/dl were subjected to a further oral glucose tolerance test and were classified as diabetic if they again met specified criteria. In addition a group of previously diagnosed and treated diabetics was included in the study. Table 1 shows the frequency of a positive family history for diabetes given by men in the three groups, "nondiabetic", "newly found diabetics" (i.e., the upper range of the frequency distribution) and "known diabetics".

Table 1. Age and percentage of family history of diabetes mellitus (D.M.) (Whitehall survey)

	40-49	Age 50-59	60+
Total	7628	8131	3063
Normal	13.0 %	11.0 %	8.6 %
New D.M.	12.8 %	25.0 %[a]	12.8 %
Known D.M.	26.1 %[b]	34.2 %[b]	30.8 %[b]

[a] $p<0.05$.

[b] $p<0.01$.

In the age group 40-49 and 60+ there was no indication of a difference in reported positive family histories between nondiabetics and newly found diabetics, though the latter reported positive significantly more frequently in the decade 50-59. By contrast, a positive family history in known diabetics was found two to three times more often in all age groups.

Obesity

Among the most important factors which determine the frequency of diabetes in a population is its degree of adiposity. In the Bedford Study, there was a stepwise increase in body weight and in skinfold thickness going from normoglycemic individuals (2 h post-glucose blood sugar less than 120 mg/dl), through borderline diabetics (2 h blood sugar between 120-200 mg/dl) to clearly diabetic (2 h blood sugar in excess of 200 mg/dl). Further analysis (25) suggested that adiposity was more strikingly represented among those newly found to have glucose intolerance during the middle years of life; among the youngest and oldest of the glucose-intolerant groups, other factors were probably of greater importance. The lessened representation of the more obese with increasing age may represent selective removal by death of those who are fat, diabetic, and old.

A striking portrayal of the interaction of genetic factors with obesity comes from a study made of siblings of maturity-onset diabetics by Baird (3). She showed that diabetes is five times more likely to occur in obese siblings of nonobese index cases than in nonobese siblings of obese index cases. If one assumes that genetic factors are playing a relatively larger role in causing the diabetes of the thin than of the fat index cases, then the obese siblings of the former can be supposed to carry both genetic and environmental determinants in contrast to the latter who carry neither (or at any rate less, of both).

On an international basis, the studies of West (48) emphasize the importance of overweight in determining the relative frequency of glucose intolerance from population to population. A very high degree of correlation was found between the rates of diabetic response to oral glucose tolerance tests, carried out on samples of 400-500 adult citizens of 10 countries, and the degree of overweight. In groups selected for similar degrees of adiposity, prevalence of glucose intolerance was very similar. Thus West ascribed most of the fourfold gradient in diabetes prevalence in the material he studied to the effects of adiposity. The populations he selected for study may not be universally representative and, indeed, Jackson, in a study of diabetes prevalence in racial groups in South Africa, has been unable to confirm the close relationship with obesity. His most obese group, the Bantu women, had the lowest prevalence of diabetes (21). A second question which may be raised in relation to West's studies (and also to much else discussed here) is the nature of the relationship between glucose intolerance and diabetes mellitus. Are the two synonymous? There are now several long-term, follow-up studies which demonstrate the frequent spontaneous reversion to normality of individuals found in population screening to be glucose intolerant; though like remissions nave been reported in 'clinical diabetics', they are almost certainly much less frequent.

Diet

It has been suggested that it may not be adiposity per se which determines the frequency of diabetes but that some feature of the composition

of the diet which gives rise to both. Himsworth (18) made a strong case
that the diet with a high proportion of its energy coming from fat was
diabetogenic. More recently, Yudkin (50) and Cohen (9) have presented
evidence that high sucrose intake might be the diabetogenic culprit.
The latter suggestion found little support from West who demonstrated
no clear link between sucrose consumption and diabetes frequency in
the multinational studies referred to above. Within populations, Baird
(2) was unable to show any difference in reported sucrose intake between siblings of diabetics who later themselves proved to be diabetic
and those who proved to be normal.

Similar negative conclusions regarding the role of sucrose were arrived
at by Kahn *et al.* (22) who studied the factors determining the incidence of new diabetics in a group of 10,000 Israeli Civil Servants.
Detailed dietary enquiry and oral glucose tolerance tests were performed
in 1963, and tolerance tests repeated in 1965. At the latter test, 171
men, previously with normal glucose tolerance, were adjudged to have
become diabetic. When the 1963 dietary record was consulted, there was
no hint of higher sucrose intake in those who had become diabetic than
in the rest. Our own dietary studies on normals and newly diagnosed
diabetics (24) brought us to the same negative conclusions on the diabetogenic role of sucrose intake, carbohydrate intake, and even total
calorie intake. In fact, in several of the population groups we studied,
there was a trend to improving glucose tolerance with increasing mean
reported sucrose intake.

The role of deficient dietary trivalent chromium and of vegetable fiber
has been hinted at and requires further study on an epidemiologic scale.

Parity

Finally, the frequency of childbearing seems in some societies to be
directly related to the later development of diabetes in women (38).
This is reflected in the interesting interrelation between parity and
family history of diabetes reported by Fitzgerald *et al.* (13). They
found that with increasing parity, diabetic women were progressively
less liable to give a positive family history for diabetes. Thus, of
diabetic women with one pregnancy or fewer, 37.5% give a positive family history; in diabetic women with 6 or more pregnancies, a positive
family history was found in only 21.2%. The implication is that each
pregnancy has diabetogenic potential; with increasing multiparity a
lesser genetic contribution to the diabetogenic mix is necessary. It
is perhaps not surprising that, with the wide variety of diabetogenic
factors the parity/diabetes relationship does not hold in all societies.

Conclusion

It is clear that environmental factors are of great importance in determining the frequency and time of appearance of both clinical forms of
diabetes mellitus. Changes in the conditions of life can be expected
to produce large changes in diabetes frequencies. In the noninsulin-dependent diabetic, ageing, obesity, and parity in women clearly play
a diabetogenic role. In the genesis of insulin-dependent diabetes we
must look with renewed interest at environmental factors, principally
infective ones, though it is likely that genetically determined factors
of susceptibility and response will be of decisive importance in determining a diabetic outcome.

The diabetogenic effect of adiposity is greater in those presumed to
carry increased genetic susceptibility to diabetes, but the mechanisms

of this interaction is not clear. There is no strong reason for inculpating any single major dietary component, though the possibility of an inherited 'hypersensitivity' to certain foods in particular groups of people has not been excluded; nor has the possibility of specific dietary deficiencies. On the basis of scanty evidence, the effects of parity in women and genetic factors would appear in some societies to be at least additive in provoking diabetes. The importance of genetic factors in determining the progressive loss of glucose tolerance with increasing age is uncertain. "Longitudinal" studies are required to elucidate this further.

Failure to take environmental factors into account will greatly hinder the interpretation of genetic data and invalidates the extrapolation of conclusions from one human population to another.

References

1. Ahuja, M.M.S., Sivaji, L., Garg, V.K., Mitroo, P.: Prevalence of diabetes in Northern India (Delhi area). Hormone and Metabolic Research 4, 321 (1972)

2. Baird, J.D.: Diet and the development of clinical diabetes. Acta Diabetologica Latina 9, (Suppl. 1) 621 (1972)

3. Baird, J.D.: Diabetes mellitus and obesity. Procedings of the Nutrition Society 32, 199 (1973)

4. Beardmore, M., Reid, J.J.A.: Diabetic children. Brit. Med. J. II, 1383 (1966)

5. Blood Glucose levels in adults, United States 1960 - 1962. Public Health Service Publication No. 1000, Series 11, No. 18. US Government Printing Office, Washington DC

6. Bloom, A., Hayes, T.M., Gamble, D.R.: Register of newly diagnosed diabetic children. Brit. Med. J. III, 580 (1975)

7. Cohen, A.M., Bavly, S., Poznanski, R.: Change of diet of Yemenite Jews in relation to diabetes and ischaemic heart disease. Lancet II, 1399 (1961)

8. Cohen, T., Nelken, L., Wolfsohn, H.: Juvenile diabetes mellitus in imigrant populations in Israel. Diabetes 19, 585 (1970)

9. Cohen, A.M., Teitelbaum, A., Balogh, M., Groen, J.J.: Effect of interchanging bread and sucrose as main source of carbohydrate in low fat diet on the glucose tolerance curve of healthy volunteer subjects. American Journal of Clinical Nutrition 19, 59 (1966)

10. Cudworth, A.G., Woodrow, J.C.: HL-A system and diabetes mellitus. Diabetes 24, 345 (1975)

11. De Ioysa, V.P.: Clinical variations of the diabetic syndrome in a tropical country (Ceylon). Archives of Internal Medicine 88, 812 (1951)

12. Dippe, S.E., Bennett, P-H., Miller, M., Maynard, J.E., Berquist, K.R.: Lack of causal association between Coxsackie B4 virus and diabetes. Lancet I, 1314 (1975)

13. Fitzgerald, M.G., Malins, J.M., O'Sullivan, D.J., Wall, M.: The effects of sex and parity on the incidence of diabetes mellitus. Quarterly Journal of Medicine 30, 57 (1961)

14. Fitzgerald, M.G., Keen, H.: Diagnostic classification of diabetes. Brit. Med. J. I, 1568 (1964)

15. Gamble, D.R., Taylor, K.W.: Seasonal incidence of diabetes mellitus. Brit. Med. J. III, 631 (1969)

16. Goto, Y., Nakayama, Y., Yagi, T.: Influence of World War II food shortage on the incidence of diabetes mellitus in Japan. Diabetes 7, 133 (1958)

17. Harris, H., McArthur, N.: Changes in sex incidence of diabetes mellitus. London: Annals of Eugenics 16, 109 (1912-1947)

18. Himsworth, H.P.: Diet in the aetiology of human diabetes. Proceedings of the Royal Society of Medicine 42, 323 (1949)

19. Histocompatibility Testing. Copenhagen: Munksgaard 1972

20. Jackson, W.P.U.: Diabetes mellitus in different countries and different races. Prevalence and major features. Acta Diabetologica Latina 7, 361 (1970)

21. Jackson, W.P.U.: Diabetes and related variables among the five main racial groups in South Africa: Comparisons from population studies. Postgraduate Medical Journal 48, 391 (1972)

22. Kahn, H.A., Herman, J.B., Medalie, J.H., Neufeld, H.N., Riss, E., Goldbourt, U.: Factors related to diabetes incidence: a multivariate analysis of two years observation on 10,000 men. The Israeli ischaemic heart disease study. Journal of Chronic Disease·23, 617 (1971)

23. Kaufman, B.J., Grant, D.R., Moorhouse, J.A.: An analysis of blood glucose values in a population screened for diabetes mellitus. Canadian Medical Association Journal 100, 692 (1969)

24. Keen, H.: Diabetes and sugar consumption. In: Is the risk of becoming diabetic affected by sugar consumption? S.S. Hillebrand (ed.) International Sugar Research Foundation, USA

25. Keen, H.: The incomplete story of obesity and diabetes. In: Recent Advances in Obesity Research. Edited by A. Howard. London: Newman Publishing Ltd., 116 1975

26. Lauvaux, J.P., Staquet, M.: The oral glucose tolerance test: a study of the influence of age on the response to the standard oral 50g glucose load. Diabetologia 6, 414 (1970)

27. Lendrum, R., Walker, G., Gamble, D.R.: Islet-cell antibodies in juvenile diabetes mellitus of recent onset. Lancet I, 880 (1975)

28. Malins, J.M., Fitzgerald, M.E., Wall, M.: A change in the sex incidence of diabetes mellitus. Diabetologia 1, 121 (1965)

29. Marine, N., Vinik, A.I., Edelstein, I., Jackson, W.P.U.: Diabetes, hyperglycaemia and glycosuria among Indians, Malays and Africans (Bantu) in Cape Town. Diabetes 18, 840 (1969)

30. Menser, M.A., Forrest, J.M., Honeyman, M.C.: HL-A antigens and congenital rubella. Lancet IV, 1508 (1974)

31. Miller, M., Bennett, P.H., Burch, T.A.: Hyperglycaemina in Pima Indians: A preliminary appraisal of its significance. In: Biomedical challenges presented by the American Indians. Washington DC.: Scientific Publication No. 165, Pan American Health Organization

32. Mouratoff, G.J., Carroll, N.V., Scott, E.M.: Diabetes mellitus in Eskimos. Journal of the American Medical Association 199, 107 (1967)

33. Nerup, J., Platz, P., Anderson, O.O., Christy, M., Lyngsøe, J., Poulson, J.E., Ryder, L.P., Nielsen, L.S., Thomsen, M., Svejgaard, A.: HL-A antigens in diabetes mellitus. Lancet II, 864 (1974)

34. Poon-King, T., Henry, M.V., Rampersand, F.: Prevalence and natural history of diabetes in Trinidad. Lancet I, 155 (1968)

35. Prior, I.A.M.: Diabetes in the South Pacific. In: Is the risk of becoming diabetic affected by sugar consumption? S.S. Hillebrand (ed.). International Sugar Research Foundation, USA, p. 4 (1974)

36. Prior, I.A.M., Harvey, H.P.B., Neave, M.N., Davidson, F.: "The health of two groups of Cook Islands Maoris". New Zealand Department of Health Special Report Series, No. 26 (1966)

37. Prosnitz, L.R., Mandell, G.L.: Diabetes mellitus among Navajo and Hopi Indinas: the lack of vascular complications. American Journal of Medical Science 253, 700 (1967)

38. Pyke, D.A., Please, N.W.: Obesity, parity and diabetes. Journal of Endocrinology 15, 26 (1957)

39. Reid, D.D., Brett, G.Z., Hamilton, P.J.S., Jarrett, R.J., Keen, H., Rose, G.A.: Cardiorespiratory disease and diabetes among middle-aged male Civil Servants; a study of screening and intervention. Lancet I, 469 (1974)

40. Sagild, U., Littauer, S., Sand-Jespersen, C., Andersen, S.: Epidemiological studies in Greenland, 1962-4. Acta Medica Scandinavica 179, 29 (1966)

41. Sharp, C.L., Butterfield, W.J.H., Keen, H.: The Bedford Survey. Proceedings of the Roayl Society of Medicine 57, 193 (1964)

42. Steinberg, A.G., Rushfort, N.B., Bennett, P.H., Burch, T.A., Miller, M.: On the genetics of diabetes mellitus. In: Pathogenesis of diabetes mellitus. Nobel Symposium 13. Stockholm: Almqvist and Wiksell, p. 237 1970

43. Steinke, J., Taylor, K.W.: Viruses and the etiology of diabetes. Diabetes 23, 631 (1974)

44. Sultz, H.A., Schlesinger, E.R., Mosher, W.E.: The Erie County survey of long term childhood illness: II Incidence and prevalence. American Journal of Public Health 58, 491 (1968)

45. Tattersall, R.B., Pyke, D.A.: Diabetes in identical twins. Lancet II, 1120 (1972)

46. Wada, S., Toda, S., Omori, Y., Yamakido, M., Blackard, W.G.: The clinical features of diabetes mellitus in Japan as observed in a hospital out-patient clinic. Diabetes 13, 485 (1964)

47. Wadsworth, M.E.J., Jarrett, R.J.: Incidence of diabetes in the first 26 years of life. Lancet IV, 1172 (1974)

48. West, K.M.: Epidemiological evidence linking nutritional factors to the prevalence and manifestations of diabetes. Acta Diabetologica Latina 9, (Suppl. 1) 405 (1972)

49. West, K.M.: Substantial differences in the diagnostic criteria used by diabetes experts. Diabetes 24, 641 (1975)

50. Yudkin, J.: Patterns and trends in carbohydrate consumption and their relation to disease. Proceedings of the Nutrition Society 23, 149 (1964)

51. Zammit Maempel, J.V.: Diabetes in Malta. Lancet II, 1197 (1965)

14. Diabetes Mellitus and Impaired Glucose Tolerance in Diseases with Chromosomal Aberrations

K. Schöffling and Ch. Schade

Three years after Tjio and Levan (46) established the correct number of
human chromosomes, the three chromosome aberrations with the highest
frequency in humans were described: Down's syndrome (19), Turner's syndrome (16), Klinefelter's syndrome (12). With further improvements in
methodology in the following year, it became possible to investigate
groups and collectives and to search for correlations between specific
chromosome aberrations and typical diseases. As will be explained later,
the question of a correlation between chromosome aberrations and diabetes mellitus has been successfully pursued only with the three diseases mentioned above.

Patients with Down's syndrome, which is easy to recognize, have a reduced life expectancy, but many do reach maturity. The frequency of
this syndrome in newborns is about 1.5 0/00. In most cases the chromosome complement has one additional small acrocentric autosome; there
is trisomy for chromosome No. 21.

The second disease, Turner's syndrome, is not as frequent as Down's
syndrome. Malformations, growth retardation, and primary amenorrhea are
the main reasons for undergoing diagnostic procedures. Maturity can be
reached if the syndrome is not accompanied by severe malformations.
The frequency in newborns is about 0.4 0/00. This disease may result
from several different chromosome aberrations. Loss of one X chromosome
in all cells or in a part of them is one cause as is load of the short
arm of one of the two X's.

In most cases, hypogonadism, gynecomastia, and/or reduced intelligence
are the symptoms leading to the suspicion of a Klinefelter's syndrome.
Since other organ malformations are rare, life expectancy is not markedly reduced. The frequency of this disease is about 2 0/00 of the male
population. Diagnosis can be made by means of the X and Y chromatin
tests. All chromosome complements or a large part of them have a XXY
karyotype.

Investigation of metabolic or hormonal disorders in series of patients
with other chromosome aberrations has not been rewarding to date since
the other different changes of gonosomes or autosomes are very rare,
difficult to recognize, or often characterized by a high letality.

The variability of the three well-defined diseases, Down's, Turner's,
and Klinefelter's syndrome, is also very high. Therefore, it is difficult to demonstrate correlations between the severity of the diseases
and the dimension of the chromosome aberrations. Chromosome analysis
is still a very protracted method. Thus it is difficult to get a sample
without selection. Other factors like intensity of clinical investigation, research field, and investigator's speciality render this type
of survey also difficult.

The first observation of diabetes mellitus in patients with chromosome aberrations was made by Farquhar (9). Among diabetic children in Scotland he observed mongolism 4-5 times more frequently than could be expected. On the other hand, White (49) found a relation of 1:1000 among 6200 children from the Joslin Clinic up to the age of 15, which seems to be the "normal relation." Generally, it is difficult or even impossible to draw correlations in the different age groups, since 60% of mongoloid children die in the first 10 years of their lives (4). The reduced resistance against infectious diseases is the main cause of death after the first birthday.

During an extensive inquiry made by Milunsky and Neurath (24), 88 diabetics were found among 20,362 patients with Down's syndrome in the United Kingdom and in the USA. Of these patients, 42 or half of them, were younger than 20 years. Using the age distribution of mongoloids in Australia, they calculated the prevalence of diabetes in the institutionalized Down's syndrome population and compared it to that in the general population. In the age group from 0-20 years the difference was significant.

Jeremiah *et al.* (17) reported similar findings, demonstrating diabetes mellitus in 6 out of 404 individuals with Down's syndrome. Burch and Milunsky (2) calculated a peak age of juvenile diabetics at 8 years in contrast to 14 years in the general population.

In the series of Milunsky and Neurath (24), 65 out of the 88 diabetics received insulin, 11 were treated with oral antidiabetic drugs, and 12 could be controlled by diet alone. This study does not include statements about age, dosage of insulin, other diseases, or complications. Therefore, it is not possible to conclude that most of the patients are typical early-onset insulin-deficient diabetics.

Runge (35) carried out intravenous glucose tolerance tests in 123 patients with Down's syndrome. According to her criteria abnormal curves were found in 30-90% of the patients, more in the older age groups. Sutnick *et al.* (45) described glucose tolerance tests made in 67 mongoloid patients. They suggested that an impaired absorption from the gastrointestinal tract may be the cause of these curves.

Milunsky *et al.* (25), Serrano-Rios *et al.* (42), and Raiti *et al.* (31) included some glucose tolerance tests with insulin determinations in their studies of patients with Down's syndrome. The first research group did not find any differences in mongoloid children when compared to normals. The second group described only minimum differences, whereas the third group stated a low glucose assimilation coefficient (K value) with an abnormal insulin response only in 1 out of 8 patients.

All data obtained from diabetics with Down's syndrome or from mongoloids with an impaired glucose tolerance are very poor and incomplete. Thus we are of the opinion that we cannot draw final conclusions today or make serious speculations in this research field.

Forbes and Engel (11) were the first to recognize a high prevalence of diabetes mellitus in patients with gonodal dysgenesis. In a group of 41 patients they observed 6 persons with clinical diabetes: 2 out of 11 (18%) were between 35 and 44 years of age, 1 out of 9 (11%) between 45 and 54 years and, finally, 3 out of 6 (50%) between 55 and 64 years. This investigation needs some clarifications.

The study includes all patients with gonodal dysgenesis seen by the authors; 60% of them are older than 35, an age distribution not found in any other study. It cannot be assumed that these patients came to medical attention only on account of their short stature, primary amenorrhea, or malformation. In our opinion, comparisons with the general population are therefore not justified.

The study includes each type of gonadal dysgenesis, also those without chromosome aberrations. In a second investigation, Engel and Forbes (8) described 8 diabetics with gonadal dysgenesis. Only 4 of them demonstrated chromosome aberrations, 2 had normal karyotypes, 1 patient was chromatin-positive, and the last one was not tested.

Patients with Turner's syndrome very often suffer from congenital malformations. About 20% of all abortions with chromosome aberrations are the consequence of an XO chromosome complement (47). The low percentage of Turner's syndrome among the other newborns with chromosome aberrations may be due to this fact.

We have no knowledge about the distribution of Turner patients among the different age groups in the general population, nor do we know exactly the life expectancy of all patients and the number of complications, including obesity. It also seems possible to us that diabetes and impaired glucose tolerance may be the consequence of complications and malformations.

In Table 1 we have compiled the results of publications referring to age of onset of diabetes in Turner's syndrome. It seems remarkable that 55 out of 64 patients (86%) were below the age of 30 and that 35% of the patients between 11 and 20 years are diabetics. This demonstration is incomplete, since it was not possible to correlate age to clinical symptoms and to the different chromosome aberrations. The data of the 27 patients described by Rimoin (32) are not known. He stated only that 77% of the XO patients between 16 and 27 years demonstrated an impaired glucose tolerance.

Table 1. Age distribution of "diabetics" among 64 patients with Turner's syndrome (compiled from literature)

Age groups	number of patients	total "diabetics"	manifest diabetics
0 - 10			
11 - 20	34	12 (35 %)	1 (3 %)
21 - 30	21	3 (14 %)	1 (5 %)
31 - 40	6	3 (50 %)	
41 - 50	2	2 (100%)	1 (50%)
51 - 60	1	1 (100%)	
61 - 80			

Jackson *et al.*, 1966; Menzinger *et al.*, 1966; Lindsten *et al.*, 1967; Cassano *et al.*, 1967; Schöffling *et al.*, 1968; Nielsen *et al.*, 1969.

Nielsen (28) defines the degree of diabetes as mild. Most of the patients with clinical diabetes received insulin (11,21,40,41,30).

Insulin secretion after glucose load has varied in the studies published up to now. Lindsten *et al.* (20) observed a delayed and diminished insulin response in patients with normal glucose tolerance in spite of a higher blood glucose level than normal. Similar results were obtained by Van Campenhout *et al.* (3) in patients with pathologic glucose tolerances. Jackson *et al.* (14) as well as Nielsen *et al.* (29) by contrast describe a brisk rise of insulin and a delayed decrease.

- We observed a normal increase of insulin up to subnormal values and a normal decline in patients with and without diminished K values (40,41) (Fig. 1). From the metabolic point of view our clinical diabetics did not show differences in any direction compared to other diabetic patients.

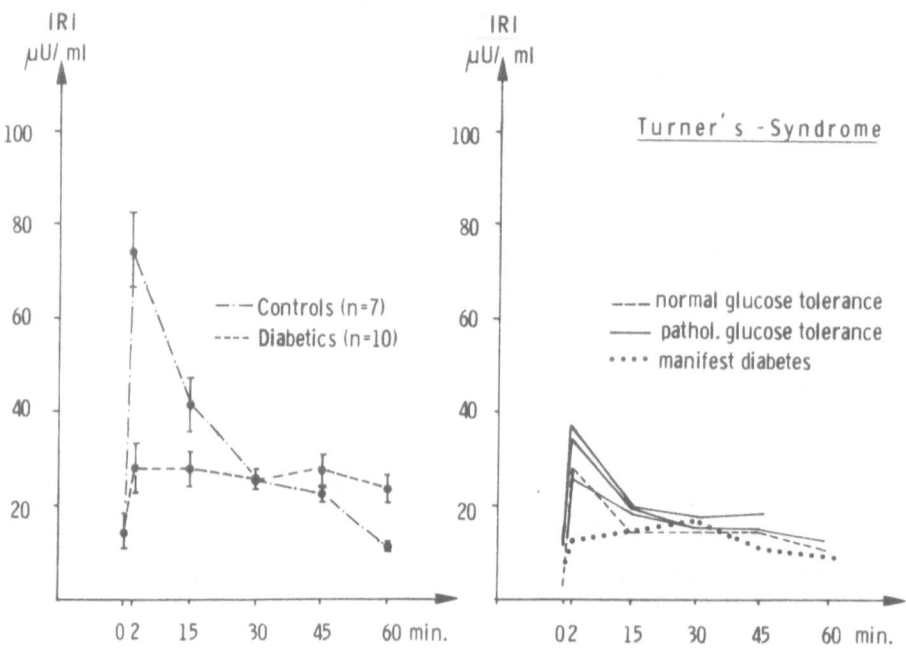

Fig. 1. Insulin secretion (IRI) in 5 patients with Turner's syndrome during i.v. glucose tolerance tests (Schöffling *et al.*, 1968)

As to Klinefelter's syndrome, we would like first to report the summarized results from the literature (Table 2). Of 215 patients with Klinefelter's syndrome described in various studies up to 1973, 17 had a manifest diabetes mellitus. A subclinical diabetes was observed in 28 out of 106 patients tested for glucose tolerance.

Cytogenetic examinations carried out by us in our endocrinologic and not in our diabetes unit revealed 54 patients with XXY Klinefelter's syndrome, all of them being nondiabetic. Two further patients were known diabetics. The mean age of all patients was 28 years.

Schade *et al.* (38) have reported the results of extensive internal investigations, examinations of carbohydrate metabolism and insulin secretion during three loading tests, and intensive inquiries of family history in 20 nondiabetic patients. Only one obese patient with positive family history concerning diabetes revealed pathologic results in two or more tests. Therefore, the diagnosis "subclinical diabetes" seems to be justified only in this single case.

Contradictory data have also been obtained with regard to insulin secretion. Nielsen (27) found elevated insulin levels in patients with impaired glucose tolerance; Serrano-Rios *et al.* (42) reported a decreased insulin secretion in nonobese patients with pathologic glucose

Table 2. Klinefelter's syndrome and diabetes mellitus. Summarized results from literature and own results (Schade *et al.*, 1973)

	Summarized results from literature	own results
Number of Klinefelter patients	215	54 + 2
Manifest diabetics	17 (7,9%)	2[a]
Patients tested for glucose tolerance	106	20
Subclinical diabetics	28 (26,4%)	1 (5%)

Authors: Rohde 1963: Wais and Salvati 1966: Becker *et al.*. 1966: Jackson *et al.*. 1966; Cassano *et al.*, 1967; Zuppinger *et al.*, 1967; Mirouze *et al.*, 1967; Nielsen *et al.*, 1969; Rubin *et al.*, 1970; Serrano Rios *et al.*, 1972.

[a] Patients from diabetes unit.

tolerance. In our investigations elevated serum insulin levels were observed. Due to the great differences between the results of various investigators, we tried to identify groups of Klinefelter patients among our sample the results on whom would allow us to confirm the findings of other authors or to give a new interpretation.

First we differentiated the subjects into obese and nonobese persons and into those with or without pathologic or suspect tolerance tests (Table 3). The high body weight of the obese patients with pathologic values, and the fact that the normal weight subjects without pathologic values were the youngest patients of our collective are noteworthy. The two patients with suspect or pathologic values demonstrated very small differences in three out of four tests, thus giving no reason for the diagnosis "subclinical diabetes." Positive or negative family histories concerning diabetes were taken as criteria for the following groups (Table 4). It is remarkable that patients with a positive family history of diabetes have a higher body weight than those without.

Table 3. Results of diabetes tests in 20 patients with Klinefelter's syndrome differentiated according to body weight (Schade *et al.*, 1973)

Groups of Klinefelter patients	mean age	values of % Broca	normal results	suspect or pathol. values in 1		2	3	values tests
Normal weight (n = 12)	19,3	82,6						
without pathol. values	17,0	86,0	7					
with pathol. values	22,6	77,8		4		1		
Overweight (n = 8)	27,3	121,4						
without pathol. values	27,4	116,8	5					
with pathol. values	27,0	129,0		1		1	1	
Total group (n = 20)	22,5	98,1	12	5[a]		2[b]	1	

Very small differences in [a] 2 out of 5 tests,
[b] 3 out of 4 tests.

We find significant differences of the mean values among the different groups of Klinefelter patients in comparison to controls (Fig. 2). In respect to the blood glucose examinations there are only small variations to be seen, and no group was found to have differences in each of the three tests. Very different insulin levels became obvious in the

Table 4. Results of diabetes tests in 20 patients with Klinefelter's syndrome differentiated into persons with negative or positive family history of diabetes mellitus (Schade *et al.*, 1973)

Groups of Klinefelter patients	mean age	values of % Broca	normal results	suspect or pathol. values in	1	2	3	tests
Negative family history of D.m. (n = 12)	22,5	91,2	7	5				
Positive family history of D.m. (n = 8)	22,5	108,5	5			2	1	
Total group (n = 20)	22,5	98,1	12	5[a]		2[b]	1	

Very small differences in [a] 2 out of 5 tests,
[b] 3 out of 4 tests.

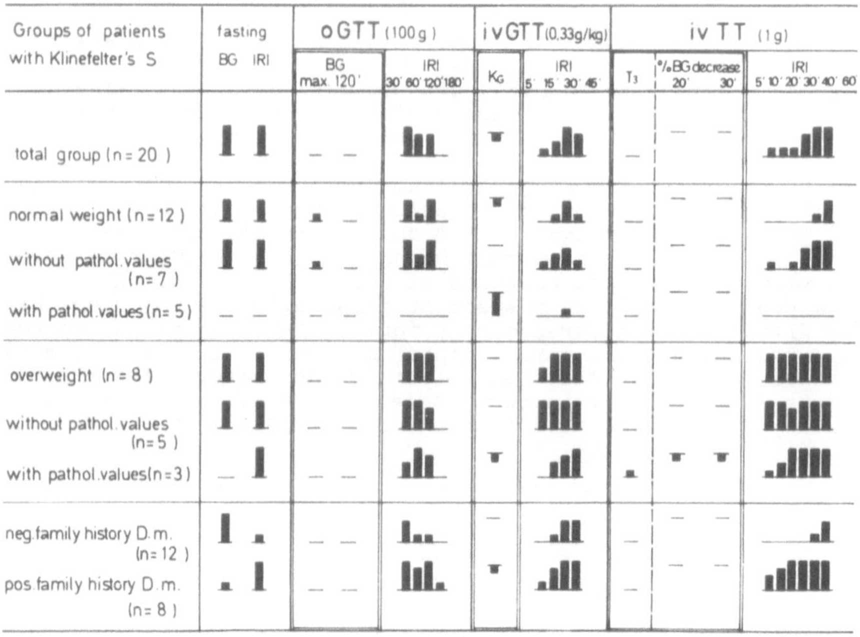

Groups of patients with Klinefelter's S	fasting BG IRI	oGTT (100g) BG max. 120'	oGTT IRI 30' 60' 120'180'	ivGTT(0.33g/kg) KG	ivGTT IRI 5' 15' 30' 45'	iv TT (1g) T₃	iv TT %BG decrease 20' 30'	iv TT IRI 5' 10' 20' 30' 40' 60'
total group (n = 20)								
normal weight (n = 12)								
without pathol. values (n = 7)								
with pathol. values (n = 5)								
overweight (n = 8)								
without pathol. values (n = 5)								
with pathol. values (n = 3)								
neg. family history D.m. (n = 12)								
pos. family history D.m. (n = 8)								

Fig. 2. Different groups of Klinefelter patients in relation to normal weight non-diabetic controls. Demonstration of the significant differences of mean values of blood glucose (BG) and serum insulin (IRI) during diabetes tests (Schade *et al.*, 1973)
(•p<0.05, ▮p<0.01, ▮p<0.005, ▮p<0.001)

overweight patients and in the group with a positive family history of diabetes, in keeping with the higher body weight, as could be expected from our observations in "normal" diabetics.

Our study further demonstrates that the mean values of insulin levels in obese and normal weight patients are different (Fig. 3). The shadows

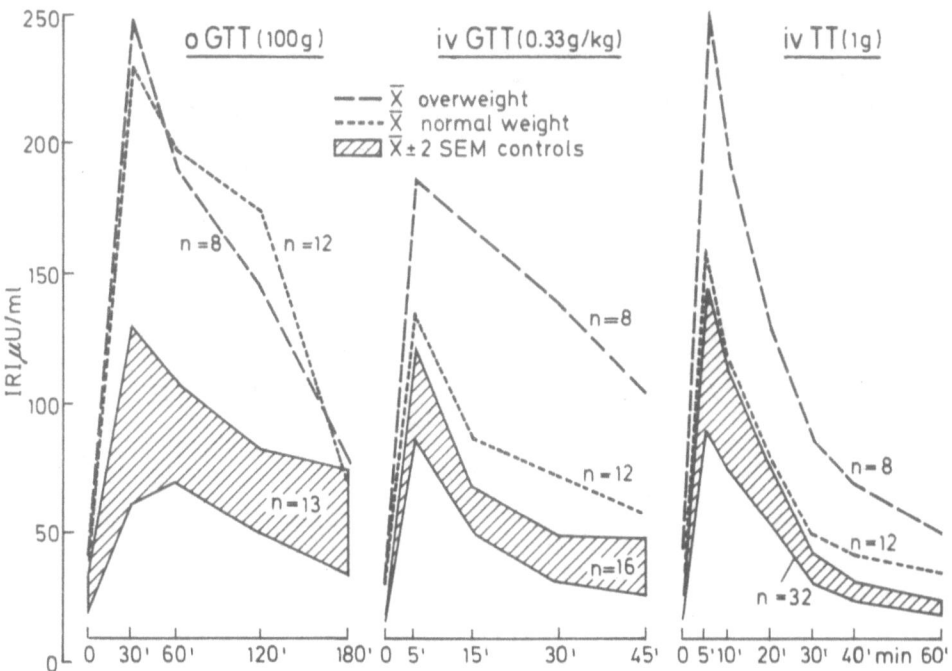

Fig. 3. Insulin secretion (IRI) in overweight and normal weight patients with Kline-felter's syndrome during glucose tolerance and tolbutamide tests (Schade *et al.*,1973)

indicate the range of mean values of the controls. The differences between the two Klinefelter groups with negative and positive family histories of diabetes also seems to be important (Fig. 4). But there are only very few differences in insulin levels, of low significance (Fig. 5).

On the basis of these observations it can be stated that obesity is responsible for the high insulin levels. Interesting is the elevated insulin of the youngest patients, with absolutely normal glucose tolerance. In our study we could neither find a high tendency to a diabetic glucose tolerance nor to diminished insulin levels.

Comparison of these data with the results obtained by other investigators using single and different tests revealed distinct differences. The lower rate of manifest diabetics and of patients with a pathologic glucose tolerance can be explained primarily by the lower age of our patients, i.e., 28 and 22.5 years, respectively. A second and, in our opinion, essential conclusion can be drawn from a review of the publications. Whereas our patients are generally healthy with the exception of obesity and disturbances due to Klinefelter's syndrome, severe diseases were described frequently with respect to alcoholism, and chronic gastrointestinal and pulmonary diseases. Looking through the literature we recognized that the diseases were not considered in those "diabetics" who had been diagnosed by a single glucose loading test.

Therefore, we have divided the data of 104 XXY patients into age groups using known body weight of them all and case histories of 40 patients (Table 5). Patients with pathologic glucose tolerance and with known obesity and/or associated diseases were correlated to the number of subjects of the corresponding age group. As could be expected, the rate of suspect cases of diabetes increases according to advancing age; on the other hand, the rate of obese or ill patients also increases.

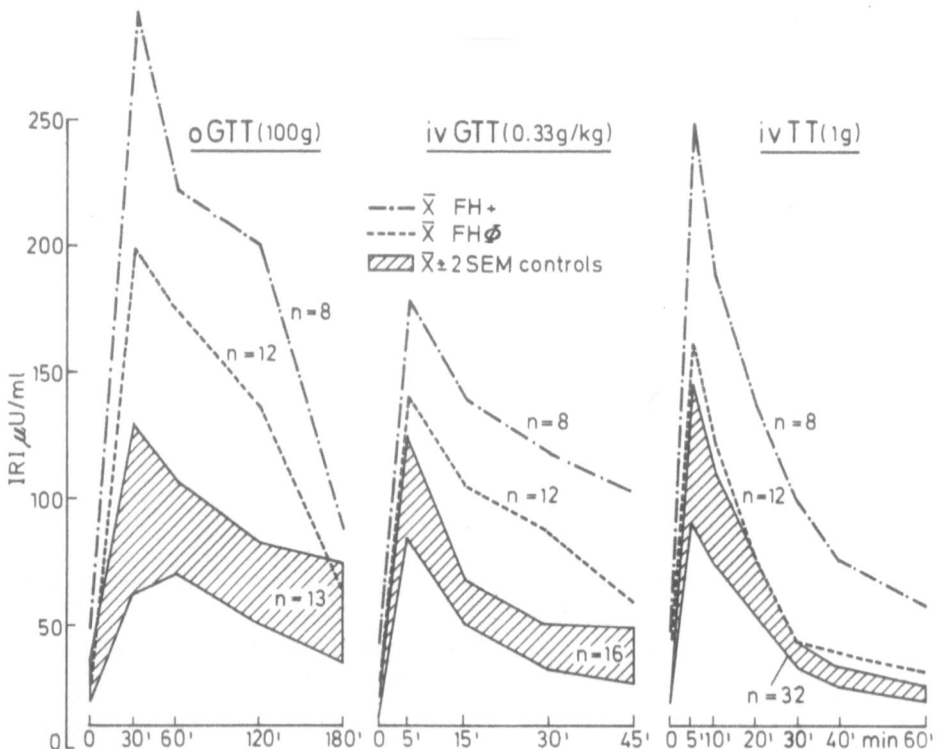

Fig. 4. Insulin secretion (IRI) in Klinefelter patients with positive (FH +) and negative (FH Ø) family history of diabetes mellitus during glucose tolerance and tolbutamide tests (Schade *et al.*, 1973)

Table 6 reveals that 72% of the suspect diabetics exhibited adiposity and/or associated diseases. If we consider the fact that we could not obtain data about possible associated diseases from 64 patients, an even higher rate has to be assumed. We suppose that at least in some of these patients there does not exist a typical diabetic glucose tolerance.

Jackson (15), Klotz (18), Rubin (34) and their coworkers observed increased insulin levels in the youngest subjects, too. Our patients were 12-21 years old; 4 out of 7 had open epiphyseal cartilages; insulin hypoglycemia revealed a normal growth hormone secretion in each of them. Grant (13) reported increased fasting insulin levels in children at age 12-15 years in contrast to younger children and to adults. We did not find reports on comparative studies upon insulin secretion in children, adolescents, and adults during glucose tolerance tests. We suppose that insulin secretion is elevated during puberty in a physiologic way.

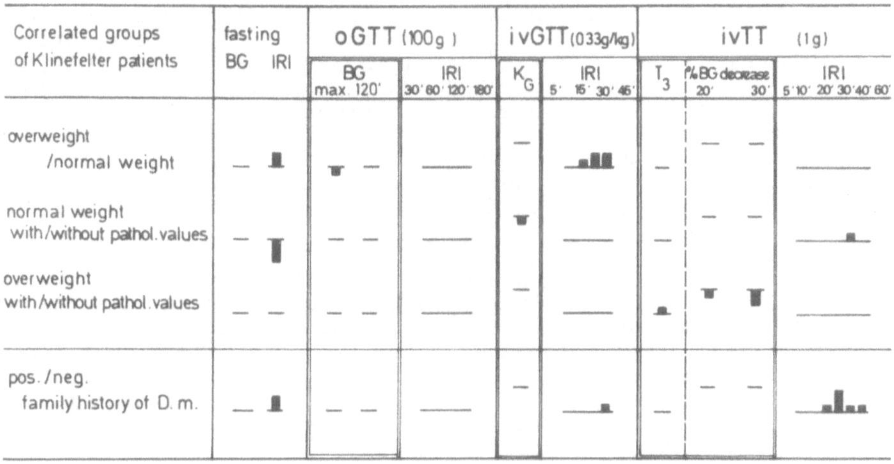

Correlated groups of Klinefelter patients	fasting BG IRI	oGTT (100g) BG max 120'	oGTT IRI 30' 60' 120' 180'	ivGTT (0.33g/kg) K_G	ivGTT IRI 5' 15' 30' 45'	ivTT (1g) T_3	ivTT % BG decrease 20' 30'	ivTT IRI 5' 10' 20' 30' 40' 60'
overweight /normal weight								
normal weight with/without pathol. values								
overweight with/without pathol. values								
pos./neg. family history of D. m.								

Fig. 5. Demonstration of the significant differences of mean values of blood glucose (BG) and serum insulin (IRI) during diabetes tests in correlated groups of Klinefelter patients (Schade *et al.*, 1973)
(● p<0.05 ▮ p<0.01 ▮ p<0.005 ▮ p<0.001)

Table 5. Age distribution of diabetics and patients with obesity and/or associated diseases among 104 Klinefelter patients using body weight of all and 40 case histories (compiled from literature; Schade *et al.*, 1972)

age groups	number of patients	"diabetics"	patients with obesity and/or associated diseases
11 – 20	13	2 (15 %)	3 (23 %)
21 – 30	29	4 (14 %)	9 (31 %)
31 – 40	20	7 (35 %)	8 (40 %)
41 – 50	20	9 (45 %)	13 (65 %)
51 – 60	16	7 (44 %)	12 (75 %)
61 – 80	6	3 (50 %)	3 (50 %)

Jackson *et al.*, 1966; Cassano *et al.*, 1967; Zuppinger *et al.*, 1967; Mirouze *et al.*, 1967; Nielsen 1969; Nielsen *et al.*, 1969; Rubin *et al.*, 1970.

Table 6. Age distribution and rate of "diabetics" with obesity and/or associated diseases among 32 patients with Klinefelter's syndrome and "diabetes" (compiled from literature; Schade *et al.*, 1972)

age groups	"diabetics" total	"diabetics" with obesity and/or associated diseases
11 – 20	2	1
21 – 30	4	3
31 – 40	7	4
41 – 50	9	8
51 – 60	7	5
61 – 80	3	2
	32	23 (72 %)

Growth hormone determinations after glucose, insulin, and arginine
load in patients with Down's, Turner's, and Klinefelter's syndrome have
revealed normal values in most cases (7,20,24,25,30,31,36,39,40,41,50).
Lindsten et al. (20) and Nielsen, Johansen, and Yde (29) found in some
patients with Turner's syndrome a paradoxically early hyper-response
after glucose administration. Our investigations (39) revealed an age-
dependence of growth hormone response to hypoglycemia in Klinefelter
patients with increased body height. Again, the number of observations
is too small for these results to be correlated to the findings obtained from the glucose tolerance tests.

Engel and Forbes (8,11), Nielsen et al. (29,30), Rimoin et al. (32) and
Milunsky (22) observed also in the families of patients with chromosome
aberrations a higher number of diabetics than could or should be expected. Therefore, they speculated about the possibility that diabetes
or the diabetic genotype may be responsible for the chromosome aberration. After having summarized the results from the literature, we
found in 30-35% of the patients with Turner's and Klinefelter's syndrome close relatives with diabetes (40,41,37).

Nielsen (28) summarized only the data of the parents and obtained a
result of 7-10%. In patients with Down's syndrome Milunsky (22) stated
a percentage of about 50 of the relatives. Fialkow (10) did not observe
an increase in comparison to a control group.

More than 50% of the parents of Rimoin's patients with Turner's syndrome
(32) demonstrated an impaired glucose tolerance. The same could be observed in 20-30% of the parents of patients with Down's syndrome (32,
22).

Burch and Milunsky (2) made some interesting speculations about the
etiology of these combinations. They seem to be of the opinion that a
genetic disposition to autoimmune diseases could be responsible for
diabetes and the chromosome aberrations, respectively. Stoller and
Collmann (44) found some hints that virus infections play a role in
the development of Down's syndrome.

Summarizing the results of these different research groups and our own
investigations, the following conclusions can be drawn:

1. Impaired glucose tolerance and diabetes mellitus seem to be more
   frequent in patients with chromosome aberrations than in other persons.
2. With rising severity of chromosome aberrations (gonosomal trisomy
   ⟶ gonosomal monosomy ⟶ autosomal trisomy) impaired glucose tolerance seems to be more frequent and seems to occur at an earlier
   age.

These data may be influenced by the following factors: Family history
of diabetes mellitus and early manifestation of this metabolic disease,
or impaired glucose tolerance due to obesity; complications caused by
malformations, infections, and other severe diseases. At present it
seems reasonable to assume that these investigations do not reveal a
causative connection between diabetes and the kind of chromosome aberrations. All findings should be interpreted with reservations until
it is possible to study unselected samples comprising a great number
of persons with chromosome abnormalities. A further elucidation of the
complex syndrome diabetes mellitus and its mode of inheritance today
and in the future may also help us to draw final conclusions.

References

1. Becker, K.L., Hoffmann, D.L., Albert, A., Underdahl, L.O., Mason, H.L.: Klinefelter's syndrome. Clinical and laboratory findings in 50 patients. Arch. Intern.
Med. 118, 314 (1966)

2. Burch, P.R.J., Milunsky, A.: Early-onset diabetes mellitus in the general and
Down's syndrome populations. Genetics, aetiology and pathogenesis. Lancet I,
554 (1969)

3. Campenhout, J. van, Antaki, A., Rasio, E.: Diabetes mellitus and thyroid autoimmunity in gonadal dysgenesis. Fertil. Steril. 24, 1 (1973)

4. Carter, C.O.: A life-table for mongols with the causes of death. J. Ment. Defic.
Res. 2, 64 (1958)

5. Cassano, C., Andreani, D., Falluca, F., Menzinger, G.: Le métabolisme glucidique
dans les dysgénésies gonadiques et dans le syndrome de Klinefelter. Actual. Endocrinol. 8, 287 (1967)

6. Collmann, R.D., Stoller, A.: A life-table for mongols in Victoria, Australia.
J. Ment. Defic. Res. 7, 53 (1963)

7. Donaldson, C.L., Wegienka, L.C., Miller, D., Forsham, P.H.: J. Clin. Endocr.
Metab. 28, 383 (1968)

8. Engel, E., Forbes, A.P.: Cytogenetic and clinical findings in 48 patients with
congenitally defective or absent ovaries. Medicine 44, 135 (1965)

9. Farquhar, J.W.: Diabetic children in Scotland and the need for care. Scott. med.
J. 7, 119 (1962)

10. Fialkow, P.J., Thuline, H.C., Hecht, F., Bryan, J.: Familial predisposition to
thyroid disease in Down's syndrome: Controlled immunoclinical studies. Amer. J.
Hum. Genet. 23, 67 (1971)

11. Forbes, A.P., Engel, E.: The high incidence of diabetes mellitus in 41 patients
with gonadal dysgenesis and their close relatives. Metabolism 12, 428 (1963)

12. Ford, C.E., Jones, K.W., Polani, P.E., de Almeida, J.C., Briggs, J.H.: A sex-
chromosome anomaly in a case of gonadal dysgenesis (Turner's syndrome). Lancet
I, 711 (1959)

13. Grant, D.B.: Fasting serum insulin levels in childhood. Arch. Dis. Childh. 42,
375 (1967)

14. Jackson, I.M.D., Buchanan, K.D., McKiddie, M.T., Prentice, C.R.M.: Carbohydrate
metabolism and pituitary function in gonadal dysgenesis (Turner's syndrome). J.
Endocrin. 34, 289 (1966)

15. Jackson, I.M.D., Buchanan, K.D., McKiddie, M.T., Prentice, C.R.M.: Carbohydrate
metabolism in Klinefelter's syndrome. J. Endocrin. 35, 169 (1966)

16. Jacobs, P.A., Strong, J.A.: A case of human intersexuality having a possible
XXY sex-determining mechanism. Nature (Lond.) 183, 302 (1959)

17. Jeremiah, D.E., Leyshon, G.E., Rose, T., Francis, H.W.S., Elliott, R.W.: Down's
syndrome and diabetes. Psychol. Med. 3, 455 (1973)

18. Klotz, H.P., Boiffin, A., Mignot, J., Larget, B., Lelievre, H.: Maladie de Klinefelter chez deux jumeaux monozygotes. Etude clinique et biologique. Ann. Endocrinol. 30, 86 (1968)

19. Lejeune, J., Turpin, R., Gautier, M.: Le mongolisme: premier exemple d'aberration
autosomique humaine. Ann. Génét. 1, 41 (1959)

20. Lindsten, J., Cerasi, E., Luft, R., Hultquist, G.: The occurrence of abnormal
insulin and growth hormone (HCG) responses to sustained hyperglycemia in a disease
with sex chromosome aberrations (Turner's syndrome). Acta endocrinol. 56, 107 (1967)

21. Menzinger, G., Fallucca, F., Andreani, D.: Gonadal dysgenesis and diabetes. Lancet I, 1269 (1966)

22. Milunsky, A.: Glucose intolerance in the parents of children with Down's syndrome. Amer. J. Ment. Defic. 74, 475 (1970)

23. Milunsky, A., Marks, V., Samols, E.: Insulin and glucose response to glucagon in Down's syndrome. Lancet II, 1093 (1967)

24. Milunsky, A., Neurath, P.W.: Diabetes mellitus in Down's syndrome. Arch. Environ. Health 17, 372 (1968)

25. Milunsky, A., Lowy, C., Rubinstein, A.H., Wright, A.D.: Carbohydrate tolerance, growth hormone and insulin levels in mongolism. Develop. Med. Child. Neurol.10, 25 (1968)

26. Mirouze, J., Jaffiol, C., Orsetti, A., Bernard, R.: L'équilibre glycémique dans le syndrome de Klinefelter. Actualité Endocrinologique 8, 276 (1967)

27. Nielsen, J.: Klinefelter's syndrome and the XYY syndrome. Acta psychiatr. Scand. 45 Suppl. 209 (1969)

28. Nielsen, J.: Diabetes mellitus in patients with aneuploid chromosome aberrations and in their parents. Humangenetik 16, 165 (1972)

29. Nielsen, J., Johansen, K., Yde, H.: The frequency of diabetes mellitus in patients with Turner's syndrome and pure gonadal dysgenesis. Acta endocrinol. 62, 251 (1969)

30. Nielsen, J., Johansen, K., Yde, H.: Frequency of diabetes mellitus in patients with Klinefelter's syndrome of different chromosome constitutions and the XYY syndrome. Plasma insulin and growth hormone level after a glucose load. J. Clin. Endocr. Metab. 29, 1062 (1969)

31. Raiti, S., Lifschitz, F., Trias, E., Sigman, B.: Down's syndrome. Study of carbohydrate metabolism. Acta endocrinol. 76, 506 (1974)

32. Rimoin, D.L., Harder, E., Whitehead, B., Packman, S., Peake, G.T., Sly, W.S.: Clin. Res. 18, 395 (1969)

33. Rohde, R.A.: Chromatin-positive Klinefelter's syndrome: clinical and cytogenetic studies. J. chron. Dis. 16, 1139 (1963)

34. Rubin, P., Mattei, A., Vague, P., Jubelin, J., Vague, J.: Exploration du métabolisme glucidique dans 22 cas de maladie de Klinefelter. Ann. Endocrinol. 31, 1003 (1970)

35. Runge, G.H.: Glucose tolerance in mongolism. Amer. J. Ment. Defic. 63, 822 (1959)

36. Ruvalcaba, R.H.A., Thuline, H.C., Kelley, V.C.: Plasma growth hormone in patients with chromosomal anomalies. Arch. Dis. Childh. 47, 307 (1972)

37. Schade, C., Simrock, R., Meixner, P., Neubauer, M., Beyer, J., Schöffling, K.: Untersuchungen des Glukosestoffwechsels und der Insulinsekretion bei Patienten mit Klinefelter-Syndrom. Vortrag VII. Kongr. Dtsch. Diabetes-Ges., Bad Nauheim, 1972

38. Schade, C., Simrock, R., Meixner, P., Neubauer, M., Beyer, J., Althoff, P.H., Schöffling, K.: Carbohydrate metabolism and insulin secretion in Klinefelter's syndrome. VIII. Congr. Internat. Diabetes Federation. Excerpta Medica, Internat. Congr. Ser. No. 280, Abstract No. 89, Brussels, 1973

39. Schade, C., Meixner, P., Althoff, P.H., Simrock, R., Neubauer, M., Beyer, J., Schöffling, K.: Age-dependence of growth hormone response to hypoglycemia in Klinefelter patients with increased body height. Acta endocr. (Kbh.) Suppl. 184, 12 (1974)

40. Schöffling, K.: Über Störungen im Kohlenhydratstoffwechsel und Wachstum bei Kranken mit Turner- und Klinefelter-Syndrom. Vortrag: VI. Karlsburger Symposium über Diabetes-Fragen, 1968

41. Schöffling, K., Neubauer, M., Melani, F., Pfeiffer, E.F.: Über die Sekretion von Insulin und Wachstumshormon beim Turner-Syndrom. Therapiewoche 18, 2045 (1968)

42. Serrano-Rios, M., Hawkins, F.G., Escobar, F., Mato, J.M., Larrodera, L., de Oya, M., Rodriguez-Minon, J.L.: Insulin secretion in Klinefelter's syndrome. The effect of testosterone. Abstract No. 246 NOVO Service. 8th Ann. Meet. Eur. Assoc. Study of Diabetes, Madrid, 1972

43. Serrano-Rios, M., San Roman Cos Gayon, C., Sordo, M.T., Rodriguez-Minon, J.L.: Insulin secretion in Down's syndrome. Diabetologia 9, 50 (1973)

44. Stoller, A., Collman, R.D.: Virus aetiology for Down's syndrome (mongolism). Nature 208, 903 (1965)

45. Sutnick, A.I., London, W.T., Gerstley, B.J.S., Coyne, V.E., Blumberg, B.S., Lustbader, E.D.: Glucose tolerance in Down's syndrome. Res. Commun. Chem. Pathol. Pharmacol. 8, 471 (1974)

46. Tjio, J.H., Levan, A.: The chromosome number of man. Hereditas (Lond.) 42, 1 (1956)

47. Valenti, C.: Alcune considerazioni citogenetiche sull'aborto. Minerva Med. 59, 1058 (1968)

48. Wais, S., Salvati, E.: Klinefelter's syndrome and diabetes mellitus. Lancet II, 747 (1966)

49. White, P.: Personal communication 1967; see Milunsky, A., Neurath, P.W.: Diabetes mellitus in Down's syndrome. Arch. Environ. Health 17, 372 (1968)

50. Wolf, H., Stubbe, P., Ammermann, M., Eberle, P.: Stoffwechseluntersuchungen und Wachstumshormonbestimmung bei Patienten mit atypischem Turner-Syndrom (XO/XX/ XXX-Mosaik, XO/XX-Mosaik). Mschr. Kinderheilkunde 117, 99 (1969)

51. Zuppinger, K., Engel, E., Forbes, A.P., Mantooth, L., Claffey, J.: Klinefelter's syndrome, a clinical and cytogenetic study in 24 cases. Acta endocrinol. 54 Suppl. 113 (1967)

15. Diabetes Mellitus and Hyperlipidemias

W. Fuhrmann

The one generally accepted definition of diabetes mellitus is hyperglycemia inappropriate to the existing environmental and nutritional
state. However, this symptom is only one of many endocrine and metabolic alterations present in clinically overt diabetes, among which
disturbances in lipid metabolism are most important. Perhaps the oldest
notion of the associated appearance of diabetes mellitus and hyperlipemia is, according to a quotation by Eggstein, a statement of Mariet
in 1799 (22), and in 1917 Joslin (18) stated: "with an excess of fat
diabetes begins and from an excess of fat diabetics die." In the earlier part of this century most authors apparently agreed that the extent of hyperlipemia depended largely on the severity of active diabetic symptoms and that the blood-lipid concentration represented the
most reliable prognostic criterion for the diabetic patient (6,18).
This was contradicted, however, by several authors and in Germany among
others by Katsch (19), who in 1938 expressed the view that the extent
of disturbance of lipid metabolism was not generally related to the
severity of diabetes, although in the mean blood lipids tended to rise
with acute diabetic decompensation and to fall again with recompensa-
tion. The moderately to strongly elevated blood-lipid concentration in
well-adjusted diabetics was judged by him to represent a personal characteristic of the individual patient. Katsch and Krainick (19) already
distinguished the reversible hyperlipemia accompanying the acute diabetic decompensation from the irreversible, permanent hyperlipemia of
well-adjusted diabetics. In 1955 Adlersberg and Wang (1) delineated
the combined appearance of mild diabetes mellitus and severe idiopathic
hyperlipemia as a distinct syndrome, which has previously been noted
by Thannhauser (36) and therefore is referred to by some as the Thann-
hauser-Adlersberg or Adlersberg-Wang syndrome and by others as the
"diabetic-hyperlipemic syndrome" (23).

While the justification for calling this a syndrome has been questioned,
later work (17) confirmed that one may distinguish two classes of hyperlipidemias in diabetic patients:

1. Secondary hyperlipidemia due to the disturbed metabolism in diabetes
   mellitus.
2. Primary hyperlipidemias associated with diabetes.

In neither type is the pathogenesis completely understood. Obviously
the increase may be due to overproduction of lipids, to impaired removal
from the bloodstream, or to the combined effect of both. Factors known
to influence the hepatic input of lipoproteins into the bloodstream
are the insulin lack in juvenile diabetes, obesity, glucagon, and hyperinsulinemia in adult-onset diabetes (11,12,21,23,24,26,31,37,38). Insulin resistance followed by hyperinsulinemia has been incriminated
as the primary factor in endogenous hyperlipidemia in general and particularly VLDL-triglyceride synthesis and secretion (25). These may

also affect factors regulating the catabolism or outflow of lipoproteins, as, for example, lipoproteinlipase activity. Individual differences of blood lipid levels appear to be as large in diabetics as in the nondiabetic population.

While primary and secondary hyperlipidemias in diabetics may be differentiated quite clearly in a larger sample, it may become difficult to discriminate between them in individual patients. The best available criterion so far is the disappearance of secondary hyperlipemia after control of the diabetic metabolic state and its persistence in the primary forms. This criterion, however, can only be applied if metabolic correction of the diabetes has been optimal for a prolonged period and if, on the other hand, the diet has been sufficient calorically and no weight loss has occurred.

Most available studies of the incidence of hyperlipidemia in diabetics do not consider these facts sufficiently. They tend to comprise a greater number of patients from a diabetic clinic with great variability in individual diabetic control. Moreover, various subforms of diabetes mellitus usually are not separately evaluated, methods of chemical determination differ, and the limits to define normality have varied. These limits, however, are crucial for the percentages of abnormals noted. My attempt to prepare a table comparing the data of several authors on the incidence of the various forms of hyperlipidemias in diabetics could not but fail for these reasons. However, in examination of the distribution of total lipids, cholesterol, and triglycerides, certain trends can be recognized:

All authors agree that triglycerides are more frequently elevated than cholesterol and to a higher degree (4,8). Particularly in diabetic keto-acidosis triglycerides may be increased tenfold or more above the limit of normal levels, and cholesterol may reach twice or more the level subsequently found in the same individual. Both may decrease rapidly under active treatment of the diabetic state.

In a group of diabetic children, studied before instituting therapy, Chance *et al.* (10) found serum total lipids elevated in 64% of patients and total cholesterol in 43%. Triglycerides were not reported separately in this study. Children with normal and abnormal lipid levels as a group did not differ in their clinical features. Serum lipid levels reached extreme values in some of these children and in all reverted to normal after insulin treatment within several weeks.

Particular attention has been paid to serum lipids in adult-onset diabetes, since it was hoped to gain a better understanding of the interaction of diabetes and hyperlipidemia as risk factors of atherosclerosis (3,4,14,20,29,32). Most studies agree that serum free fatty acid levels are elevated in all diabetics. Triglyceride levels were increased in some 30-40% of patients studied, if a limit of more than 200mg/100ml was accepted. There was a positive correlation between triglyceride levels and diabetes decompensation. Values concerning cholesterol differ considerably, in part due to the different "cut-off" points chosen. Remarkable is the strong positive correlation, which has been found between triglyceride levels and body weight and also between triglyceride levels and the quality of control of the diabetes achieved in the particular patients judged by the fasting blood sugar level. Wahl *et al.* (40) found positive correlations also with age in female patients and with type of therapy in males. No correlation was noted to the duration of diabetes in both sexes. Cholesterol was correlated only to body weight in males and females and somewhat to age in females. The introduction of a classification of hyperlipidemias by Fredrickson and Levy (15) stimulated new interest and gave hope for an easier discrimination of primary and secondary forms of hyperlipidemias among diabetics. This, too, proved disappointing: of the various lipoprotein classes, particularly the very low density lipoprotein (VLDL) fraction was found to be increased in diabetic hyperlipoproteinemia. Low-density lipoproteins (LDL) as well as high density lipoproteins (HDL) have a relatively higher triglyceride content.

As suggested by Vogelberg and Gries (39) one might distinguish an exogenous from an endogenous type, and also a mixed form of diabetic hyperlipoproteinemia. The exogenous type is characterized by hyperchylomicronemia and an electrophoretic pattern similar to type I of Fredrickson. It is fairly common in decompensated diabetes on a high-fat diet. Pathogenetically, a decreased utilization of chylomicron VLDL in peripheral tissues is assumed, which may be caused by a deficiency of insulin-dependent lipoprotein lipase. In the endogenous type the pre-beta-lipoproteins are increased. This type is less dependent on diet and resembles type IV in Fredrickson's scheme. It is the type predominant in adult-onset diabetes that may persist in well-controlled diabetics. The commonly found mixed type, resembling type V hyperlipoproteinemia, combines both characteristics.

In all adult series type IV hyperlipoproteinemia was found to be most common, with an incidence of some 20-50% among all diabetics, but this held true equally for decompensated as for well-compensated diabetes mellitus (7,27,42). Types I and III were uniformly rare or absent, but incidence figures for type IIa, IIb, and V differed grossly. Generally triglycerides were more commonly found elevated than cholesterol.

In unselected samples of the general population type IV also proved to be the most common type of hyperlipoproteinemia, and, as for example also in the diabetic group studied by Wahl *et al.* (40), males are more commonly affected than females. For example: Brown *et al.* (9) found type IV in Albany, New York, in a random sample of the population with a frequency of 26% in males and 8% in females. A type II pattern was seen in his sample of blood donors in 8.7 and 10.4% respectively. His figures seem unusually high, due to the low cut-off points used (for triglycerides p.e. 160 mg/100 ml). Wood *et al.* (43), using a cut-off point for triglycerides of 200 mg/100 ml and for cholesterol of 275 mg/100 ml, found in a population sample in California type IV in 8.6% (13% in males, 5.8% in females) and type II in 3.7%, the latter more common in females than in men.

Thus, type IV is, apparently, more common in diabetes than in the population at large, while for the other types this cannot be said with certainty. When speaking about the frequency of various types of hyperlipoproteinemia in diabetics, the fact must also be noted that the phenotype of hyperlipoproteinemia may change in a patient within a short time, depending on his metabolic state or other factors.

One may also ask the question, whether diabetes is found more often in patients with certain types of hyperlipidemia and among their relatives as compared with the general population. Statements of this kind are found frequently in the literature but rarely are they backed by sufficient statistics. Carbohydrate intolerance has been noted more frequently than to be expected by chance in patients with various types of hyperlipoproteinemia, particularly those with types IIb, IV, and V (13,16,28). In a recent study of Schoenfeld *et al.* (34,35) glucose intolerance was noted in 7 out of 9 patients studied. In type III abnormal response to glucose load was seen slightly more often than in controls. Type III, IV, and V patterns can be induced in susceptible individuals by a high carbohydrate diet. Overt diabetes has not been found unusually often in type I, II, and III patients, but is more common in patients with types IV and V (5). However, glucose intolerance, hyperinsulinism, or diabetes mellitus are not present in all patients with these types of hyperlipoproteinemia. In fact, within one family study by Schoenfeld and Kudzma (34) of two brothers with the same clinical type IV hyperlipoproteinemia only one had an abnormal glucose tolerance. While this patient was obese, his brother was not. This observation supports the conclusion that the basic inherited defect, leading to type IV hyperlipoproteinemia, is different from the carbohydrate disturbance and that obesity, decreased glucose tolerance, or even overt diabetes may only aggravate the inherited abnormality in lipid metabolism, as, on the other hand, hyperlipidemia may decrease insulin sensitivity.

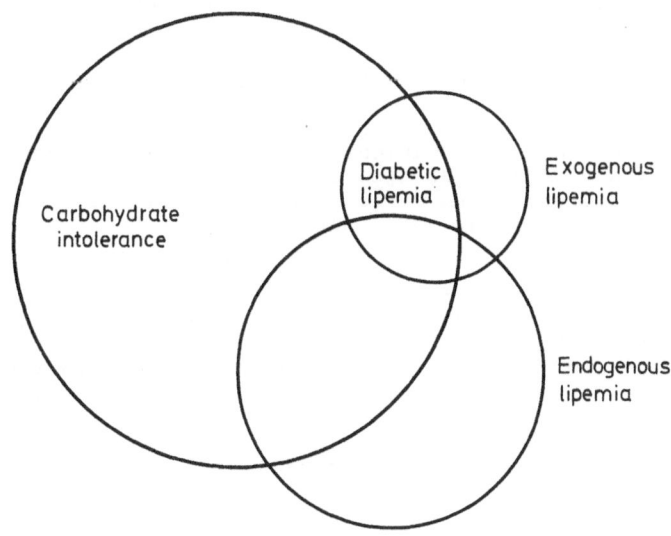

Fig. 1. The universe of carbohydrate intolerance and lipemia (from Bierman and Porter (5))

The interaction of carbohydrate tolerance and hyperlipemia has been pictured very well by Bierman and Porte (5). The question remains, why do the hyperlipoproteinemias, particularly type IV, the so-called endogenous hyperlipoproteinemias, and carbohydrate intolerance so frequently coexist? Do they have a common link? Bierman and Porte suggested, that obesity might be this link, but other authors argue against such an interpretation and think rather of insulin resistence and hyperinsulinism. Is it perhaps that diabetes acts only by aggravating and promoting the manifestation of an independently existing predisposition to a certain type of hyperlipidemia? Or is it that the hyperlipidemia types IIa, IIb, and possibly III in diabetics represent coexisting diseases due to chance and only between type IV and V and diabetes does some interaction or causal relatioship exist?

A possible step towards an answer to this problem could be a systematic study of close relatives of diabetics with various types of hyperlipoproteinemias. To my knowledge such a study has not been done so far, although Chance et al. (10) have mentioned an unpublished observation of abnormalities in the lipid metabolism in parents of diabetic children with hyperlipidemias.

The interpretation of any such information obtained or even the building of models will be extremely difficult as long as we have no further information on the genetics of diabetes mellitus as well as the hyperlipidemias. Both represent metabolic anomalies that are largely quantitatively defined, with unclear borderlines, open to definition. Both depend in their development to some degree on age, moreover, both most probably represent heterogeneous groups for whose further subdivision available biochemical methods do not suffice. Furthermore, diabetes mellitus as such in all probability has a multifactorial genetic background as is true also of the more common types of hyperlipoproteinemias, particularly of the so-called type IV in Fredrickson's definition, whose system in its original definition was introduced to represent phenotypes not genotypes, a fact frequently overlooked.

With this state of affairs it is risky to develop a hypothesis to explain the interaction of both metabolic disturbances on a genetic level. Separate genetic determination is strongly suggested by the facts that many, but not all, patients with comparable diabetes show different forms and degrees of hyperlipidemia and that, on the other hand, comparable patients with various forms of hyperlipidemias show different degrees of carbohydrate inducibility of their hyperlipidemia and various degrees of carbohydrate intolerance and diabetes.

One may assume that in any diabetic, hyperlipoproteinemia will develop, if he decompensates and becomes ketoacidotic. His genetic make-up in regard to hyperlipoproteinemia may decide, though, how easily this might happen and possibly to some degree also, which type of hyperlipidemia he may develop. Whereas in some the exogenous type with chylomicronemia will develop, an underlying predisposition to endogeneous hyperlipidemia in another may in otherwise the same circumstances, determine the manifestation of exogenous-endogenous mixed type, type V. At another level of decompensation one patient might show outright endogenous hyperlipidemia, type IV, while another has not yet any gross hyperlipidemia at all. In yet another group hyperlipidemia type IV persists even if diabetes is well controlled, perhaps documenting a specific genetic predisposition to this type of hyperlipidemia. Hence, inasmuch as a certain persistent type of hyperlipoproteinemia in a diabetic patient is genetically determined per se, one may expect to find in first-degree relatives the same type preferentially.

While quantitative data for a more general analysis and particularly for a unifying hypothesis are missing, expected distributions in relatives may be analyzed with respect to general trends under certain simplified assumptions, adapting a model developed by Saddi and Feingold (30) for hemochromatosis and diabetes: If we assume that diabetes is determined by a multifactorial genetic system which defines a predisposition distributed as a continuous variable, and if we further simplify the picture by postulating a sharp threshold beyond which each individual will develop diabetes by the age of 50 (curve a), and that having genetically determined hyperlipoproteinemia lowers the threshold for diabetes, then, due to some interference with carbohydrate metabolism, diabetes should be considerably more frequent among hyperlipidemic persons than in the general population (curve b). While the distribution of predisposition to diabetes remains the same, the threshold is shifted to the left. Looking at first-degree relatives of the first group, we will find the distribution shifted to the right according to the rules set forth by Carter and others, diabetes being more frequent among them (curve c). The same trend should be found among first-degree

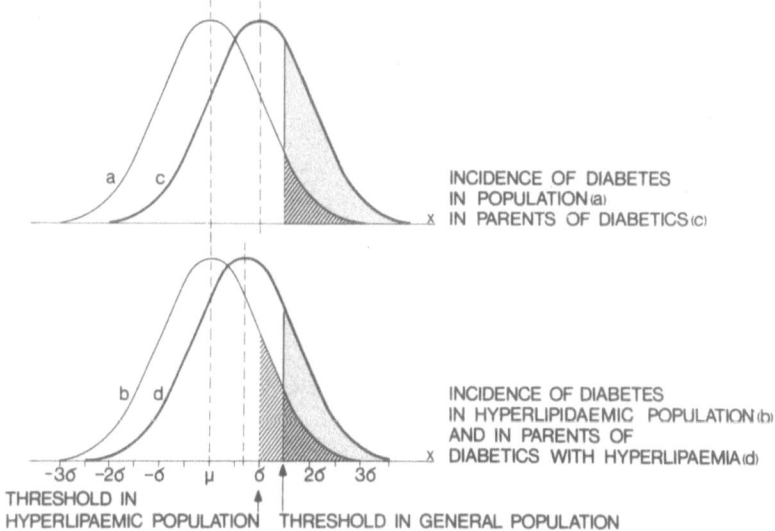

Fig. 2. A model of possible influence of hyperlipoproteinemia on incidence of diabetes mellitus: (a) general population; (b) individuals with hyperlipoproteinemia;
(c) and (d) first-degree relatives (parents) of (a) and (b) respectively
Hatched area = incidence of diabetes in probands
gray area   = incidence of diabetes in first-degree relatives (parents)
Scale represents S.D. from the mean

relatives of hyperlipidemic diabetics (curve d), but comparing both
groups we should expect that first-degree relatives of the nonlipidemic
diabetics would have a higher increase in diabetes frequency than first-
-degree relatives of the hyperlipidemic diabetics, as set out before,
the mean value of the genetic predisposition for diabetes in the proband group should be lower among hyperlipidemic diabetics than among
nonhyperlipidemic diabetics.

The same considerations could be made vice versa regarding the frequency of hyperlipidemia in the diabetic and nondiabetic population:
carbohydrate intolerance and diabetes, by shifting the threshold for
overt hyperlipidemia to the left, increase the frequency of persistent
hyperlipoproteinemia among diabetics above that seen in the general
population (curve b, compared to curve a), and again the frequency of
hyperlipoproteinemia among parents of nondiabetic hyperlipoproteinemic
patients (curve c) should be higher than among parents of hyperlipoproteinemic diabetics (curve d).

To my knowledge, no data are available to test these predictions. A
large number of observations may be necessary. Moreover, neither diabetes nor hyperlipidemias represent genetically homogeneous diseases,
nor are both determined in a simple multifactorial fashion with a sharp
all-or-none threshold. Interaction must be assumed to be complex at
various levels and different in various types of both diseases. Of interest in this regard may be observations of special forms of hyperlipidemia in diabetics, such as that of Wille *et al.* (41), who described hitherto unobserved hyper-alpha-lipoproteinemia associated with
a slow-moving pre-beta-lipoprotein in 3 out of 83 patients with maturity-onset type diabetes.

143

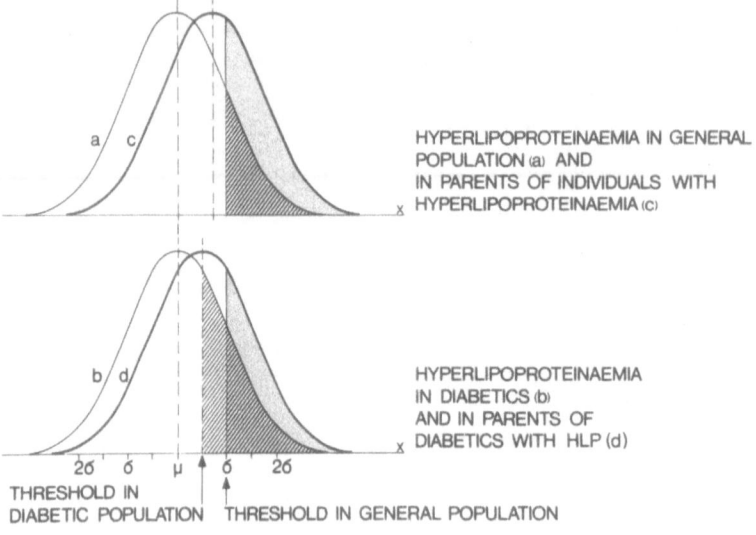

Fig. 3. Model of possible influence of diabetes on incidence of hyperlipoproteinemia:
(a) general population; (b) diabetics; (c) and (d) first-degree relatives (parents)
of (a) and (b) respectively
Hatched area = incidence of hyperlipoproteinemia in probands
gray are   = incidence of hyperlipoproteinemia in first-degree relatives (parents)

In conclusion: The task remains, first to disentangle the genetics and
pathogenesis of either disease and only then to analyze the interaction
of recognized subgroups or disease entities. It may be of some practical and theoretical advantage, though, to conduct pilot studies with
groups defined in a preliminary fashion.

References

1. Adlersberg, D., Wang, C.: Syndrome of idiopathic hyperlipemia, mild diabetes mellitus, and severe vascular damage. Diabetes 4, 210 (1955)

2. Adlersberg, D., Eisler, L.: Circulating lipids in diabetes mellitus. JAMA 170,
   1261 (1959)

3. Albrink, M.J., Lavietes, P.H., Man, E.B.: Vascular disease and serum lipids in
   diabetes mellitus. Observations over 30 years (1931-1961). Ann. Int. Med. 58,
   305 (1963)

4. Bergqvist, N.: Serum lipids in an ambulatory diabetic clientele. Acta med. scand.
   187, 213 (1970)

5. Bierman, E.L., Porte, D.: Carbohydrate intolerance and lipemia. Ann. Int. Med.
   68, 926 (1968)

6. Bloor, W.R.: The lipoids ("fat") of the blood in diabetes. Journ. Biol. Chem. 26,
   417 (1916)

7. Borrie, P., Slack, J.: A clinical syndrome characteristic of primary type IV-V
   hyperlipoproteinemia. Brit. Journ. Dermatology 90, 245 (1974)

8. Braunsteiner, H., Sailer, S., Sandhofer, F.: Plasmalipide bei Patienten mit Diabetes mellitus. Klin. Wschr. 44, 116 (1966)

9. Brown, D.F., Daudiss, K.: Hyperlipoproteinemia. Prevalence in a free-living population in Albany, New York. Circulation XLVII, 558 (1973)

10. Chance, G.W., Albutt, E.C., Edkins, S.M.: Serum lipids and lipoproteins in untreated diabetic children. Lancet I, 1126 (1969)

11. Eaton, R.P., Schade, D.S.: Glucagon resistance as a hormonal basis for endogenous hyperlipemia. Lancet I, 973 (1973)

12. Ford, S., Bozian, R.C., Knowles, H.C.: Interactions of obesity, and glucose and insulin levels in hypertriglyceridemia. Amer. Journ. Clin. Invest. 21, 904 (1968)

13. Glueck, C.J., Levy, R.I., Fredrickson, D.S.: Immunoreactive insulin. glucose tolerance, and carbohydrate inducibility in types II, II, IV, and V hyperlipoproteinemia. Diabetes 18, 739 (1969)

14. Gries, F.A., Engelhardt, A., Cramer, M., Jahnke, K.: Metabolite des Fett- und Kohlenhydratstoffwechsels bei normgewichtigen Stoffwechselgesunden sowie bei Adipösen und Diabetikern. Verhandl. Deutsch. Ges. Inn. Med. 76, 371 (1970)

15. Fredrickson, D.S., Levy, R.: Familial hyperlipoproteinemia. In: The Metabolic Basis of Inherited Disease, 3rd ed.. Stanbury, J.B., Wyngaarden, J.B., Fredrickson, D.S. (eds.). New York: Mc Graw Hill, 1972

16. Jacobsen, B.B.: Type V hyperlipoproteinemia. Atherosclerosis 17, 471 (1973)

17. Jahnke, K.: Störungen des Fettstoffwechsels. Ärztl. Praxis 26, 4438 (1974)

18. Joslin, E.P., Bloor, W.R., Gray, H.: The blood lipoids in diabetes. Journ. Amer. Med. Ass. 69, 375 (1917)

19. Katsch, G., Krainick, H.G.: Zur Physiologie und Pathologie des intermediären Fettstoffwechsels. Klin. Wschr. 18, 436 (1939)

20. Levy, R.I., Glueck, C.J.: Hypertriglyceridemia, diabetes mellitus, and coronary vessel disease. Arch. Intern. Med. 123, 220 (1969)

21. Man, E.B., Albrink, M.J.: Serum lipids in different phases of carbohydrate metabolism. Yale J. Biol. Med. 29, 316 (1956)

22. Mariet (1799). Cited by M. Eggstein: Diabetes und Fett. Med. Welt 18, 843 (1967)

23. Nikkilä, E.A.: Plasma triglycerides in human diabetes. Proc. Royal Soc. Med. 67, 662 (1974)

24. Nikkilä, E.A.: Control of plasma and liver triglyceride kinetics by carbohydrate metabolism and insulin. Advances Lipid. Res. 7, 63 (1969)

25. Olefsky, J.M., Farquhar, J.W., Reaven, G.M.: Reappraisal of the role of insulin in hypertriglyceridemia. Amer. Journ. Med. 57, 551 (1974)

26. Reaven, G.M., Lerner, R.L., Stern, M.P., Farquhar, J.W., Nakanishi, R.: Role of insulin in endogenous hypertriglyceridemia. Journ. Clin. Invest. 46, 1756 (1967)

27. Reimer, F., Kremer, G.J., Müller, D.: Häufigkeit von Fettstoffwechselstörungen bei asymptomatischen und manifesten Diabetikern. Klin. Wschr. 51, 973 (1973)

28. Rose, H.G., Kranz, P., Weinstock, M., Juliano, J., Haft, J.I.:Combined hyperlipoproteinemia. Evidence for a new lipoprotein phenotype. Atherosclerosis 20, 51 (1974)

29. Righetti, A., Scherrer, J.R., Micheli, H., Pometta, D.: Etude clinique des relations entre le diabète, les hyperlipoprotéinémies et l'athéromatose. Schweiz. med. Wschr. 103, 668 (1973)

30. Saddi, R., Feingold, J.: Idiopathic hemochromatosis and diabetes mellitus. Clin. Genet. 5, 242 (1974)

31. Sailer, S., Bolzano, K., Sandhofer, F., Spath, P., Braunsteiner, H.: Triglyceridspiegel und Insulinkonzentration im Plasma nach oraler Glukosegabe bei Patienten mit primärer kohlenhydratinduzierter Hypertriglyceridämie. Schweiz. Med. Wschr. 98, 1512 (1968)

32. Santen, R.J., Willis, P.W., Fajans, S.S.: Atherosclerosis in diabetes mellitus. Correlations with serum lipid levels, adiposity, and serum insulin level. Arch. Intern. Med. 130, 833 (1972)

33. Schlierf, G., Weinans, G., Weinans, T., Reinheimer, W., Kahlke, W.: Häufigkeit und Typenverteilung von Hyperlipoproteinämien bei stationären Patienten einer Medizinischen Klinik. Dtsch. Med. Wschr. 97, 1371 (1972)

34. Schonfeld, G., Kudzma, D.J.: Type IV hyperlipoproteinemia, a critical appraisal. Arch. Intern. Med. 132, 55 (1973)

35. Schonfeld, G., Birge, C., Miller, P., Kessler, G., Santiago, J.: Apolipoprotein B levels and altered lipoprotein composition in diabetes. Diabetes 23, 827 (1974)

36. Thannhauser, S.J.: New Engl. J. Med. 237, 515 (1947). Cited by Nikkilä, 1974

37. Tiengo, A., Muggeo, M., Fedele, D., Marchior, E., Crepaldi, G.: Insulin-secretion in hyperlipoproteinemias. Act. Diabet. 11, 149 (1974)

38. Tzagournis, M., Chiles, R., Ryan, J.M., Skillman, T.G.: Interrelatioships of hyperinsulinism and hypertriglyceridemia in young patients with coronary heart disease. Circulation 38, 1156 (1968)

39. Vogelberg, K.H., Gries, F.A.: Hyperlipoproteinämie bei Diabetes Mellitus. Münchn. Med. Wschr. 115, 650 (1973)

40. Wahl, P., Hasslacher, Ch., Vollmar, J.: Diabetes und Hyperlipoproteinämien. Dtsch. Med. Wschr. 99, 2158 (1974)

41. Wille, L.E., Aarseth, S.: Demonstration of hyper-α-lipoproteinemia in three diabetic patients. Clin. Genet. 4, 281 (1973)

42. Wilson, D.E., Schreibman, P.H., Day, V.C., Arky, R.A.: Hyperlipidemia in an adult diabetic population. J. Chron. Dis. 23, 501 (1970)

43. Wood, P.D.S., Stern, M.P., Silvers, A., Reaven, G.M., Groeben, J. von der: Prevalence of plasma lipoprotein abnormalities in a free-living population of the Central valley, California. Circulation XLV, 114 (1972)

44. Wollenweber, J., Christl, H.L., Schlierf, Chr., Wohlenberg, H.: Hyperlipoproteinämien bei ambulanten Patienten. Dtsch. Med. Wschr. 98, 463 (1973)

16. Genetic Syndromes Associated with Lipatrophic Diabetes

J. KÖBBERLING

On searching for examples of the heterogeneity of diabetes mellitus,
lipatrophic diabetes is an example of an instance where it is easy to
separate out a special type of diabetes on clinical grounds. Lipatrophic diabetes is not a genetic entity. It is a special type of diabetes
occurring in different, well-defined, genetic as well nongenetic syndromes. The terminology in this field is very conflicting; a vast number
of synonyms have been proposed in the literature, which is difficult to
disentangle.

There are two early descriptions of probable lipatrophic diabetes by
Ziegler (48) and by Hansen and McQuarrie (19). Lawrence in 1946 (26)
presented an excellent and comprehensive case report, including post-
morten findings. The patient was a young woman, who, as in both earlier
descriptions, suffered from the acquired form of the disease. In this
paper Lawrence first introduced the term "lipatrophic diabetes." It
has been proposed to use the term "Lawrence type of diabetes" for the
lipatrophic diabetes (41). The following symptoms are associated with
lipatrophic diabetes (Lawrence type of diabetes):

1. Partial or total absence of adipose tissue
2. Severe hyperlipidemia
3. Insulin-resistant diabetes
4. Lack of ketoacidosis in spite of poor control of blood glucose levels
5. Hepatomegaly
6. An elevated basal metabolic rate without hyperthyroidism

Lipatrophic diabetes is frequently used synonymously with generalized
lipodystrophy. Since diabetes may be absent in generalized lipodystrophy, at least for many years, this term should be avoided. Furthermore, cases of typical lipatrophic diabetes are known in which the
loss of fat has not affected the whole body. Lipatrophic diabetes should
be used to designate the characteristic type of insulin-resistant diabetes which may follow extensive loss of fat, whether this is generalized or not.

I. Recessively Inherited Congenital Generalized Lipodystrophy

This type was first described by Berardinelli (3) in a 2-year-old boy,
a product of consanguineous marriage. Familial occurrance was first
described by Seip (40). The syndrome is now called the Berardinelli-
Seip syndrome by most authors. Forty-two cases in 31 families were
summarized by Seip in 1971 (41), and a further case was subsequently
described by Gordon et al. (16). The frequency of affected males and
females is about equal. A variety of sibling cases have been described
(1,6,8,23,36,40,45). In one family as many as five out of a total of
twelve siblings were affected (7). Consanguinity among parents has been

documented in 9 families (3,6,12,29,31,37,40,42). There is thus no doubt that this syndrome is inherited as an autosomal recessive trait.

The main clinical picture is an extreme paucity of fat in adipose tissue. This is not confined to the subcutis; adipose tissue is also absent in the whole body including the perirenal, retroperitoneal, mesenteric, and epicardial areas, and in the bone marrow. Even the Bichat's fat pad in the cheeks is lacking, leading to the characteristic appearance. Adipocytes can be demonstrated on microscopic examination but they contain very little fat. In almost all cases the lipodystrophy is permanent.

The growth velocity in patients with congenital generalized lipodystrophy is increased during the first 4 years (42), and at the end of this period the height is generally well above the 97th percentile. Then follows a period of normal growth and, due to the lack of pubertal growth spurt, the adult height is normal. The body build is often described as masculine with an acromegaloid pattern and muscular hypertrophy. In practically all published cases an acceleration of skeletal maturation has been observed. There is usually a moderate enlargement of the clitoris in female patients with congenital generalized lipodystrophy. Irregular menstrual bleeding and oligomenorrhea seem to be common. Breast development is often poor, although the breast is the only organ in which adipose tissue may be found.

In infancy and early childhood glucose tolerance is usually normal. Between 7 and 12 years of age a reduced glucose tolerance develops which is followed by frank diabetes. All of the cases reported in the literature so far that have been followed to adulthood have become diabetic.

The diabetes is characterized by increased plasma insulin levels, both radioimmunologically and with biological methods (rat diaphragm and epididymal fat). Intravenous insulin tolerance tests with usual doses result in negligible depression of the blood glucose. Very high insulin doses are necessary to control blood glucose levels. Ketosis is always minimal or absent. A variety of vascular complications, including peripheral vascular disease (28), diabetic retinopathy (46), and diabetic nephropathy (17) occur, as well as affections of peripheral nerves (46). The glycogen stores of the liver are usually normal or increased and muscular glycogen content is probably normal.

Severe hyperlipidemia is one of the regular findings in patients with congenital generalized lipodystrophy. The type (Fredrickson's classification, 14) is not consistent, and a marked variation in lipidemia from time to time in the same patient has been described (26,41).

Hypermetabolism in spite of normal thyroid function is found in most patients with generalized lipodystrophy. In the case described by Lawrence (26), the greatly increased basal metabolic rate (up to + 177%) has led to a thyroidectomy. After operation the basal metabolic rate fell to +38% but the patient developed signs of hypothyroidism and had to be treated with thyroid hormones. Usually the basal metabolic rate ranges between + 30 and + 60% (8,17,22,35,42,48). In some patients, however, the basal metabolic rate was found to be within the normal limits (23,31,37,39). Hyperthyroidism has never been observed.

Hepatomegaly is a constant finding in generalized lipodystrophy. The degree of liver enlargement varies greatly from a liver palpable 2-3 cm below the costal margin to enormously enlarged livers, reaching below the umbilicus. Histologically a marked fatty infiltration is the most outstanding feature.

A nearly constant finding in congenital generalized lipodystrophy is acanthosis nigricans, a peculiar skin change, mostly occurring in the flexural areas of the extremities and the neck. The brain is probably affected in all cases of congenital generalized lipodystrophy, and about half of the patients have been mentally retarded, often severely.

II. Acquired Type of Generalized Lipodystrophy

The acquired type of generalized lipodystrophy in most cases manifests itself in childhood. In 20 out of the 28 reported cases the loss of fat was observed before 15 years of age, and in all but 2 before the age of 30 years.

In approximately half of the cases a well-defined preceding illness has been observed, e.g., an infection such as whooping cough, measles, chickenpox, mononucleosis, smallpox vaccination, prolonged diarrhea, or nonspecific febrile illness (41). The disease has also been reported to start following an attack of jaundice, after a difficult delivery, or following hyperthyroidism successfully treated with propylthiouracil. In two cases an inflammatory process of the adipose tissue with tender swelling preceded the fat loss (43,48). This was diagnosed as Weber-Christian disease in biopsy. Two cases of acquired generalized lipodystrophy have been reported that developed in patients with astrocytomas of the diencephalon, close to the third ventricle (34,35). Thus, if preceding illness are of any causative importance, this is very unspecific.

In the acquired form of the disease females are more frequently affected than males (19:9). Parental consanguinity and affection of more than one sibling have not been described in this form of lipodystrophy.

The clinical and biochemical features are identical to those in the congenital type of generalized lipodystrophy. The rate of growth and skeletal maturation is greatly influenced by the time of onset of the disease. If it starts in infancy or early childhood, the pattern of growth maturation may be similar to that of congenital lipodystrophy. According to Seip (41) the liver affection may be more severe, and frank diabetes may develop more rapidly than in the congenital type. Eruptive xanthomas are reported to develop only in the acquired type (4,9,10, 26,32).

III. Partial Lipodystrophies with Dominant Inheritance

Some observations of familial lipodystrophy or lipatrophic diabetes do not fit into the given classification. The following five families all are suspect for autosomal dominant inheritance.

1. Brown and Winkelmann (5) have briefly reported a 41-year-old woman who lost subcutaneous fat at puberty. This well developed woman had a striking body habitus consisting of a large neck (which is never described in generalized lipodystrophy) and prominent body musculature. Inquiry into the family history disclosed that eight further family members in four generations all had a similar body habitus and cutaneous findings. The inheritance followed an autosomal dominant pattern. In addition, three of the aunts had diabetes but no information is given as to whether the diabetes was of the lipatrophic type. In the illustration of the patient, the face did not appear lipatrophic in a way that is characteristic for most patients with generalized lipodystrophy.

2. A second observation of this type was made by Köbberling et al. (24, 25). A 24-year-old female patient with a history of diabetes since the age of 11 exhibited the following peculiarities of body shape: There was a well-developed subcutaneous fat on the face and on the trunk. The face looked round and full which led to efforts to exclude the Cushing's syndrome. On the arms and legs, however, no subcutaneous fat was palpable and the skin folds were very thin. The appearance was thus masculine, the subcutaneous veins were visible, and the muscles looked hypertrophied. There was no clitoris enlargement. The peculiar fat distribution has been present as long as the patient can remember.

The patient had a very severe hyperlipidemia classified as Fredrickson type III. Insulin resistance was observed in an i.v. insulin tolerance test. In spite of high insulin doses the control of blood glucose levels remained poor, but even in times of very bad control or under a dietary regimen with 70% of calories given as fat, ketoacidosis has only been minimal or absent. Hepatomegaly and an elevated basal metabolic rate were also observed.

The mother and a sister of the patient exhibit the same peculiar apperance and a slight hyperlipidemia but no diabetes mellitus.

The combination of this type of partial lipodystrophy with severe hyperlipidemia, insulin-resistant diabetes mellitus without ketoacidosis, and an elevated basal metabolic rate was further observed in two unrelated patients without familial occurrence. Due to the great similarity in the symptomatology all five cases might be regarded as one syndrome although only three of them, including the two sporadic cases, had frank diabetes mellitus.

In the one family the familial pattern is suggestive of dominant inheritance (Fig. 1). It was not possible to establish if the two

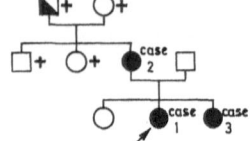

● Lipodystrophy of the ex-
tremitis and hyperlipidemia
✗ index case, lipatrophic
diabetes
◨ reported as being affected
+ deceased, not examined

Fig. 1. Pedigree of a family with partial lipidystrophy (Köbberling et al. (25))

sporadic cases are of nongenetic origin or if they are also genetic, either as a new mutation or inherited. Since nobody had previously realized the peculiar body shape (even the patient did not know for how long it had existed) it may well be that further family members exhibit the same syndrome with or without diabetes. It is assumed that the syndrome will be overlooked in most patients or regarded just as a minor peculiarity. Lipodystrophy of the face is much more impressive than lipodystrophy of the extremities.

3. Another family with dominant inheritance has been described by Ozer et al. (30). A 52-year-old woman, five of her six siblings and three of her four children were found to have a syndrome characterized by

excessive accumulation of fat on the face, neck (described as "fat neck"), shoulder girdle, axillae, back, and genitalia. In contrast, the limbs appeared devoid of fat with prominant musculature and phlebectasia. All family members have type IV hyperlipidemia, and frank diabetes was found in two, abnormal glucose tolerance in four. This was reported as a "new syndrome" and it was mentioned that a second family was under investigation.

4. Very recently a further, closely related syndrome probably with dominant inheritance has been described by Dunnigen et al. (11). Several members of two families extending over three generations were found to have symmetrical lipatrophy of the trunk and the limbs with round and full face and hyperlipidemia. As in the other families with dominant inheritance not all affected subjects were diabetic. Those subjects who were diabetic were described to be insulin-resistant and in some nondiabetic family members high plasma insulin values were found.

5. See addendum

Thus, besides the syndromes of congenital and acquired generalized lipodystrophy there seems to exist a group of syndromes which have the following in common:

1. Partial lipodystrophy with a varying pattern between the families but a constant pattern within each family
2. Hyperlipidemia
3. Lipatrophic diabetes in some, but not all affected subjects
4. Dominant inheritance

The lipatrophic diabetes is a facultative symptom in these inherited syndromes which probably arises if other endogenous or exogenous factors superimpose on the genetic background.

In three of the described families (11,25) only female patients were affected (3,5 and 6 individuals respectively). In the family of Brown and Winkelmann (5) three females and four males are affected. No sex distribution is given by Ozer et al. (30).

IV. Progressive Lipodystrophy

These syndromes of partial lipodystrophy have to be separated from another syndrome often called partial lipodystrophy. Better names for this syndrome are progressive lipodystrophy, cephalothoracic lipodystrophy, or Barraquer-Simons disease. This syndrome is somewhat more common (>200 cases published), usually develops in childhood, and has a female to male ratio of 4:1. In this syndrome quite often a definite illness precedes the onset of fat loss and there is a high incidence of various renal disorders (13,15,18,20,38,47). A defect of complement has been claimed as cause of this syndrome (27,33,38,47). Diabetes has often been described in partial lipodystrophy, but it is not nearly as common as in total lipodystrophy and is usually not characterized by the high degree of insulin resistance and the lack of ketosis. This syndrome is most probably of nongenetic origin. In three cases a familial occurrence has been claimed (2,21,44), but all of these do not stand a critical evaluation (38). This syndrome has only been mentioned to illustrate the difference between this type of partial lipodystrophy and the group of genetic syndromes given above which are associated with lipatrophic diabetes.

Summary

Lipatrophic diabetes is a clinically well-defined type of diabetes mellitus which is characterized by a partial or total absence of adipose tissue, severe hyperlipidemia, insulin-resistant diabetes without ketoacidosis, hepatomegaly and elevated basal metabolic rate. It does not represent a homogenous genetic entity but may be subdivided as follows:

1. A recessively inherited syndrome (congenital generalized lipodystrophy)
2. A nongenetic syndrome (acquired generalized lipodystrophy)
3. A group of dominantly inherited syndromes (various types of partial lipodystrophy)

References

1. Bamatter, F.: Leprechaunisme. Rec. Méd. Suisse Rom. 84, 494 (1964)

2. Barraquer Ferré, L.: Pathogenesis of progressive cephalothoracic lipodystrophy. J. Nerv. Ment. Dis. 109, 113 (1949)

3. Berardinelli, W.: An undiagnosed endocrinometabolic syndrome: report of 2 cases. J. Clin. Endocr. 14, 193 (1954)

4. Boudin, G., De Gennes, J.L., Pépin, B., Barraine, R., Saltiel, H.: Diabète lipo-atrophique avec manifestations neurologiques. Bull. Soc. Méd. Paris 114, 895 (1963)

5. Brown, J., Winkelmann, R.K.: Acanthosis nigricans: Study of 90 cases. Medicine (Baltimore) 47, 33 (1968)

6. Brubaker, M.M., Levam, N.E., Collipp, P.J.: Acanthosis nigricans and congenital total lipodystrophy. Arch. Derm. 91, 320 (1965)

7. Brunzell, J.D., Shankle, S.W., Bethune, J.E.: Congenital generalized lipodystrophy accompanied by cystic angiomatosis. Ann. Intern. Med. 69, 501 (1968)

8. Craig, J.W., Miller, M.: Lipoatrophic diabetes. In: Diabetes. Williams, R.H (ed.). New York: Hoeber, 1960

9. Davis, J., Feiwel, M.: Lipoatrophy, gigantism, and hyperlipemia with xanthomatosis and acanthosis nigricans. Brit. J. Derm. 69, 229 (1957)

10. De Gennes, J.L., Saltiel, H., Trémolières, J., Apfelbaum, M., Laudat, P.: Révision de l'exploration métabolique et endocrinienne d'un cas de diabète lipo-atrophique. Presse Méd. 75, 2605 (1967)

11. Dunnigan, M.G., Cochrane, M.A., Kelly, A., Scott, J.W.: Familial lipoatrophic diabetes with dominant transmission. J. of Med. 49, 33 (1974)

12. Fosbrooke, A.S., Segall, M.M.: Observations on fat and carbohydrate metabolism in generalized lipodystrophy. Biochem. J. 112, 33 (1969)

13. Fowler, P.B.S.: D.M. Lipodystrophia progressiva and temporary hydronephrosis. Brit. Med. J. I, 1249 (1955)

14. Frederickson, D.S., Lees, R.S.: A system for phenotyping hyperlipoproteinemia. Circulation 31, 321 (1965)

15. Gellis, S.S., Green, S., Walker, D.: Chronic renal disease in children with lipodystrophy. Amer. J. Dis. Childh. 96, 605 (1958)

16. Gordon, H., Pimstone, B.L., Leary, M., Gorson, W.: Congenital generalized lipodystrophy with abnormal growth hormone homeostasis. Arch. Derm. 104, 551 (1971)

17. Hamwi, G.J., Kruger, F.A., Eymontt, M.J., Scarpelli, D.G., Gwinup, G., Byron, R.: Lipoatrophic diabetes. Diabetes 15, 262 (1966)

18. Hamza, M., Levy, M., Broyer, M., Habib, R.: Deux cas de glomérulo-néphrite membrano-proliférative avec lipodystrophie partielle de type facio-tronculaire. J. d'Urol. Néphol. 76, 1032 (1970)

19. Hansen, A.E., McQuarrie, I.: Serum and tissue lipids in a peculiar type of generalized lipodystrophy (lipohistiodiaresis). Amer. J. Dis. Childh. 60, 754 (1940)

20. Horton, B.T., Emmett, J.L.: A typical syndrome in uremia; lipodystrophy involving lower extremities. Med. Clin. N. Amer. 15 1505 (1932)

21. Igersheimer, W.W.: Progressive lipodystrophy. Amer. J. Dis. Childh. 75, 206 (1948)

22. Jeménez-Diaz, C., Rodriguez-Minon, J.L., Arrieta, F.: El sindrome de lipodistrofia, esteatosis hepatica y diabetes resistente. Rec. Clin. Esp. 86, 9 (1962)

23. Jolliff, J.W., Craig, J.W.: Lipoatrophic diabetes and mental illness in three siblings. Diabetes 16, 708 (1967)

24. Köbberling, J., Willms, B., Kattermann, R., Creutzfeldt, W.: Diabetes mellitus und familiäre partielle Lipoatrophie. 2. Intern. Donau-Symposium über Diabetes Mellitus. Verl. d. Wien. Med. Akad., 1971, p. 427

25. Köbberling, J., Willms, B., Kattermann, R., Creutzfeldt, W.: Lipodystrophy of the extremities. A dominantly inherited syndrome associated with lipatrophic diabetes. Humangenetik 29, 111 (1975)

26. Lawrence, R.D.: Lipodystrophy and hepatomegaly with diabetes, lipaemia, and other metabolic disturbances. Lancet I, 724 (1946)

27. Ljunghall, S., Fjellström, K.E., Wibell, L.: Partial lipodystrophy and chromic hypocomplementemic glomerulonephritis. Acta Med. Scand. 195, 493 (1974)

28. Marcus, R.: Retinopathy, nephropathy, and neuropathy in lipoatrophic diabetes. Diabetes 15, 351 (1966)

29. Miyahara, R., Tsutamura, C., Sugihara, M.: A case of generalized lipodystrophy. Hiroshima J. Med. Sci. 14, 31 (1965)

30. Ozer, F.L., Lichtenstein, J.R., Kwiterovich, P.O., McKusik, V.A.: A "new" variety of lipodystrophy. Clin. Res. 21, 533 (1973)

31. Pachioli, R., Olivi, O., Genova, R.: La lipidistrofia, un quadro di paniperpituitarismo anteriore nell'infanzia. Minerva Pediat. 18, 1387 (1966)

32. Pavel, I., Cimpeanu, S., Nicolesco, M., Bonaparte, H., Petrovici, G., Stoian, N.: Le diabète lipo-atrophique est-il un diabète lipidique? Presse Méd. 71, 1279 (1963)

33. Peters, D.K., Charlesworth, J.A., Sissons, J.G.P., Williams, D.G., Boulton-Jones, J.M., Evans, D.J.: Mesangiocapillary nephritis, parital lipodystrophy, and hypocomplementemi. Lancet II, 535 (1973)

34. Pieragostini, P., Girotti, F., Midulla, M.: Lipodistrofia e gigantismo in un bambino con tumore endocranico. Minerva Pediat. 21, 1836 (1969)

35. Pierron, H., Perrimond, H., Orsini, A.: Lipoatrophie généralisée chez un enfant de trois ans par tumeur diencéphalique. Arch. Franc. Pédiat. 24, 827 (1967)

36. Reed, W.B., Dexter, R., Corley, C., Fish, C.: Congenital lipodystrophic diabetes with acanthosis nigricans. The Seip-Lawrence syndrome. Arch. Derm. 91, 326 (1965)

37. Reed, W.B., Ragsdale, W., Curtis, A.C., Richards, H.J.: Acanthosis nigricans in association with various genodermatosis. With emphasis on lipodystrophic diabetes and Prader-Willi syndrome. Acta Derm. Veneorol. 48, 465 (1968)

38. Reichel, W., Köbberling, J., Fischbach, H., Scheler, F.: Membranoprolipherative glomerulonephritis with partial lipodystrophy. Discordant occurrence in identical twins. Klin. Wschr. 54, 75 (1976)

39. Schwartz, R., Schafer, I.A., Renold, A.E.: Generalized lipoatrophy, hepatic cirrhosis, disturbed carbohydrate metabolism and accelerated growth (lipoatrophic diabetes). Amer. J. Med. 28, 973 (1960)

40. Seip, M.: Lipodystrophy and gigantism with associated endocrine manifestations. A new diencephalic syndrome? Acta Paediat. Scand. 48, 555 (1959)

41. Seip, M.: Generalized Lipodystrophy. Ergebnisse der inneren Medizin und Kinderheilkunde. Heidelberg: Springer-Verlag, 1971, Vol. XXXI, p. 59

42. Seip, M., Trygstad, O.: Generalized lipodystrophy. Arch. Dis. Childh. 38, 447 (1963)

43. Senior, B., Gellis, S.S.: The syndromes of total lipodystrophy and of partial lipodystrophy. Pediatrics 33, 593 (1964)

44. Taylor, W.B., Honeycutt, W.M.: Progressive lipodystrophy and lipoatrophic diabetes. Arch. Derm. 84, 31 (1961)

45. Torikai, T., Fukuchi, S., Sasaki, C., Ishigaki, J., Isawa, K., Suzuki, A., Namiki, T., Hashimoto, N., Hashimoto, S.: Two sibling cases with lipoatrophic diabetes. Endocr. Jap. 12, 197 (1965)

46. Tourniaire, J., Guinet, P., Mornex, R., Veyrat, A., Magnien, J.M.: Diabète lipoatrophique. Etude clinique et biologique d'un cas atypique. Bull. Soc. Méd. Paris 44, 3289 (1968)

47. Williams, D.G., Scopes, J.W., Peters, D.K.: Hypocomplementaemic membranoproliferative glomerulonephritis and nephrotic syndrome associated with partial lipodystrophy of the face and trunk. Proc. Roy. Soc. Med. 65, 591 (1972)

48. Ziegler, L.H.: Lipodystrophies: report of 7 cases. Brain 51, 147 (1928)

Addendum

After going to press a further family with partial lipodystrophy, lipatrophic diabetes, and dominant inheritance has been described (Davidson, M.B., Young, R.T.: Metabolic studies in familial partial lipodystrophy of the lower trunk and extremities. Diabetologia 11, 561 (1975)). The habitus that runs in this family and the metabolic disturbances closely resemble the syndrome described by Köbberling et al.(25). Although 5 male family members are diabetic the lipatrophic syndrome seems to be confined to 8 female patients.

17. Hereditary Hyperglycemic Syndromes in Laboratory Rodents

W. STAUFFACHER, R. KIKKAWA, M. AMHERDT, and L. ORCI

The subject of the hereditary hyperglycemic syndromes occurring in laboratory rodents and of their potential usefulness as "models" for the study of human diabetes has received much attention in recent years. Thus, at least three entire workshops and several extensive reviews were devoted to this topic during the last few years (1,2,9,14,15,17, 20). For this reason, the present discussion will be limited to a brief review of current knowledge concerning the genetic transmission of some of the animal syndromes and to a description of their clinical course and of insulin-secretory patterns and pancreatic anomalies apparently characteristic for some of them. Finally, these observations will be related to more recent findings suggesting that such apparent pancreatic anomalies need not to be the primary hereditary defect responsible for the occurrence of the syndrome but that they may merely represent a characteristic feature of the genetic background of the animal carrying the "diabetogenic" gene (9,12).

Mode of Inheritance of Hyperglycemic Syndromes

Table 1 summarizes the current understanding of the mode of inheritance of the hyperglycemic syndromes most frequently mentioned in the available literature. It shows that, in a first group of animals, a single autosomal dominant or recessive gene appears to be responsible for the occurrence of the syndrome while the interplay of a number of hereditary components seems to be necessary for hyperglycemia to occur in a second group. This has been most convincingly demonstrated for the Chinese hamster as is discussed in Chapter 19, and the metabolic fate of which appears to be governed by at least four genes, two of which are required for hyperglycemia to occur, and three or four for the development of a syndrome resembling ketosis-prone youth-onset diabetes of man. The animal most recently added to this list is the South African hamster, the syndrome of which bears some similarities with that of the Chinese hamster and seems to be inherited in a polygenic, non-sex-linked pattern (18,19).

The third group comprises animal strains in which "spontaneous" hyperglycemic syndromes occurred when they were transfered from their natural habitat in arid, semi-desert regions where food is scarce and available only at the cost of considerable physical activity, to laboratories where they were fed with calory-rich laboratory chow. Although some evidence suggests that hereditary factors may participate in the pathogenesis of these syndromes too, this has thus far not been clearly established and the type of transmission or the mode of inheritance is still entirely unknown.

Table 1. Hyperglycemic syndromes in rodents: genetic transmission[a]

Animal strain (gene denomination)	Mode of inheritance
1. Single-gene mutants	
Yellow (A^y + variants)	dominant
Obese (ob)	recessive
Adipose (ad)	recessive
Diabetes (db)	recessive
2. Inbred strains and hybrids	
New Zealand obese = NZO	polygenic
KK, Toronto - KK	polygenic
Cricetulus griseus (Chinese hamster)	polygenic
Mystromys albicaudatus (South African hamster)	polygenic
3. Hereditary (?) with strong environmental component	
Acomys cahirinus (spiny mouse)	unknown
Psammomys obesus (sand rat)	unknown
Ctenomys tolarum (tuco-tuco)	unknown

[a] Modified from (5).

The Clinical Course of the Hyperglycemic Syndromes

In Table 2 the animals are grouped according to the metabolic characteristics of their syndromes. For the sake of simplicity, and not with
the intention to imply identity, the animal syndromes are given desig-
nations usually employed in describing obesity and diabetes in man:

Table 2. Hyperglycemic syndromes in rodents: "clinical picture"

Animal strains	Type of syndrome[a]		
	O	AOD	JD
Yellow	+	−	−
Obese	+	−	−
Adipose	+	−	−
NZO	+	+	−
KK, T-KK	+	+	−
Diabetes	−	+	+
Cricetulus griseus	−	−	+
Mystromy albicaudatus	−	−	+
Acomys cahirinus	+[b]	+	+
Psammomys obesus	+	+	+
Gnenomys tolarum	+	+	+

[a] Abbreviations denoting a certain similarity of the animal syndrome with human
obesity or diabtes: O = obesity; AOD = adult-onset diabetes; JD = juvenile diabetes.
[b] Obesity apparently not associated with hyperinsulinemia.

thus, "O" stands for obesity associated with glucose intolerance or mild hyperglycemia; "AOD" stands for "adult-onset diabetes" and indicates syndromes usually, but not necessarily, associated with obesity; hyperglycemia is more consistent and more severe than in the first group, but absolute insulin deficiency and ketoacidotic decompensation do not occur. "JD" stands for juvenile diabetes and is used for those syndromes in which true insulin deficiency and ketoacidosis do occur. It may be seen that in some animal strains all three types of clinical evolution are encountered. This does not necessarily imply progression from obesity to ketosis-prone diabetes; although such progression does occur, the evolution may also come to a permanent halt at any point. Equally, JD does not imply that all animals so classified die from keto-acidosis: indeed, ketoacidosis is extremely rare in the diabetic (dbdb) mouse although the animals are usually severely hyperglycemic and loose weight; in addition, and as discussed in Chapter 19, certain sublines of Chines hamsters never do develop ketoacidosis although the animals fulfill the other criteria of juvenile diabetes, in that they are lean and markedly hyperglycemic.

In general, the observations summarized in Table 2 suggest that the currently known hyperglycemic syndromes of rodents may be subdivided into three groups: in the first, obesity is the predominant feature and severe hyperglycemia is not seen; in the second, obesity and marked hyperglycemia are frequently associated, but insulin deficiency as evidenced by the occurrence of weight loss and ketoacidosis does not occur; the third group comprises those animals in which true insulin-deficiency diabetes and ketoacidosis may occur.

Insulin Secretion and B-Cell Anomalies

In view of the obvious implication of the pancreatic B-cell in glucose homeostasis and in the pathogenesis of hyperglycemic syndromes, and since a distinct anomaly of the kinetics of insulin secretion (deficient "early phase" of insulin release) is considered by some to represent the genetic anomaly responsible for human diabetes (7), the analysis of the kinetics of insulin release in animals with spontaneously occur-ring hyperglycemic syndromes has received much attention in recent years (3,4,5,6,10,11).

Some of the more relevant data presented in these studies are summarized in Table 3, in which the obese (obob) mouse exemplifies those syndromes in which obesity is the predominant feature, the NZO mouse those in which obesity is associated with more marked hyperglycemia (AOD of Table 2), and the "misty" type of the diabetic (dbdb) mouse and those strains of Acomys Cahirinus in which true insulin deficiency does occur.

Table 3 shows that in control animals (Swiss Albino and C57BL-mice), glucose induces a rapid early phase of insulin release followed by a transient decline of insulin concentrations and a prolonged secondary rise which lasts as long as glucose concentrations are elevated. This pattern is entirely comparable to that seen in normal man. In the other animals used, distinct and reproducible patterns of insulin secretion can be observed: In the obese (obob) mouse, baseline insulin concentra-tions are elevated, insulin secretion is kinetically normal but quanti-tatively enhanced relative to the prevailing glucose concentration and to the values measured in control animals (5).

In the NZO mouse, baseline values of plasma insulin (IRI) are elevated, but glucose-induced early-phase insulin release appears to be diminished, while during the late phase, insulin concentrations rise markedly (6).

This pattern is very much reminiscent of that seen in human adult-onset diabetes.

Table 3. Plasma IRI baseline levels and glucose-induced IRI responses[a]

Animal strain	Age (weeks)	IRI levels and responses		
		Baseline	early phase	late phase
Swiss albino (control)	12	N	N	N
C-57 Bl (control)	8	N	N	N
Obese	8	+++	+++	+++
NZO	16-30	++	-	++
Diabetes (misty)	7	+	+++	++
"	12	++	++	++
"	18	++	-	+
"	30	+	-	-
Acomys cahirinus	7-20	N	-	N

[a] Legend:
  N = normal response;
  + = slightly elevated levels or exaggerated responses;
 ++ = moderately elevated levels or exaggerated responses;
+++ = greatly elevated levels or exaggerated responses;
  - = diminished response from given baseline.
(Modified from 13,14,15,16)

In the diabetic mouse (dbdb), the pattern of insulin release varies with age and with the degree of glucose intolerance: in young animals, the kinetics of insulin release are normal with a rapid early rise and a clear-cut secondary phase; as the animals becomse older, baseline insulin levels become more and more elevated, and insulin secretion above this baseline is progressively blunted. In still older animals, baseline levels of IRI decrease again but no further secretory response above this baseline can be provoked (5).

In Acomys Cahirinus, at all ages and independent of the degree of obesity, the early phase of insulin release is blunted while the secondary phase is comparable to that observed in the control mice (3,10). This pattern has recently been confirmed with in vitro studies in which isolated islets obtained from spiny mice were perfused with solutions containing various concentrations of glucose (11). In general, these data indicate that insulin secretion is kinetically normal in those syndromes of which obesity is the predominant feature and somehow defective in those syndromes in which hyperglycemia is more severe. Only in the diabetic (dbdb) and the spiny mouse have attempts been made to study insulin release during the early phases of the syndrome. These experiments have clearly shown that deficient insulin secretion is not an early feature of the diabetic syndrome of dbdb mice while, in Acomys cahirinus, it can be detected prior to the occurrence of hyperglycemia.

The ultrastructural features of the B-cells of the animal strains discussed here have been described in detail (4,16) and will only be summarized here:

The B-cells of the obese (obob) mouse show signs of high functional activity but no abnormal cytological features. In the B-cells of the diabetic (dbdb) mice a progressive dilatation of the cisternae of the rough endoplasmic reticulum (RER) becomes evident as hyperglycemia progresses and insulin release becomes abnormal. The picture seen in severely hyperglycemic animals is compatible with the existence of an imbalance between the relative functional capacities of the RER and the Golgi complex in favor of the former. It is currently unknown whether the dilatation of the RER by newly synthesized material reflects the fact that the function of the Golgi complex is normally a rate-limiting step in the elaboration of insulin, or whether an abnormal limitation of the capacity of the Golgi complex is a feature of primary pathogenetic importance for the ultimate arrest of B-cell function in the dbdb mouse. Whatever the answer may be, detailed examination at the ultrastructural level suggests that in the B-cell of the diabetic mouse, a process preceding the actual release of insulin is defective. This interpretation is compatible with the observation that, in young dbdb mice, insulin release is kinetically normal although quantitatively excessive.

The ultrastructural evidence indicative of an impairment of insulin secretion in Acomys cahirinus includes the consistent feature of high granularity of the B-cells, the frequent occurrence of lysosomal digestion of secretory granules, and the unique feature of massive glycogen infiltration of still well-granulated B-cells observed in severely diabetic spiny mice, the pancreas of which still contains considerable amounts of insulin (Table 4 and Figs. 1 and 2). The cause or causes of this impairment are still unknown and may include a lack of autonomic innervation or a deficiency in the microtubular-microfilamentous system involved in the intracellular translocation and the ultimate release of granular insulin (13). Thus, both biological and morphological evidence suggests that in spiny mice, an impairment of insulin secretion represents an early feature of the hyperglycemic syndrome and that its occurrence precedes that of hyperglycemia.

Table 4. Plasma glucose, plasma IRI, and pancreas IRI of age- and weight-matched glucosuric and nondiabetic spiny mice

	Animal No.	Body weight (g)	Plasma glucose (mg/100 ml)	Plasma IRI (µU/ml)	Pancreas IRI (mU/mg)
Controls:	1	75	142	10	83
	2	44	122	12	22
	3	77	105	15	47
	4	79	123	12	-a
	5	78	98	10	32
Glucosuric:	6	78	312	4	21
	7[b]	54	529	4	15
	8	71	463	15	20
	9[c]	80	173	12	49
	10[c]	57	120	4	26

[a] Sample lost. [b] Persistently ketonuric. [c] Glucosuric only when fed.

In view of the observations summarized here, one is tempted to conclude that the primary hereditary anomalies responsible for the occurrence of the hyperglycemic syndromes of those animals in which deficiencies of insulin secretion can be demonstrated are located within the B-cell. However, it should be remembered that hyperglycemia may be the phenotypic manifestation of a number of hereditary anomalies, the mode, manner, and time of penetrance of which may in turn be modified by genetic

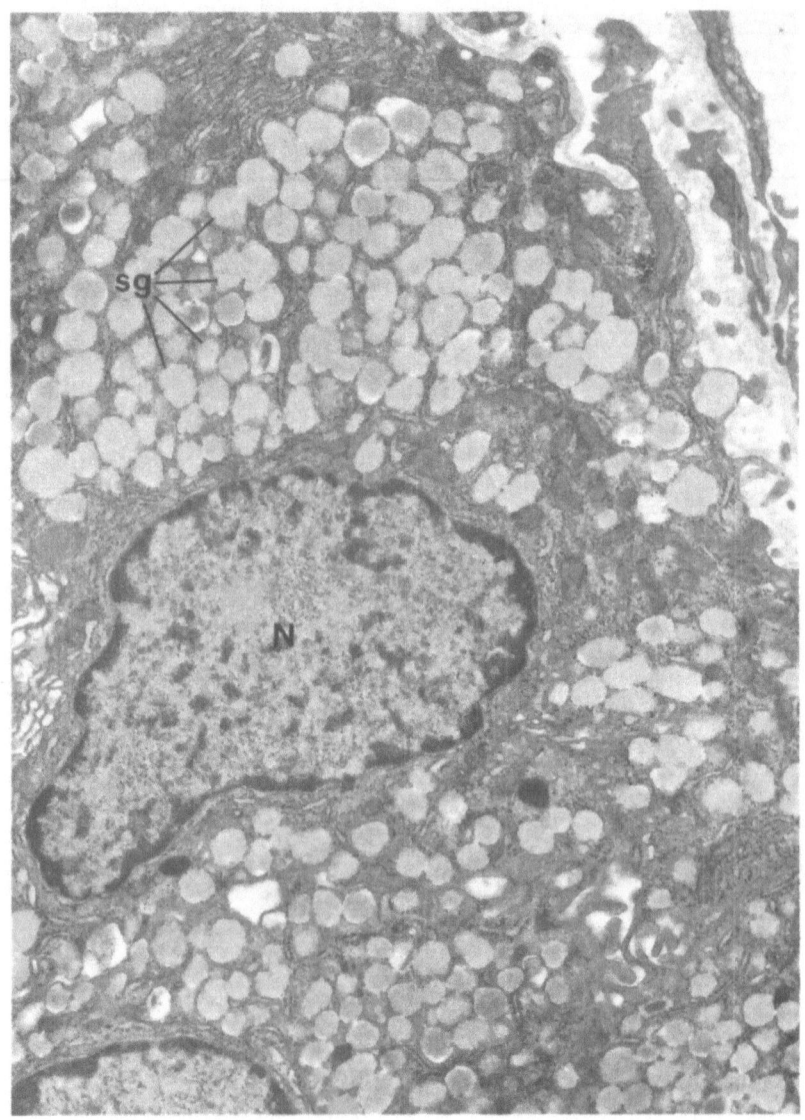

Fig. 1. B-cells of a normoglycemic spiny mouse (age 19 months). B-cells contain numerous secretory granules (sg), mostly of pale type. N = nucleus; X 9,6000

or environmental factors. Indeed, it seems that the time and manner of manifestation of an hereditary hyperglycemic syndrome as well as its clinical course are determined not only by the nature of the genetic defect but also by additional and independent components of the "genetic background" of a given organism. Thus, the experiments recently performed by Hummel and Coleman at the Jackson Laboratories and summarized in Figure 3 indicate that the capacity of the pancreas to compensate for increased insulin demand may be such a component of the genetic background rather than the primary factor responsible for the occurrence of the hyperglycemic syndrome.

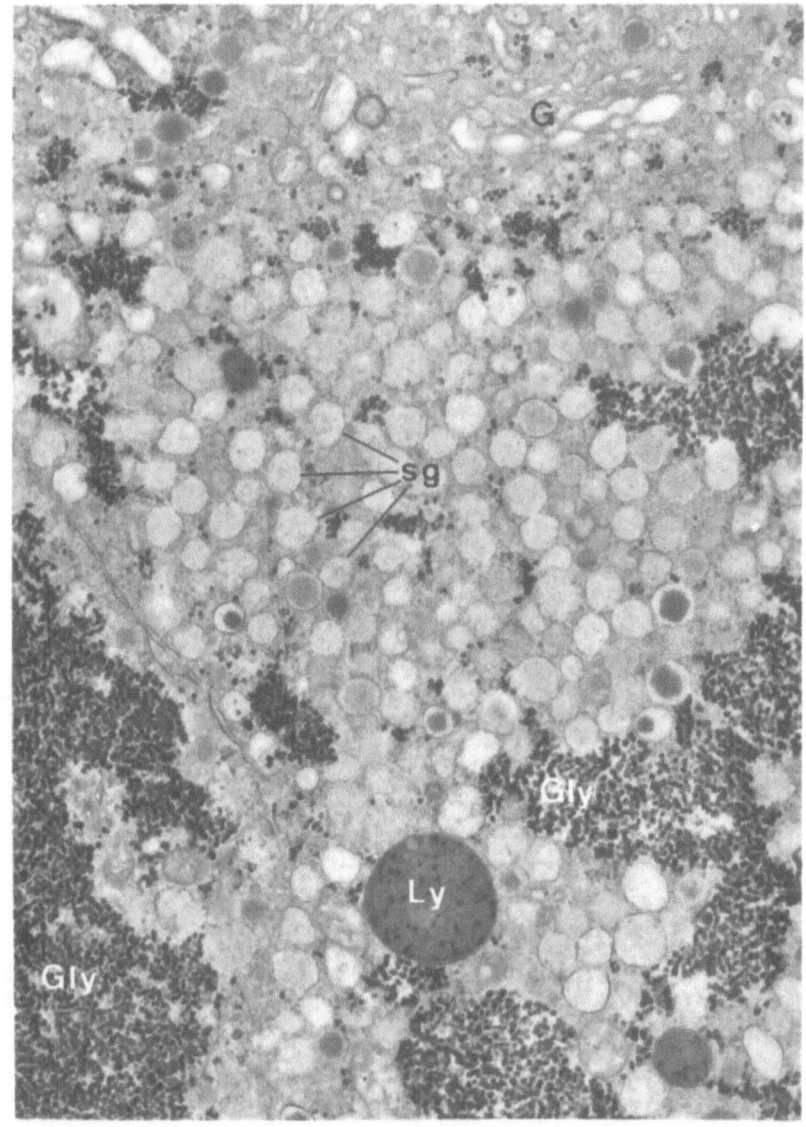

Fig. 2. B-cells of animal No. 7 of Table 4 (ketotic diabetic, age 20 months). Although infiltrated by glycogen (Gly), B-cells still contain appreciable number of secretory granules. G = Golgi comples; Ly = lysosome; X 21,200

These experiments (Fig. 3) can be described as follows: the syndrome of the obese (obob) mouse occurred first in the C57BL/6J strain of mice; the more severely hyperglycemic and insulin-deficient diabetes (dbdb)mutant was discovered in the C57BL/KsJ strain of mice. Hummel and Coleman have succeeded in transferring each of the two genes responsible for the two syndromes into the mouse-strain in which the other one was discovered, i.e., the obese gene into the C57BL/KsJ strain and vice.versa. The results showed that in the new environment the diabetes-gene induced a syndrome predominantly characterized by obesity

161

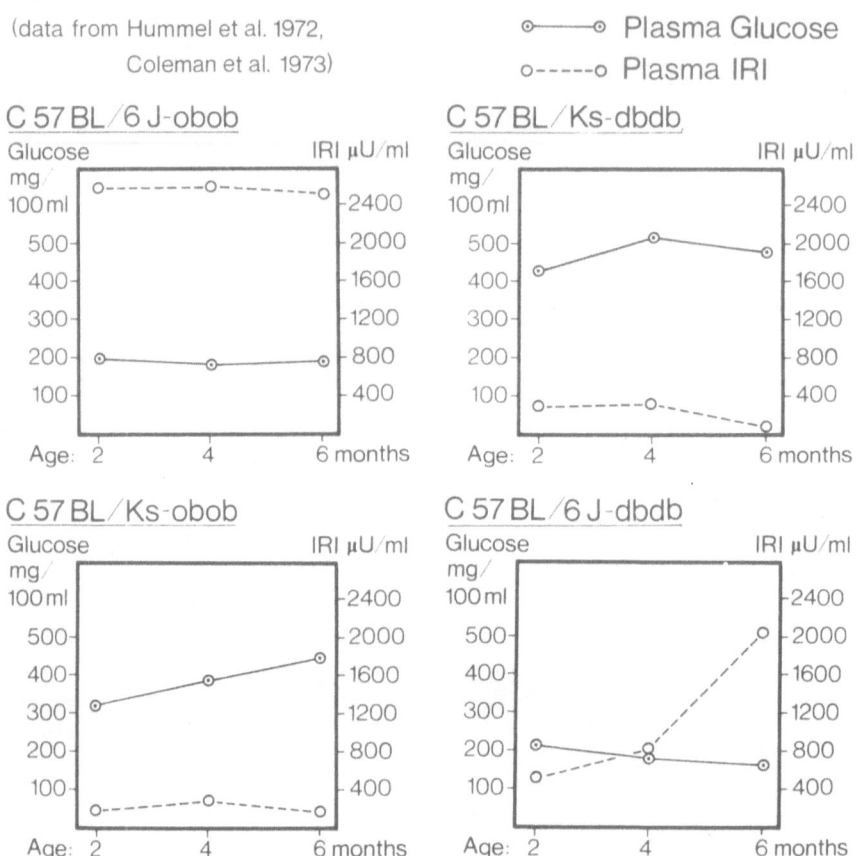

ob AND db GENES ON DIFFERENT GENETIC BACKGROUNDS

(data from Hummel et al. 1972,
Coleman et al. 1973)

o———o Plasma Glucose
o-----o Plasma IRI

Fig. 3. Fed plasma glucose and plasma IRI concentrations at different ages of *obob* (left) and *dbdb* mice when the "diabetogenic" gene develops on the genetic background of the original mouse strain (top panels) or on that on which the other syndrome was originally bred. For explanation, see text. (Redrawn from data of references 8 and 9)

and mild hyperglycemia, whereas the obese gene provoked severe insulin-deficiency diabetes once it was transferred into the C57BL/KsJ strain.

In terms of the present discussion these observations indicate that even apparently well-defined B-cell anomalies need not necessarily be a visible "marker" of a hereditary diabetogenic anomaly but that they may equally well reflect a feature of the background genome of an animal which carries a genetic anomaly imposing an excessive demand for insulin on the organism's B-cells, and which may be entirely unrelated to the pancreas.

These findings certainly do not render any more simple our concepts concerning the hereditary factors responsible for the occurrence of diabetes. However, it is likely that they are closer to the ultimate truth than the simplistic views thus far favored by most of those interested in the pathogenesis and the genetics of diabetes mellitus.

References

1. Bray, G.A., York, D.A.: Genetically transmitted obesity in rodents. Physiol. Rev. 51, 598 (1971)

2. Cameron, D.P., Stauffacher, W., Renold, A.E.: Spontaneous hyperglycemia and obesity in laboratory rodents. In: Handbook of Physiology, Section 7, Steiner, D.F., Freinkel N. (eds.). American Physiological Society, Washington, D.C., Vol. I, p. 611

3. Cameron, D.P., Stauffacher, W., Orci, L., Amherdt, M., Renold, A.E.: Defective immunoreactive insulin secretion in the acomys cahirinus. Diabetes 21, 1060 (1972)

4. Cameron, D.P., Amherdt, M., Orci, L., de Peyer, R., Stauffacher, W.: Biochemical and morphological studies of immunoreactive insulin secretion in spontaneous and acquired obesity and/or hyperglycemia in rodents. Acta Diab. Lat. 9, 89 (1972)

5. Cameron, D.P., Stauffacher, W., Amherdt, M., Orci, L., Renold, A.E.: Kinetics of immunoreactive insulin release in obese hyperglycemic laboratory rodents. Endocrinology 92, 257 (1973)

6. Cameron, D.P., Opat, F., Insch, S.: Studies of immunoreactive insulin secretion in NZO mice in vivo. Diabetologia 10, 649 (1974)

7. Cerasi, E., Luft, R.: Plasma insulin response to glucose infusion in healthy subjects and in diabetes mellitus. Acta Endocrin. 55, 278 (1967)

8. Coleman, D.L., Hummely, K.P.: The influence of genetic background on the expression of the obese (ob) gene in the mouse. Diabetologia 9, 287 (1973)

9. First Brook Lodge Workshop on Diabetes in Laboratory Animals. Diabetologia 3, 63 (1967)

10. Gutzeit, A., Rabinovitch, A., Studer, P.P., Trueheart, P.A., Cerasi, E., Renold, A.E.: Decreased intravenous glucose tolerance and low plasma insulin response in spiny mice (Acomys cahirinus). Diabetologia 10, 667 (1974)

11. Gutzeit, A., Rabinovitch, D., Karakch, C., Stauffacher, W., Renold, A.E., Cerasi, E.: Evidence for decreased sensitivity to glucose of isolated islets from spiny mice (Acomys cahirinus). Diabetologia 10, 661 (1974)

12. Hummel, K.P., Coleman, D.L., Lane, P.W.: The influence of genetic background on expression of mutations at the diabetes locus in the mouse. I C57CL/Ks3 and C57BL/6J strains. Biochem. Genetics 7, 1 (1972)

13. Renold, A.E., Cameron, D.P., Amherdt, M., Stauffacher, W., Marliss, E., Orci, L., Rouiller, C.: Endocrine-metabolic anomalies in rodents with hyperglycemic syndromes of hereditary and/or environmental origin. In: Impact of Insulin on Metabolic Pathways, Shafrir, E. (ed.). London-New York: Akademic Press, 1972, p. 15

14. Malaisse-Lagae, F., Ravazzola, M., Amherdt, M., Gutzeit, A., Stauffacher, W., Malaisse, W.J., Orci, L.: An apparent abnormality of the B-cell microtubular system in spiny mice (Acomys cahirinus). Diabetologia II, 71 (1975)

15. Second Brook Lodge Workshop on Spontaneous Diabetes in Laboratory Animals. Diabetologia 6, 154 (1970)

16. Stauffacher, W., Orci, L., Amherdt, M., Burr, I.M., Balant, L., Froesch, E.R., Renold, A.E.: Metabolic state, pancreatic insulin content and B-cell morphology of normoglycemic spiny mice (Acomys cahirinus): indications for an impairment of insulin secretion. Diabetologia 6, 330 (1970)

17. Stauffacher, W., Orci, L., Cameron, D.P., Burr, I.M., Renold, R.A.: Spontaneous hyperglycemia and/or obesity in laboratory rodents: an example of the possible usefulness of animal disease models with both genetic and environmental components. Rec. Progr. Horm. Res. 27, 41 (1971)

18. Stuhlmann, R.A., Packer, J.T., Doyle, R.E.: Spontaneous diabetes mellitus in Mystromys albicaudatus: repeated values from 620 animals. Diabetes 21, 715 (1972)

19. Stuhlmann, R.A., Srivastava, P.K., Schmidt, G., Vorbeck, M.L., Townsend, J.F.: Characterization of diabetes mellitus in South African Hamster (Mystromys albicaudatus). Diabetologia 10, 685 (1974)

20. Third Brook Lodge Workshop on Spontaneous Diabetes in Laboratory Animals. Diabetologia 10, 491 (1974)

Supported in part by the Fonds National Suisse de la Recherche Scientifique (grants Nr.3.060.73 and 3.0310.73) and by grants-in-aid through the Fondation Emile Barell, F. Hoffmann - La Roche Basel and the Fondation Sandoz for the advancement of medical research.

18. Environmental Influences on the Manifestation of Diabetes Mellitus in Chinese Hamsters

G. C. Gerritsen, M. C. Blanks, F. L. Schmidt, and W. E. Dulin

It is well known that external and internal environmental factors can influence the development of diabetes mellitus if the proper genotype is present. Such factors as obesity (6,19,43) and diet (12,13,65), as well as age, hormones, drugs, and liver disorders (57) can affect glucose tolerance. Even in monozygotic twins, who have identical genotypes, there is a high degree of discordance in a variety of parameters associated with diabetes (7,36-39,47,54,63,64).

Studies on the interaction of environmental and genetic factors in man are difficult since diabetes is difficult to predict because the basic genetic lesion or lesions are unknown and environmental factors are difficult to control. The Chinese hamster may be a useful tool since it exhibits many of the characteristics of human diabetes mellitus, as shown in Table 1. If we can understand the genetic contribution to hyperglycemia in the hamster and determine the environmental factors which contribute to the pathogenesis of diabetes, it may give us valuable information for planning human studies.

Methods

Various types of Chinese hamsters used for the studies reported in this paper are defined in Table 2. All animals were maintained on Purina mouse breeder chow ad lib. and housed individually. Starting at 15 days of age, hamsters are continuously tested for glycosuria by Testape monthly (biweekly prior to 1973). After a maximun 4+ testape test, animals were tested biweekly for ketonuria by Ketostix.

Bleeding techniques, blood sugar determination, and oral glucose tolerance testing (1.5 g/kg) have been described (29).

The effect of diet composition and restriction on blood sugar and body weight was studied in diabetes. One diet was Purina mouse chow, which had 12.4% fat, 16.3% protein, and 56% carbohydrate with a caloric value of 4.0 cal/g. The other diet was Purina rat chow which had a lower fat content, of 7.1%. In addition it contained 29.2% protein and 42.4% carbohydrate, with a caloric values of 3.5 cal/g. These diets were fed ad lib and at restricted levels of 2.5 g/day. During ad lib. feeding food consumption was measured by the difference between food placed in cage and food not consumed.

Identification of the prediabetic newborn Chinese hamster and hyperphagia (40% increase in food consumption) in this animal prior to development of glycosuria have been described (30,31). The effect of diet limitation on hyperphagic prediabetic Chinese hamsters has been reported (32,35). All prediabetics used in these studies had ketotic dams and sires while nonprediabetic control pups were as defined in Table 2. In initial studies, prediabetic and nonprediabetic controls of similar

Table 1. Summary of Changes in Diabetic Chinese Hamsters

Parameters	Results	Reference Numbers
Blood sugar	Variable	29
OGTT	Abnormal	29
Responses to Sulfonylureas	Mild yes, Severe no	28
Ketosis	Yes	29
Onset	Variable	56
Plasma insulin	Decreased	20
Pancreatic insulin	Decreased	20
Insulin release in vitro	Decreased	8,27,37
Insulin synthesis in vitro	Decreased	8
B-cell granulation	Decreased	5,45
Glucose production from pyruvate	Increased	9
Hepatic gluconeogenic enzymes	Increased	9
Hepatic glycolytic enzymes	Decreased	9
Glucose utilization fat	Normal	29
Glucose utilization muscle	Normal	29
Insulin sensitivity	Normal	22
Body composition	Not obese	33,34
Retinal lesions	Yes	26,60,61
Kidney lesions	Yes	61,58,17
Neurologic lesions	Yes	46,55
Sorbitol in lens and nerve	Elevated	40
Vascular changes	Yes	16,11,49
Mode of inheritance	Any 2 of 4 homozygous recessive genes	3,4
Sexes affected	Both	34
Prediction of diabetes	Yes	30

Table 2. Definitions of Chinese Hamsters

Stage Inbreeding F >	Type	Definitions
9	Nondiabetic	No. + Testape results; no diabetic relatives for > 8 inbred generations
8	Aglycosuric	No. + Testape results but diabetic siblings
8	Trace	Intermittant 1 + testape
12	Diabetic	Consistent 4 + Testape for >4 months
-	Ketonuric	Consistent Ketostix rating of "large" for >2 months
-	Prediabetic	Animals which are genetically diabetic but have not exhibited glycosuria or hyperglycemia but ultimately will

birth weight and litter size were compared for growth rate, blood sugar, plasma insulin, and pancreatic insulin. Fat, protein, and solids were also determined on eviscerated carcasses at 15 and 25 days of age. The specific methods for these determinations have been reported (35). In all studies, weights of dams were similar (±2 g) as were weights of all sires (±2 g). This was important since large parents tend to have larger pups than small parents.

The effect of hyperphagia on the change from the prediabetic to the diabetic state was studied by limiting the diet of prediabetics from: (1) birth to 150 days, (2) birth to weaning, and (3) weaning to 30 months of age. Food intake was limited during the preweaning period by fostering one-half of each prediabetic litter into nondiabetic litters to make large heterogeneous litters consisting of 2 prediabetic plus 5 nondiabetic pups. Prediabetic litters averaged 4 pups while nondiabetic litters were adjusted to 5. Thus, 2 prediabetics were fostered into the nondiabetic litters and forced to compete with the 5 nondiabetic pups, while their 2 prediabetic siblings were left with their natural mother and did not have to compete for available nutrition. After weaning, diet limitation to within normal range was accomplished by feeding fostered prediabetics 2.5 g/day of Purina mouse chow. Nonfostered prediabetic siblings were allowed food ad lib.

In the initial fostering and diet limitation studies, prediabetics were switched from 2.5 g/day to nonrestricted feeding at 150 days of age. This was done to prove that they were actually prediabetic, since it had been shown that Chinese hamsters in the Upjohn colony either develop glycosuria by 5 months or remain free of it for life (33,56).

In order to study the possible effect of the ketotic uterine environment on the development of diabetes in the prediabetic Chinese hamster pup, ovarian transplant techniques were developed by one of us (56a). The ovary of the ketotic was transplanted to a nondiabetic. The nondiabetic with the genetic ketotic ovary was bred to a ketotic male to produce pups with a diabetic genotype from the normal uterine environment. These animals have been compared with similar genotypes born from the ketotic uterus for growth rate, food consumption, onset of glycosuria, and ketonuria.

Results

Since it was unrealistic to make repetitive blood sugar measurements on large numbers of very small animals, testing for glycosuria was used as an end point for genetic studies and classification of animals. It appears that glycosuria is an acceptable end point since it correlates well with blood sugar (Table 3).

In Figure 1, the offspring of F-2 diabetic siblings of the PG subline were diabetic, trace, and nondiabetic. Similar phenotypes were also produced by crosses of F-2 nondiabetic siblings of the PG sublines and F-5 siblings of the L subline (Fig. 2).

Due to the heterogeneity observed within litters regardless of parent type, selection against diabetes and inbreeding was done. The results presented in Figure 3 show that nondiabetic sublines of Chinese hamsters have been produced by continuous brother-sister mating for 10 and 12 generations. These animals have no glycosuria in their lines for the past 10 generations. They breed true for the nondiabetic trait. However, at comparable stages of inbreeding, diabetic-producing sublines still display considerable phenotypic heterogeneity in offspring (Fig. 4).

However, those animals identified as aglycosurics (Fig. 4) had abnormal
glucose tolerance.

Table 3. Correlation of blood sugar with glycosuria and ketonuria in the Chinese
hamster (reproduced from Dulin and Gerritsen (1972))

No. of animals	Urine test[a] by TesTape and Ketotix	Fasting blood sugar[b] (mg%)	Range
155	negative	96 ± 12	60.132[c]
46	4+glycosuria	243 ± 11	128.383[d]
50	heavy ketonuria	326 ± 8	226.428

[a] Tested every 2 weeks.
[b] Tested when glycosuric and/or ketonuric.
[c] All but 7 were less than 120 mg %.
[d] All but 3 were greater than 150 mg %.

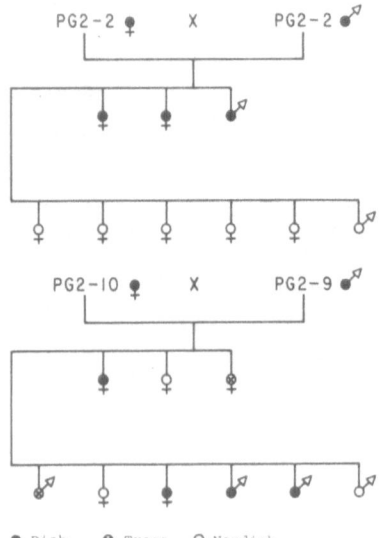

● Diab.   ◉ Trace   ○ Nondiab.

Fig. 1. Type of offspring from diabetic X diabetic cross
(reproduced from Gerritsen *et al.*, 1970)

It was possible that environmental factors such as diet might play a
role in the phenotypic heterogeneity observed in litters from inbred
diabetic parents such as those presented in Figure 4. Blood sugar of
diabetic Chinese hamsters was decreased when caloric intake was reduced
by: (1) limiting the diet to 2.5 g of mouse chow, (2) ad lib. rat chow,
or (3) 2.5 g of rat chow per day (Fig. 5). The fall in blood sugar was
more rapid in the animals fed rat chow ad lib. than in those fed 2.5 g
of mouse chow even though the caloric intake in the group on ad lib.
rat chow was 50% greater (Fig. 5). The greatest blood sugar decrease
was observed in the group on 2.5 g rat chow per day. It should be noted
that caloric intake was lowest in this group. Further, it should be
pointed out that blood sugar was reduced but not normalized by caloric
restriction.

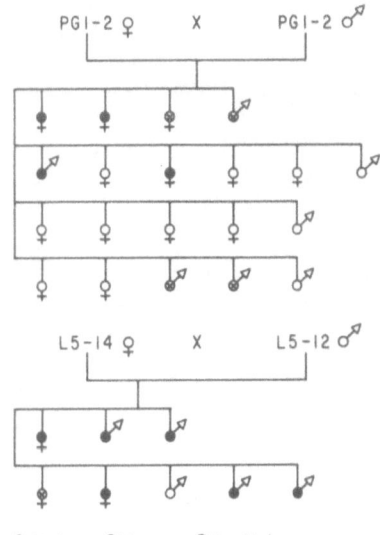

Fig. 2. Type of offspring from nondiabetic X
nondiabetic cross (reproduced from Gerritsen
et al., 1970)

● Diab. ● Trace ○ Nondiab.

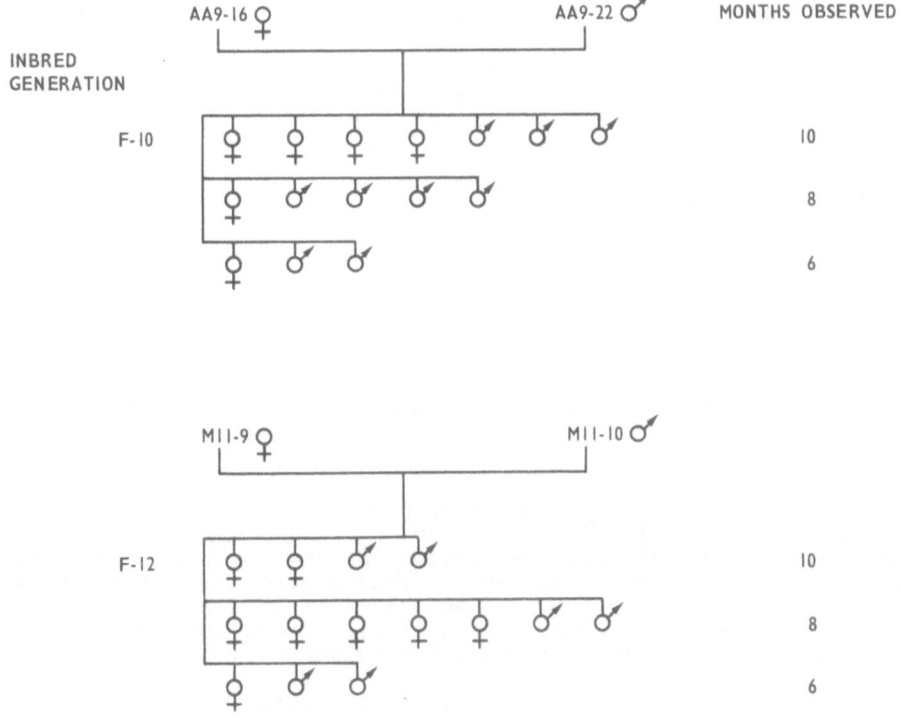

O = NONDIABETIC

Fig. 3. Crosses of inbred nondiabetic Chinese hamsters resulting in all nondiabetic
offspring

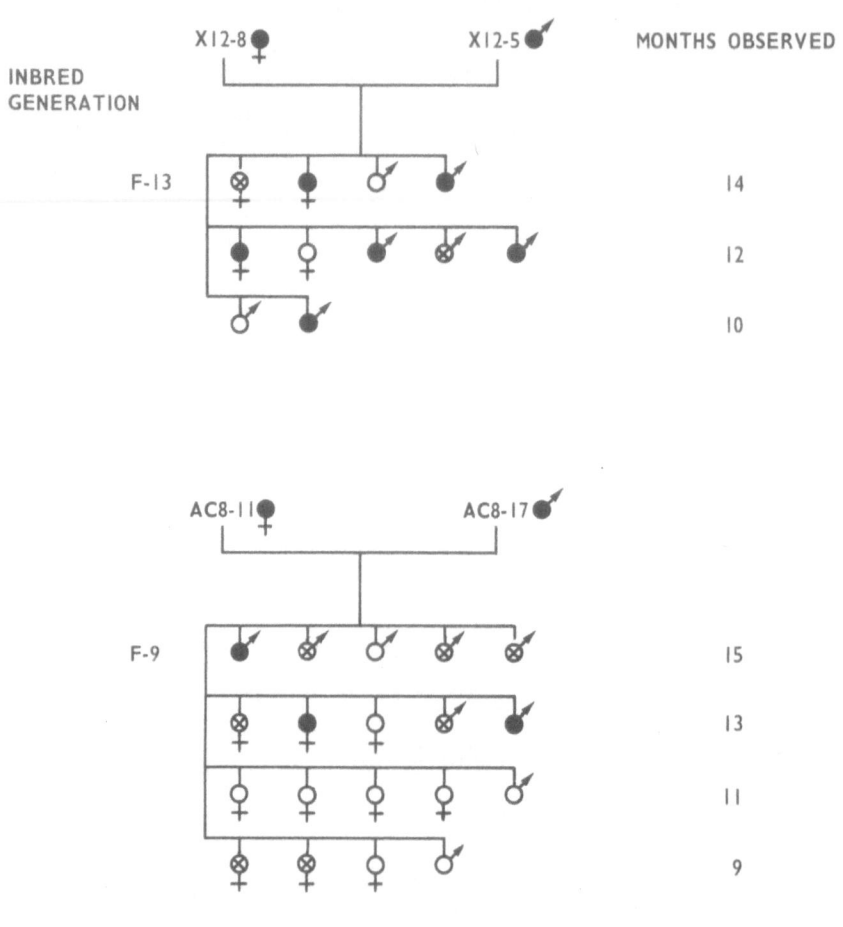

Fig. 4. Crosses of inbred diabetic Chinese hamsters resulting in aglycosuric, trace, and diabetic phenotypes

In the L subline, inbreeding has progressed to the 26th generation (Fig. 6). It was interesting to note that the phenotypic heterozygosity persisted through the 22nd generation. However, starting with the F-24 generation, the Chinese hamsters in this subline have bred true for 4+ glycosuria as shown for F-26 animals (Fig. 6). Over 90% of the F-24 generation were diabetic by 6 and all by 11 weeks, and 90% of F-26 hamsters were diabetic by 4 and all by 7 weeks of age.

When ketotic diabetics were mated, all offspring became diabetic (30). During the past 6 years, 160 offspring from ketotic parents were weaned.

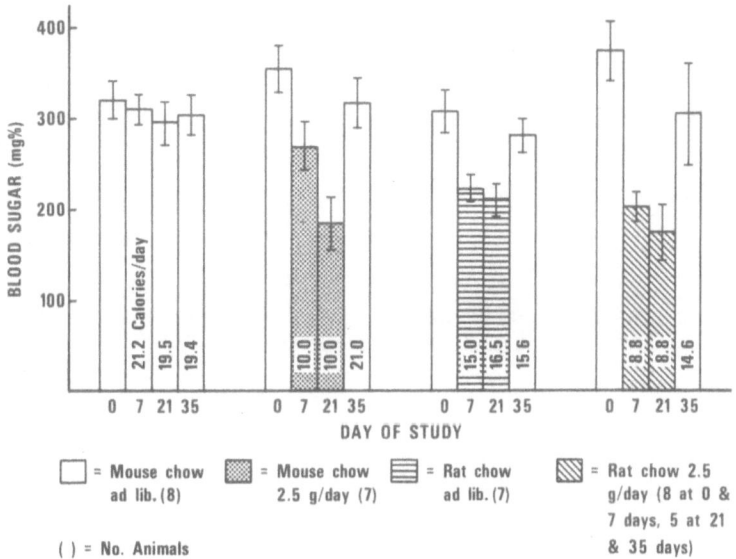

Fig. 5. Effects of diet on blood sugar of diabetic hamsters. Diets were changed at 0 and 21 days
P values at 7 days = 0.025 between mouse chow ad lib. and 2.5 g mouse chow; 0.005 between mouse chow ad lib. and rat chow ad lib.; 0.001 between mouse chow ad lib. and 2.5 g rat chow; 0.05 change from 0 day between rat chow 2.5 vs. rat chow ad lib.; 0.05-0.1 change from 0 day between mouse chow 2.5 vs. 2.5 g rat chow.
P values at 21 days = <0.05 between mouse chow ad lib. and rat chow ad lib.; <0.005 between mouse chow ad lib. and 2.5 g mouse chow, 2.5 g rat chow and rat chow ad lib.; <0.05 change from 0 day between rat chow ad lib. and 2.5 g rat chow; Number in bars = calories/day. (Reproduced from Gerritsen and Blanks, 1974)

All 160 developed diabetes and about 50% also became ketotic (Table 4). It was apparent that pups resulting from the cross of two ketotic parents could be identified as prediabetic at birth. The most significant observation made on these animals was that they were hyperphagic prior to onset of glycosuria (31). Subsequent studies indicated that prediabetics with ketotic parents were hyperphagic from birth (Table 5). Birth weights of prediabetics and nonprediabetic control hamsters were similar. At 15 and 25 days, prediabetics were significantly heavier than controls when both types were raised in equal-sized litters. Fasting blood sugar, plasma insulin, and pancreatic insulin levels of prediabetics did not differ from nonprediabetics at either 15 or 25 days of age. Total lipids and solids were significantly increased in the eviscerated carcasses of prediabetics at 15 and 24 days.

Table 4. Type of Offspring from Mating Ketotic X Ketotic Diabetic Chinese Hamsters. (Reproduced from Dulin and Gerritsen, 1972)

No. offspring	No. diabetic	No. ketotic
160	160	75

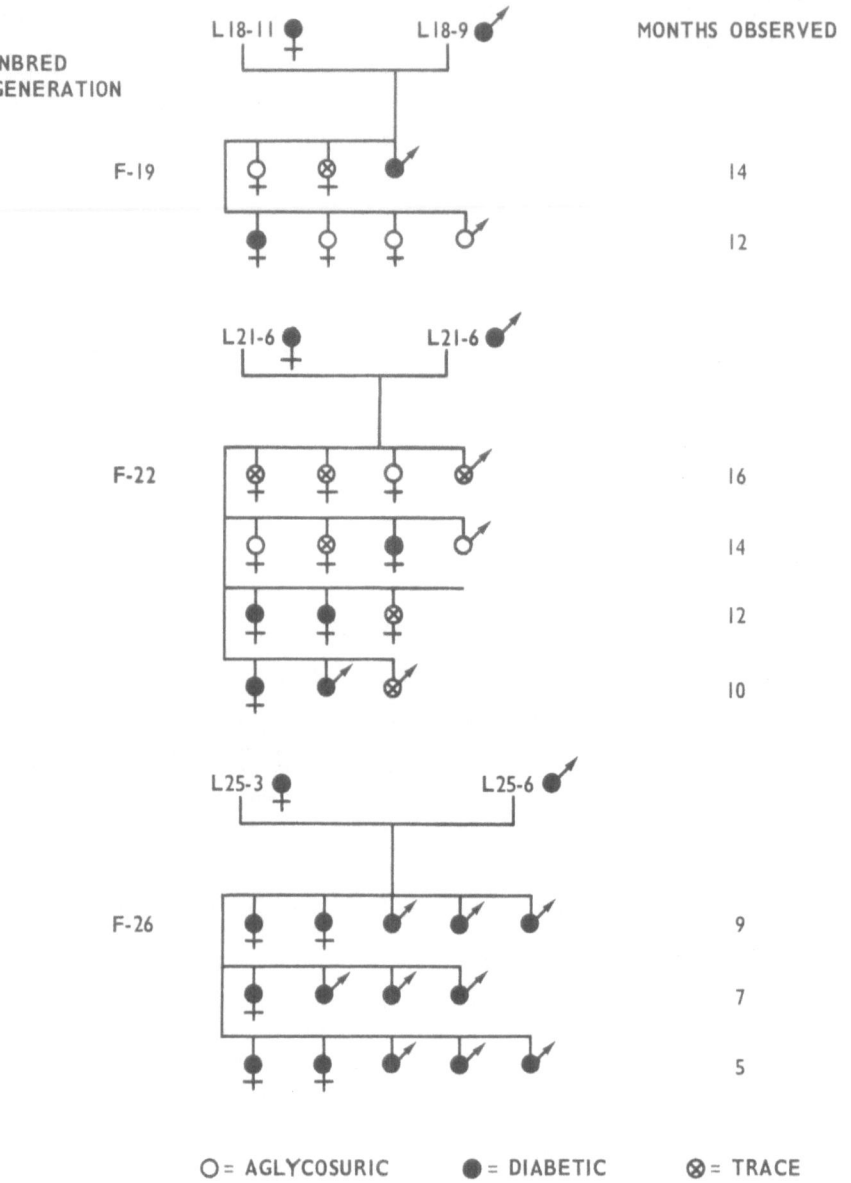

Fig. 6. Crosses of highly inbred Chinese hamsters from subline L (reproduced from Dulin and Gerritsen, 1972)

In order to study the effect of hyperphagia on subsequent development of diabetes, prediabetic newborns were fostered into large litters. Fostering prediabetics into large litters was an effective procedure for limitation of dietary intake since body weight of the fostered prediabetics was significantly less than their nonfostered siblings at 15 days (Fig. 7). The significant difference in body weight of the fostered and nonfostered prediabetics was maintained during the last 9 days of suckling but growth rates during this period appear to be simi-

Table 5. Comparison of fasted prediabetic with nonprediabetic Chinese hamster pups of similar litter size and parent weight (mean values ± S.E.M.) (Reproduced from Gerritsen, Blanks *et al.*, 1974)

Measurement	Newborn		15 Days old		25 Days old	
	Nonprediabetic	Prediabetic	Nonprediabetic	Prediabetic	Nonprediabetic	Prediabetic
Number	15	18	9	9	6	9
Body weight (g)	1.6±0.2	1.75±0.2	5.9 ±0.2	7.9±0.4[a]	9.8±0.4	12.2 ±0.03[a]
Blood sugar (mg/100 ml)	–	–	85 ±4.6	88 ±5.0	89 ±4.3	94 ±4.5
Plasma insulin (U/ml)	–	–	3.2 ±1.0	5.1±1.6	9.3±5.0	8.7 ±4.6
Pancreatic insulin (U/g.)	–	–	0.86±0.07	0.69±0.08	0.55±0.1	0.49 ±0.001
Carcass lipids (%)	–	–	1.1 ±0.06	2.3±0.2[a]	2.9±0.8	4.3 ±0.1[a]
Carcass solids (%)	–	–	21.6 ±0.2	25.2±0.8[a]	27.3±1.7	33.0 ±0.4[a]
Carcass proteins (%)	–	–	14.9 ±1.8	16.5±1.5	19.0±1.0	19.2 ±1.0

[a] $p < 0.01$.

lar since the slopes of the curves are similar. Even though the two fostered prediabetics had significantly lower body weight at 15 days than their own natural nonfostered siblings, they still gained significantly more weight that the five nonprediabetic offspring of their foster mothers.

The significant difference in weaning body weights of nonfostered and fostered prediabetics was maintained by limiting the diet of fostered pups to an intake of 2.5 g/day (Fig. 8). The fostered prediabetics were maintained at a significantly lower body weight than their nonfostered and ad lib. fed siblings for the entire 150 days of diet limitation. The only exception was at 94 days, which is the time of sexual maturity in the Chinese hamster. The diet-limited animals had a rapid growth spurt after the switch to a nonrestricted feeding, so that after 14 days they were no longer significantly lighter than siblings fed ad lib. The growth rate of the prediabetics limited to 2.5 g/day was normalized as shown in Figure 9. Growth curves of nondiabetic weanlings fed ad lib were similar to those of the prediabetics limited to 2.5 g/day and of similar initial weights. The mean daily food consumption for the nondiabetics was 2.45 g/day.

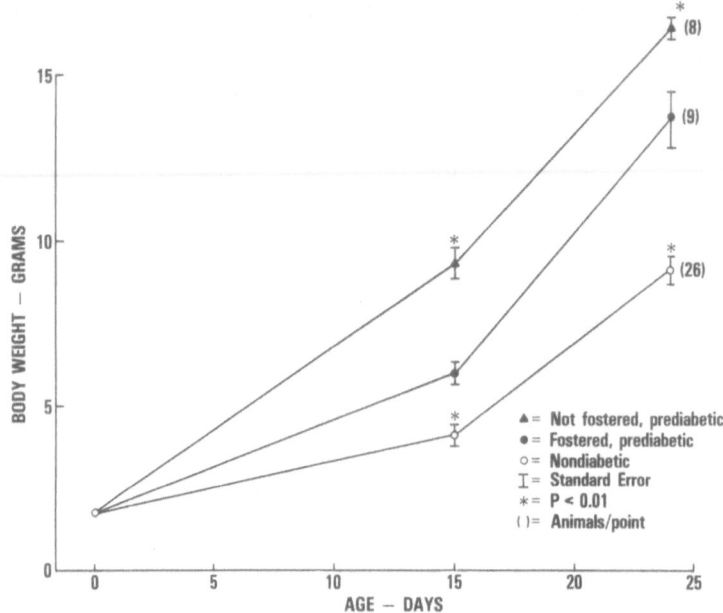

Fig. 7. Preweaning Chinese hamsters body weights of nonfostered prediabetics of litter size 2 and fostered prediabetics with nonprediabetics of total litter size 7

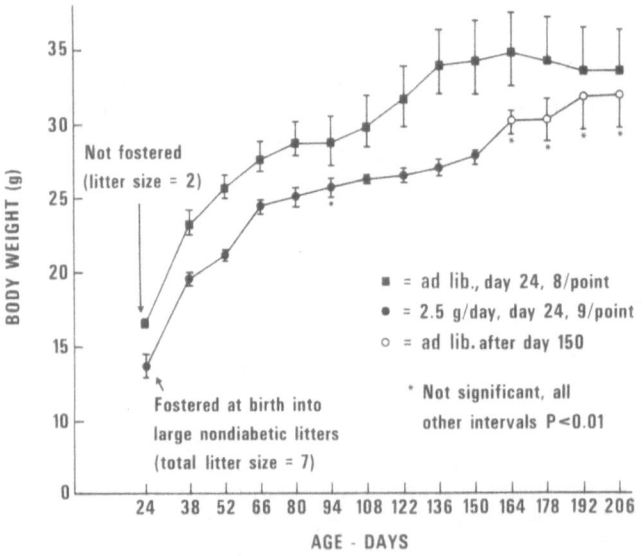

Fig. 8. Effects of food restriction on body weights of prediabetic Chinese hamsters (reproduced from Gerritsen, Blanks *et al.*, 1974)

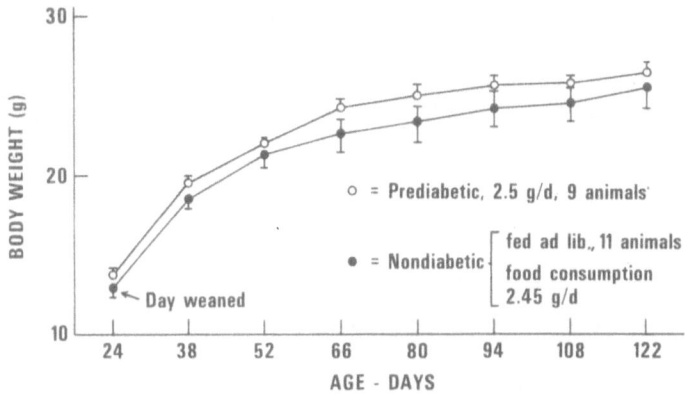

Fig. 9. Comparison of growth rates of nondiabetic Chinese hamsters fed ad lib. and prediabetics limited to 2.5 g of food/day (reproduced from Gerritsen and Dulin, 1972)

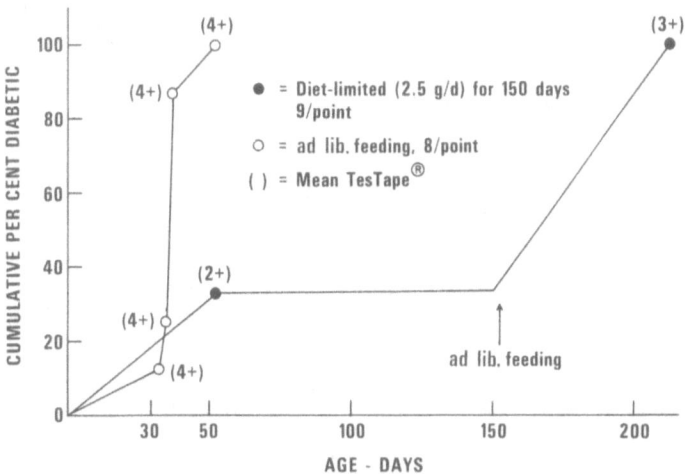

Fig. 10. Difference in age of onset and severity of diabetes in diet-limited and ad lib. fed prediabetic Chinese hamsters (reproduced from Gerritsen and Dulin, 1972)

Diabetes developed very rapidly in the prediabetic Chinese hamster pups which were not limited to a normal food intake (Fig. 10). At 40 days of age, 7 of 8 prediabetics on nonrestricted food intake had developed glycosuria (4+ TesTape value). In contrast, only 3 of the 9 prediabetics which were limited to a normal quantity of food developed mild glycosuria (2+ TesTape) by 50 days of age and remained at 2+, but when switched to nonrestricted feeding, glycosuria increased to 4+ within a few days. The other 6 prediabetics which were fostered and subsequently limited to 2.5 g/day did not develop glycosuria as long as they were limited to this quantity of food intake. However, within 50 days after these animals were placed on nonrestricted diet they all showed mild glycosuria (2+ to 3+). Further, these animals remained very mild diabetics for their entire life span.

Seven out of the eight hamsters fed ad lib. also developed ketonuria, but ketonuria never developed in their siblings which were diet-limited for the first 150 days (Fig. 11).

It was also observed that 5 of 8 of the hamsters fed ad lib. died prior to 300 days of age (Fig. 12). The 3 that survived beyond 300 days died

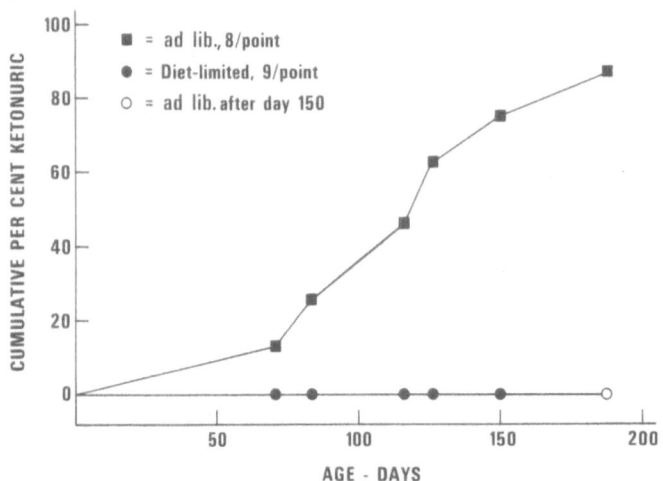

Fig. 11. Incidence of ketonurics in ad lib. fed versus diet-limited Chinese hamsters (reproduced from Gerritsen and Dulin, 1972)

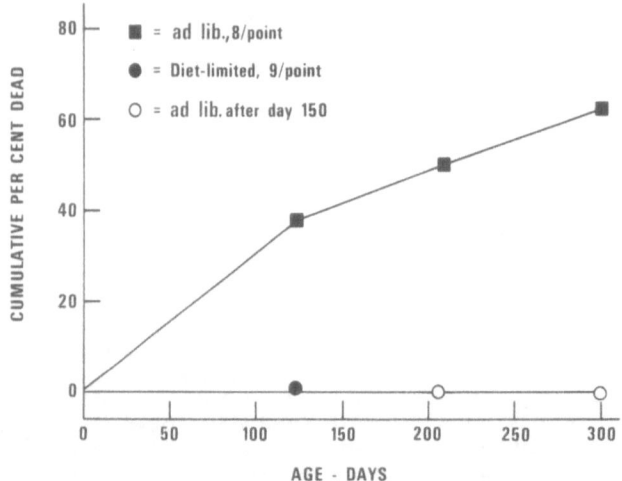

Fig. 12. Mortality in ad lib. fed versus diet-limited Chinese hamsters (reproduced from Gerritsen and Dulin, 1972)

prior to 18 months of age. In contrast, all the siblings which were diet-limited for the first 150 days survived beyond 2 years.

In other studies, preweaning diet-limitation alone had no significant effect on onset of severity or diabetes or survival. The results were similar to data shown for ad lib. fed animals in Figures 10-12. Limitation of diet to 2.5 g/day after weaning resulted in a reduced growth rate, but by 200 days of age, body weights were no longer significantly different. Again, all the siblings fed ad lib. developed diabetes very rapidly but only 3 of the 12 animals which were kept on 2.5 g/day for 30 months showed trace glycosuria which was intermittent. They never progressed to consistent mild glycosuria and the other 9 have never shown any glycosuria.

It is interesting to note that prediabetics (defined retrospectively), born from the cross of two nonketotic diabetics were not hyperphagic (34) and did not show faster than normal growth rate during the prediabetic phase. This observation suggested an environmental effect of the uterus of a ketotic mother on the prediabetic offspring.

Growth rates of hamsters of the diabetic genotype from normal and ketoacidotic uteri are compared in Figure 13. The normal uterine environment was obtained by ovarian transplantation. There was a slight but significant increase in the growth rate of pups derived from the ketotic dams. Food consumption was significantly elevated in pups with ketotic dams during the prediabetic state (Fig. 14). Onset of diabetes was rapid in pups from ketotic dams compared with those born out of the normal uterus. Further, the severity as judged by Testape tests was considerably reduced (Fig. 15). Development of Ketonuria was also markedly retarded and less severe in animals from the nondiabetic uterus (Fig. 16).

Discussion

It is recognized that the title of this paper may be inappropriate since diabetes mellitus in the Chinese hamster has been defined by the criteria of glycosuria and ketonuria. Therefore, it is possible that the genetics of glycosuria and the interaction of environmental factors has been studied. It is well recognized that a parameter such as glycosuria is far from the genome. However, it is generally accepted that diabetes can, in part, be defined as inappropriate hyperglycemia. The data in Table 3 show an excellent correlation between glycosuria and hyperglycemia in this animal.

The family histories presented suggest the genetic liability for diabetes in the Chinese hamster. A tremendous amount of data similar to that presented in Figures 1 and 2 were analyzed by Butler (34). The simplest hypothesis consistent with the data was that there are a minimum of four genes which influence development of glycosuria in the Chinese hamster. When any combination of two out of the four genes are in the homozygous recessive state, diabetes may result. It is recognized that other hypotheses could be proposed such as the various ones proposed for man, one of which is multigenic inheritance (51,59).

The observation that all offspring of two ketotics develop diabetes suggested a different genotype for ketonuric diabetics. The data are consistent with the hypothesis that when any three of the four genes are in the homozygous recessive state a ketonuric animal may result. If this hypothesis is correct, then offspring from the cross of two ketotics must have at least two recessive genes and therefore can be defined as genetic prediabetics at birth. It has been reported that onset of glycosuria has become quite uniform but the onset of ketosis has remained variable despite continued inbreeding by brother-sister mating (33).

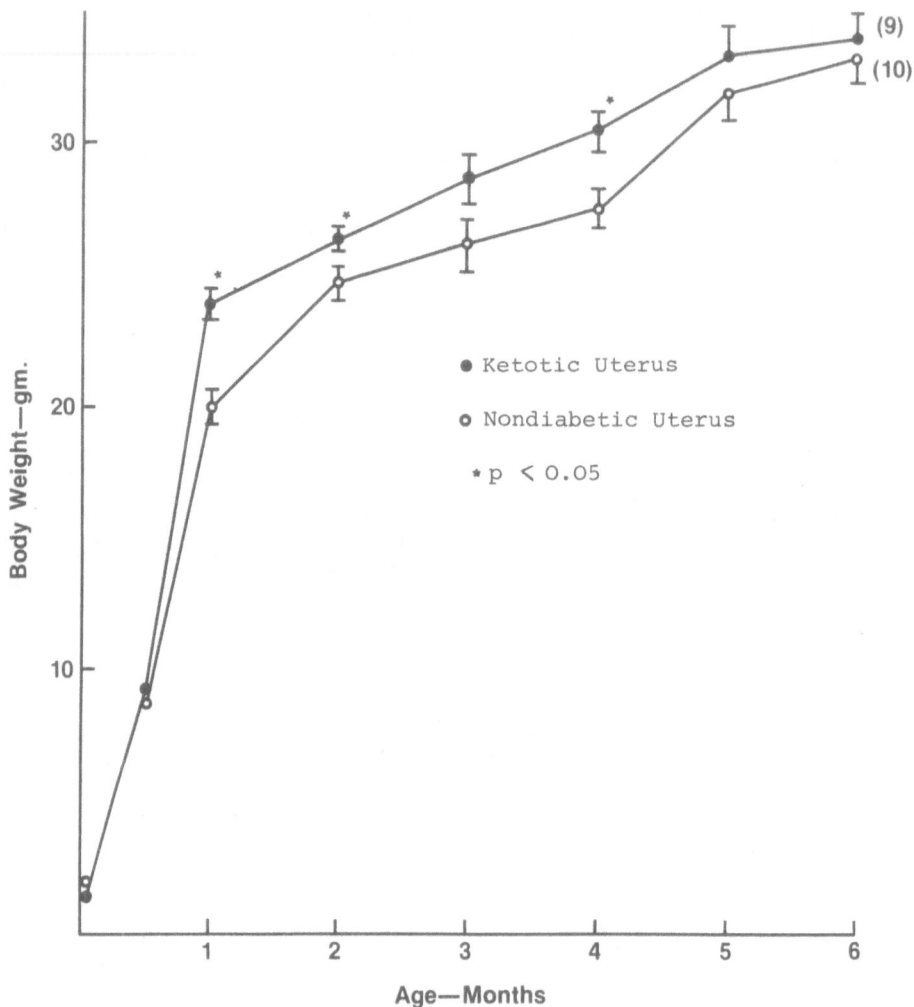

Fig. 13. Effect of uterine environment on growth of Chinese hamsters with similar diabetic genotype. ( ) = number of hamsters (reproduced from Gerritsen and Dulin, 1972)

These observations suggest that onset of ketonuria may be more susceptible to environmental influences. This is supported by Grodsky's observation that ketonuria disappeared when ketotic diabetic Chinese hamsters were placed on low fat diet (4% fat) in San Francisco (37). This observation has recently been confirmed in our laboratories.

As previously mentioned there is considerable discordance among monozygotic human twins with a diabetic genotype. Evaluation of Chinese hamster pedigrees show a similar phenomenon (Figs. 4 and 6). These

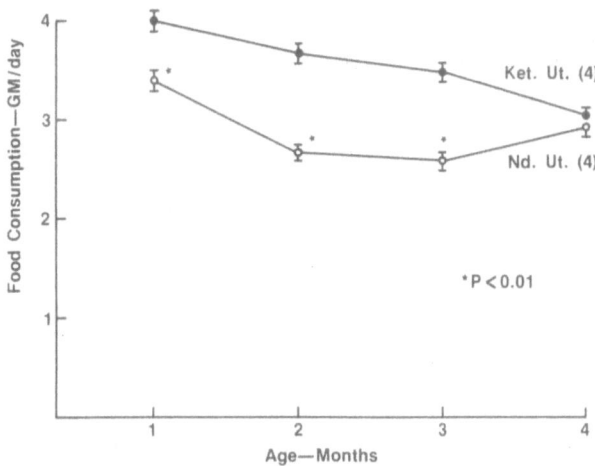

Fig. 14. Effect of uterine environment on food consumption during the prediabetic phase. ( ) = number of hamsters

litters result from 10-22 generations of continuous brother-sister mating. Therefore 90 to greater than 99% of their genetic material should be homozygous (23). However, the degree of concordance within litters does not approach the calculated degree of genetic homozygosity. Therefore one interpretation is that there must be environmental factors influencing these phenotypes. It is interesting to note that F-10 or later nondiabetics (lines AA and M) do breed true (Fig. 3) suggesting that environmental factors do not appear to alter the phenotype of the genetic nondiabetic, at least with regard to glycosuria. However, in the sublines which produce diabetics that are inbred less than 22 generations (Figs. 4 and 6, Y, AC and L lines), there was considerable heterogeneity of phenotype within litters. It is clear from the abnormal results of the glucose tolerance tests that aglycosurics have a defect in their ability to cope with a glucose load. Further, Grodsky *et al*. perfused the pancreata of aglycosurics and reported a defect in insulin secretion similar to that observed in diabetic Chinese hamsters (37). These observations suggest that diabetic, trace, and aglycosuric siblings had genetic homogeneity. Therefore, it is difficult to understand why they had phenotypic heterogeneity. It is possible that the entire genetic background of the siblings was still variable enough so that one diabetic genotype was expressed as glycosuria while another was not. The concept of genetic background variability even after 20 generations of inbreeding is supported by the observations that after 23 generations of inbreeding in the L subline, Chinese hamsters breed true for diabetes. This suggests that at F-24 the entire genetic make up of all the animals within a litter is so uniform that expression of the genes responsible for diabetes is constant and all animals show early glycosuria. The concept that genetic background can contribute to phenotypic heterogeneity at stages of inbreeding less than F-23 in the Chinese hamster is supported by the classic experiments of Coleman and Hummel (14,15,41). They placed the ob gene and the db gene on different genetic backgrounds in highly inbred mouse strains C57BL/KsJ and C57BL/6J and found that the phenotype varied depending on the background. If our proposed genetic hypothesis is correct, it is possible that in animals with two homozygous recessive genes for diabetes one was buffered (24) to a greater extent than its siblings, and thus the defect was expressed as glycosuria in one sibling but not in the other. Also, the possibility exists that

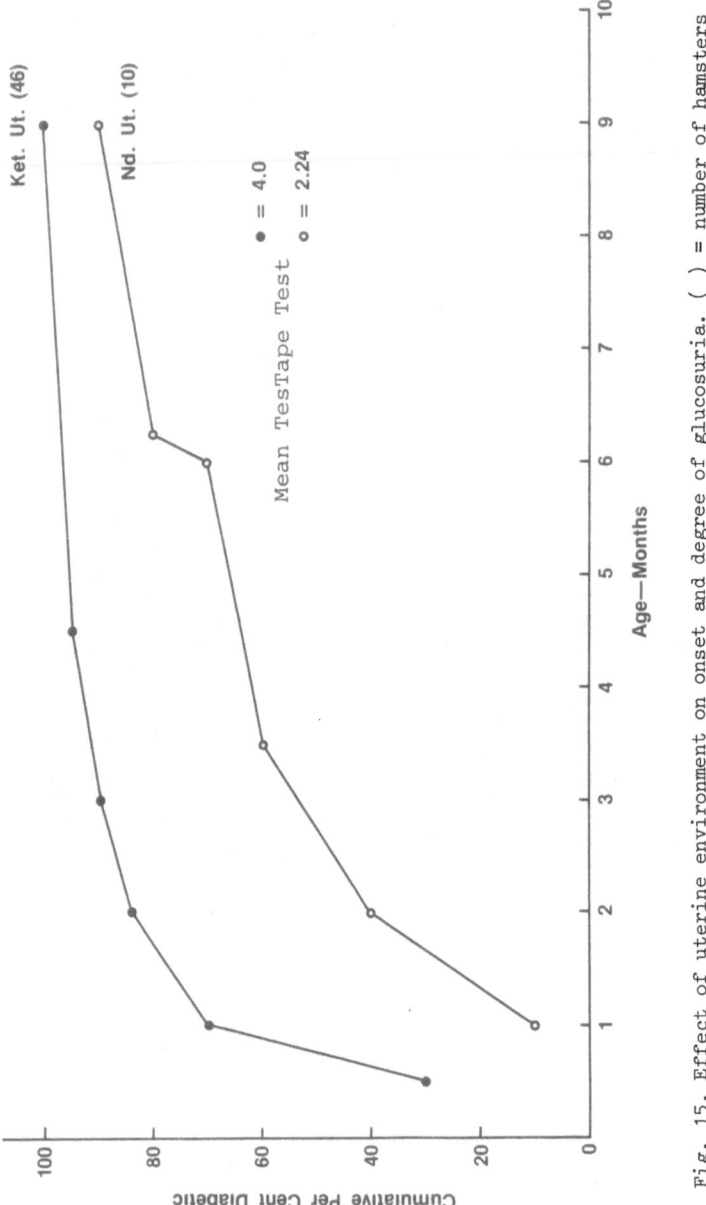

Fig. 15. Effect of uterine environment on onset and degree of glucosuria. ( ) = number of hamsters

a natural selection against genetic homogeneity could have influenced the data since half of the female breeders are infertile or cannibalistic.

It appears that caloric restriction and/or reduction of fat in the diet will decrease blood sugar levels of the markedly hyperglycemic hamster without weight loss. However, it should be pointed out that blood sugar could not be normalized by severe caloric restriction (8.8 cal/day).

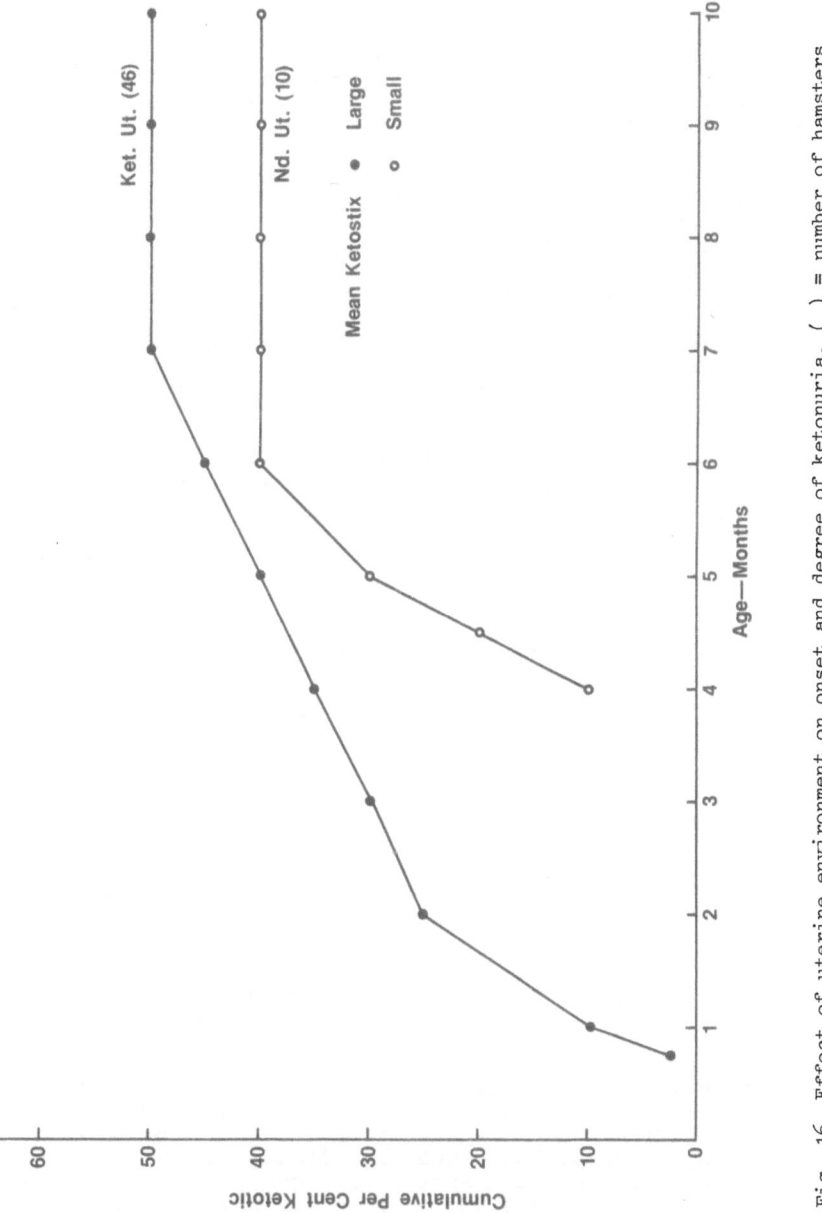

Fig. 16. Effect of uterine environment on onset and degree of ketonuria. ( ) = number of hamsters

This procedure resulted in significant weight loss and in a few cases mortality from starvation. These diet studies suggest that once the genetic mutation has been expressed as hyperglycemia and glycosuria in the Chinese hamster, it cannot be reversed by dietary manipulation. Whether increasing caloric intake in aglycosurics of diabetic genotype will cause hyperglycemia remains to be determined.

The significant increase in body weight and carcass fat suggests that prediabetic Chinese hamsters overeat starting at birth. These results support and extend the previously observed hyperphagia of prediabetics following weaning (31). Since plasma insulin levels were not elevated in the prediabetics, it can be concluded that hyperphagia was not due to hyperinsulinism, which would be expected to increase food intake (48), and that the increased body fat did not influence plasma insulin levels of the prediabetic.

It is apparent that the fostering procedure was effective in limiting food intake prior to weaning since the prediabetic pups did not grow as rapidly as their nonfostered siblings. The appetite drive, however, of the fostered prediabetics was greater than their foster mother's own pups since they gained significantly more weight. In the fostered litters (Fig. 7) growth rates were similar for both fostered and non-fostered prediabetic pups from 15-24 days since the slopes of the growth curves are similar. This may be explained by the observation that mothers with large litters have been known to soften food by chewing it and then force feeding their pups from 13 days until they are weaned.

It should be pointed out that fostering prediabetics into large litters and subsequent limitation of food to 2.5 g/day mormalized body weight at weaning time and subsequent growth rate compared with nondiabetics from litters and parents of similar size.

This is shown in Figure 9 where weaning weights of nondiabetic pups and subsequent growth curves are similar to the food-limited predia-betics. When prediabetics were switched from limited to nonrestricted feeding their food consumption increased to 3.0-3.5 g/day. It is in-teresting to note that their food consumption remained at this level for the rest of their lives (over 2 years) and never increased to the expected level of 4-5 g/day normally consumed by diabetics (33). This observation suggests that the diet limitation for the first 150 days of life has a prolonged effect on food intake.

The data show that limiting food intake of the hyperphagic prediabetic hamster to the lower limit of normal (2.5 g/day) results in a milder diabetes and retards the onset of glycosuria. Further, diet limitation for only 150 days eliminated development of ketonuria which under nor-mal circumstances would have been expected in some of these prediabe-tics (21,30). In addition, all the prediabetics fed ad lib. died prior to 18 months, while all their siblings whose diet was limited to 150 days, survived for just over 2 years. These observations are consistent with epidemiologic findings from the Upjohn colony (34,56). Limitation of diet only during the preweaning period did not alter the develop-ment of diabetes, suggesting that diet limitation must persist beyond the weaning age of 24 days. Diet limitation to 2.5 g/day from weaning for 30 months resulted in a slower growth rate in the prediabetics compared with their ad lib. fed siblings, but they eventually attained similar body weights. Prolonged diet limitation, however, essentially prevented development of diabetes in these prediabetics and their life expectancy was normalized (34). Since dietary restriction for long periods of time is difficult, it will be of interest to determine if diet limitation from weaning to 100 days of age or the advent of sexual maturity will be sufficient to retard onset and reduce the severity of diabetes in prediabetic Chinese hamsters.

If prediabetics from ketonuric parents are allowed food ad lib., they develop glycosuria very early, which is generally followed by ketosis and premature death in many of them. These observations lend conside-rable confidence to the concept that environmental modification can alter the course of a genetically influenced syndrome such as diabetes.

However, it must be re-emphasized that once marked hyperglycemia has developed, diet-limitation did not normalize the animal (Fig. 5). This suggests that modification of the environment, in this case diet, must be done very early, prior to interactions with the genes which are responsible for hyperglycemia.

Whether the early increase in body weight and lipid content prior to hyperglycemia contributes to early development of diabetes is not known. This, however, is possible, since obesity has been implicated in the development of spontaneous diabetes in other laboratory animals (16, 50) and also of maturity-onset diabetes in man (1,42). In addition, there appears to be a positive correlation between obesity, carbohydrate intolerance and hyperinsulinism in childhood (62). This concept is supported by the observation that after switching the animals which had been on a limited diet to nonrestricted feeding, they gained weight prior to onset of glycosuria. Their food consumption, however, did not become so excessive that they progressed to severe diabetes, as evidenced by a lack of ketonuria and premature death.

Unfortunately, there has been no report in the literature as to the effects of diet limitation on human prediabetics. There is, however, a suggestion that emotional problems and stress during the prediabetic years may lead to poor nutritional habits which may have an effect on development of diabetes (62). Other circumstantial evidence suggests that severe caloric restriction during wars can decrease the prevalence of diabetes (2,53).

The observation that prediabetic Chinese hamsters have preweaning hyperphagia suggests that appetite control was abnormal at birth in these animals. It is not clear if this resulted from genetic or environmental influence. Since all the prediabetics had ketotic dams, the intrauterine environment may be an important factor influencing the preweaning food intake. It is generally agreed that, in man and animals, glucose crosses the placental barrier, and that although fetal blood sugar levels are lower than maternal levels, there appears to be a significant correlation (44,52). There is also evidence to suggest that elevated fetal blood sugar levels can produce relative fetal hyperinsulinism (18,25). Furthermore, it is possible that the high levels of maternal blood ketone bodies may pass the placental barrier. Thus abnormal blood levels of glucose, insulin, and ketone bodies, alone or in combination, may influence the developing appetite control mechanisms of the prediabetic Chinese hamster in utero. Another possibility is that genes, alone or in combination with factors emanating from the maternal environment, may influence these developing appetite control mechanisms. It should be pointed out that only offspring from two ketonuric Chinese hamsters are hyperphagic and that offspring of two nonketotic diabetic parents inbred less than 22 generations do not all develop diabetes. Further, it has been postulated that ketonuric, diabetic hamsters have a different genotype than nonketonuric, diabetic hamsters. The possibility that genetic background and maternal ketonemia may influence appetite control mechanisms in the prediabetic Chinese hamster neonate is supported by recent observations that "hybrid prediabetics" from nonketonuric diabetic parents of two different inbred sublines did not display accelerated growth or hyperphagia during their prediabetic phase (34).

Data from the ovarian transplant studies must be considered preliminary but they do support the contention that the ketonemic maternal environment plays a role in the development of hyperphagia. This conclusion is supported by observations that prediabetics born to a ketotic dam are hyperphagic but prediabetics born from a nondiabetic uterus (transplant derived) or prediabetics from a diabetic dam (defined in retrospect) are not hyperphagic. The data strongly suggest that the environmental factor of ketonemia in the pregnant Chinese hamster is related to hyperphagia in the offspring. However, the remote possibility does exist that maternal ketone bodies circulating in the fetus caused a genetic mutation which was expressed as hyperphagia in the offspring.

The results of the diet limitation studies of prediabetics born to ketotic dams and the ovarian transplant experiment are remarkably similar. Again, this points to the importance of the maternal environment.

In conclusion: It is evident that hyperglycemia, glycosuria, and ketonuria in the Chinese hamster are the result of interaction of the diabetic genetic mutation and environment. It is highly probable that there are many factors which remain obscure but it is equally probable that nutrition and maternal environment interact with the diabetic genotype.
Once the diabetic genotype has been expressed as hyperglycemia, it may be impossible to completely normalize the individual. Thus identification of the prediabetic and intervention or manipulation of environmental factors during the prediabetic phase are of primary importance. It may be concluded from the diet-limitation studies in prediabetics that normalizing food intake of the hyperphagic prediabetic Chinese hamster has a marked influence on onset and severity of the disease. The increase in longevity suggests the benefits of delaying the development and/or reducing the severity of the disease. It appears that continued diet limitation will essentially keep the prediabetic free of clinical symptoms of diabetes and normalize life span.

The data presented suggest that, if genetic and environmental factors can be understood and manipulated properly, the clinical symptoms and, perhaps, the consequences of abnormal metabolism may be prevented.

References

1. Allison, R.S.: Carbohydrate tolerance in overweight and obesity. Lancet 1, 537 (1927)

2. Bouchardat, H.: De la Glucosurie du Diabète Sucré. Paris, 1883. Cited by: Renold, A.E., Burr, I., Stauffacher, W.: On the pathogenesis of diabetes mellitus: Possible usefulness of spontaneous hyperglycemic syndromes in Animals. In: Nobel Symposium 13. Pathogenesis of Diabetes Mellitus. Cerasi, E., Luft, R. (eds.). New York-London: John Wiley, 1969

3. Butler, L.: The inheritance of diabetes in the Chinese hamster. Diabetologia 3, 124 (1967)

4. Butler, C., Gerritsen, G.C.: A comparison of the modes of inheritance of diabetes in the Chinese hamster and the KK mouse. Diabetologia 6, 163 (1970)

5. Carpenter, A-M., Gerritsen, G.C., Dulin, W.E., Lazarow, A.: Islet and beta cell volumes in diabetic Chinese hamsters and their nondiabetic siblings. Diabetologia 3, 92 (1967)

6. Cerasi, E., Luft, R.: Plasma insulin response to sustained hyperglycemia induced by glucose infusion in human subjects. Lancet II, 1359 (1963)

7. Cerasi, E., Luft, R.: Insulin response to glucose infusion in diabetic and nondiabetic monozygotic twin pairs. Genetic control of insulin response? Acta Endocr. (Kbh) 55, 330 (1967)

8. Chang, A.Y.: The structure and metabolism of the pancreatic islets. Wenner-Gren Symposium No. 16. Falkurez, S., Hellman, B., Taljedal, I.B. (eds.). New York: Pergamon Press, 1970, p. 515

9. Chang, A.Y., Schneider, D.I.: Metabolic abnormalities in the pancreatic islets and livers of the diabetic Chinese hamster. Diabetologia $\underline{6}$, 180 (1970)

10. Chobanian, A.V., Gerritsen, G.C., Brecher, P.I., McCombs, L.: Aortic glucose metabolism in the diabetic Chinese hamster. Diabetologia $\underline{10}$, 589 (1974)

11. Chobanian, A.V., Gerritsen, G.C., Brecher, P.I., Kessler, M.: Cholesterol metabolism in the diabetic Chinese hamster. Diabetologia $\underline{10}$, 595 (1974)

12. Cohen, A.M., Bavly, S., Poznanski, R.: Change of diet of Yemenite Jews in relation to diabetes and ischemic heart disease. Lancet $\underline{II}$, 1399 (1961)

13. Cohen, A.M., Bavly, S., Poznanski, R.: The prevalence of diabetes among different ethnic groups in Israel. Metabolism $\underline{10}$, 50 (1961)

14. Coleman, D.L., Hummel, K.P.: The influence of genetic background on the expression of the obese (ob) gene in the mouse. Diabetologia $\underline{9}$, 287 (1973)

15. Coleman, D.L., Hummel, K.P.: Hyperinsulinemia in pre-weaning diabetes (db) mice. Diabetologia $\underline{10}$, 607 (1974)

16. Coleman, D.L., Hummel, K.P.: Studies with the mutation-diabetes in the mouse. Diabetologia $\underline{3}$, 238 (1967)

17. Conforti, A.: Ultrastruttura del rene nel diabete spontaneo dell'hamster cinese (*Cricetulus griseus*). Acta diabet. lat. $\underline{9}$, 655 (1972)

18. Cornblath, M., Joassen, G., Weisskopf, B., Swiatek, K.R.: Hypoglycemia in the newborn. Pediat. Clin. N. Amer. $\underline{13}$, 905 (1966)

19. Ditschuneit, H.: Diabetes. Proceedings of the XVII. Cong. Inter. Diabetes Fed. Rodriguez, R.R., Vallance-Owen, J. (eds.). Amsterdam: Excerpta Medica, 1971, p. 526

20. Dulin, W.E., Chang, A.Y. and Gerritsen, G.C.: Spontaneous diabetes in the Chinese hamster. In: Les Mutants Pathologiques Chez L'Animal, leur intérêt dans la recherche bio-médicale. Sabourdy, M. (ed.). Paris: Centre National de la Recherche Scientifique, 1970, p. 133

21. Dulin, W.E., Gerritsen, G.C.: Interaction of genetics and environment on diabetes in the Chinese hamster as compared with human and other diabetic animal species. Acta diabet. lat. (Suppl. 1) $\underline{9}$, 48 (1972)

22. Dulin, W.E., Gerritsen, G.C.: Experimental models for investigation of diabetic therapeutic problems. In: Metabolic Regulation, Insulin Metabolism and Diabetes. Academic Press. In press.

23. Falconer, D.S.: The UFAW Handbook on the Care and Management of Laboratory Animals. 3rd ed. Lane-Petter, W., Worden, A.N., Hill, B.F., Patterson, J.S., Ververs, H.G. (eds.). Kent: The Courier Printing and Publishing Co., Ltd., 1966, p. 72

24. Falconer, D.S.: Introduction to Quantitative Genetics. New York: Ronald Press, 1960, p. 129

25. Farquhar, J.W.: The significance of hypoglycemia in the newborn infant of the diabetic woman. Arch. Dis. Childh. $\underline{31}$, 203 (1956)

26. Federman, J.L., Gerritsen, G.C.: The retinal vasculature of the Chinese hamster: A preliminary study. Diabetologia $\underline{6}$, 186 (1970)

27. Frankel, B.J., Gerich, J.E., Hagura, R., Fanska, R.E., Gerritsen, G.C., Grodsky, G.M.: Abnormal secretion of insulin and glucagon by the *in vitro* perfused pancreas of the genetically diabetic Chinese hamster. J. Clin. Invest. $\underline{53}$, 1637 (1974)

28. Gerritsen, G.C., Dulin, W.E.: Serum proteins of Chinese hamsters and response of diabetics to tolbutamide and insulin. Diabetes $\underline{15}$, 331 (1966)

29. Gerritsen, G.C., Dulin, W.E.: Characterization of diabetes in the Chinese hamster. Diabetologia $\underline{3}$, (1967)

30. Gerritsen, G.C., Needham, L.B., Schmidt, F.L., Dulin, W.E.: Studies on the prediction and development of diabetes in offspring of diabetic Chinese hamsters. Diabetologia 6, 158 (1970)

31. Gerritsen, G.C., Blanks, M.C.: Preliminary studies on food and water consumption of prediabetic Chinese hamsters. Diabetologia 6, 177 (1970)

32. Gerritsen, G.C., Dulin, W.E.: Effect of diet restriction on onset of development of diabetes in prediabetic Chinese hamsters. Acta diabet. lat. (Suppl. 1) 9, 597 (1972)

33. Gerritsen, G.C., Blanks, M.C.: Characterization of Chinese hamsters by metabolic balance, glucose tolerance and insulin secretion. Diabetologia 10, 493 (1974)

34. Gerritsen, G.C., Johnson, M.A., Soret, M.G., Schultz, J.R.: Epidemiology of Chinese hamsters and preliminary evidence for genetic heterogeneity of diabetes. Diabetologia 10, 581 (1974)

35. Gerritsen, G.C., Blanks, M.C., Miller, R.L., Dulin, W.E.: Effect of diet limitation on the development of diabetes in prediabetic Chinese hamsters. Diabetologia 10, 559 (1974)

36. Gottlieb, M.S., Root, H.F.: Diabetes mellitus in twins. Diabetes 17, 693 (1968)

37. Grodsky, G.M., Frankel, B.J., Gerich, J.E., Gerritsen, G.C.: The diabetic Chinese hamster: In vitro insulin and glucagon release; the "Chemical Diabetic"; and the effect of diet on ketonuria. Diabetologia 10, 521 (1974)

38. Harvald, B.: Genetic prespectives in diabetes mellitus. Acta Med. Scand. (Suppl. 476) 17, (1967)

39. Harvald, B., Hauge, M.: Hereditary factors elucidated by twin studies. Genetics and epidemiology of chronic disease. U.S. Pub. Health Services Publ. 1163, 1 (1965)

40. Holcomb, G.N., Klemm, L.A., Dulin, W.E.: The polyol pathway for glucose metabolism in tissues from normal, diabetic and ketotic Chinese hamsters. Diabetologia 10, 549 (1974)

41. Hummel, K.P., Coleman, D.L., Lane, P.W.: The influence of genetic background on expression at the diabetes locus in the mouse. I. C57BL/KsJ and C57BL/6J strains. Biochem. Genet. 7, 1 (1972)

42. Joslin, E.P., Dublin, L.T., Marks, H.H.: Studies in diabetes mellitus. IV. Etiology. Amer. J. Med. Sci. 192, 9 (1936)

43. Karam, J.H., Grodsky, G.M., Forsham, P.H.: Excessive insulin response to glucose in obese subjects as measured by immunochemical assay. Diabetes 12, 197 (1973)

44. Krauer, F., Joyce, J., Young, M.: The influence of high maternal plasma glucose levels and maternal blood flow on the placental transfer of glucose in the guinea pig. Diabetologia 9, 453 (1973)

45. Luse, S.A., Caramia, F., Gerritsen, G.C., Dulin, W.E.: Spontaneous diabetes mellitus in the Chinese hamster: an electron microscopic study of the islets of Langerhans. Diabetologia 3, 97 (1967)

46. Luse, S.A., Gerritsen, G.C., Dulin, W.E.: Cerebral abnormalities in diabetes mellitus: an ultrastructural study of the brain in early onset diabetes mellitus in the Chinese hamster. Diabetologia 6, 192 (1970)

47. Malins, J.M., Cassar, J., Pyke, D.A.: Diabetes in a pair of identical twins. Diabetes 19, 878 (1970)

48. May, K.K., Beaton, J.R.: Hyperphagia in the insulin-treated rat. Proc. Soc. Exp. Biol. (N.Y.) 127, 1201 (1968)

49. McCombs, L., Gerritsen, G.C., Dulin, W.E., Chobanian, A.V.: Morphologic changes in the aorta of the diabetic Chinese hamster. Diabetologia 10, 607 (1974)

50. Nakamura, M., Yamada, K.: Studies on a diabetic KK strain of mouse. Diabetologia 3, 212 (1967)

51. Neel, J.V., Fajans, S.S., Conn, J.W., Davidson, R.T.: Genetics and the epidemiology of chronic diseases. Neel, J.V., Shaw, M., Schull, W. (eds.). U.S. Pub. Health Service Publ. 1163, 1965, p. 105

52. Oakley, N.W., Beard, R.W., Turner, R.C.: Effect of sustained maternal hyperglycaemia on the fetus in normal and diabetic pregnancies. Brit. Med. J. 1, 466 (1972)

53. Pyke, D.A.: Clinical diabetes and its biochemical basis. Oakley, W.G., Pyke, D.A., Taylor, K.W. (eds.). London: Blackwell, 1968, p. 245

54. Pyke, D.A., Tattersall, R.B.: Diabetic retinopathy in identical twins. Diabetes 22, 613 (1973)

55. Schlaepfer, W.W., Gerritsen, G.C., Dulin, W.E.: Segmental demyelination in the distal peripheral nerves of chronically diabetic Chinese hamsters. Diabetologia 10, 541 (1974)

56. Schmidt, F.L., Leslie, L.G., Schultz, J.R., Gerritsen, G.C.: Epidemiological studies·of the Chinese hamster. Diabetologia 6, 154 (1970)

56a.Schmidt, F.L., Miller, R.L., Peterson, T., Soret, M.G.: A microsurgical technique for orthotopic ovarian transplantation in the Chinese hamster. Surgery. (In press)

57. Seltzer, H.S.: Diabetes Mellitus: theory and practice. (Ellenberg, M., Rifkin, H. (eds.). New York: McGraw Hill, 1970, p. 453

58. Shirai, T., Welsh, G.W., 3rd, Sims, E.A.H.: Diabetes mellitus in the Chinese hamster. II. The evolution of renal glomerulopathy. Diabetologia 3, 266 (1967)

59. Simpson, N.E.: Multifactorial Inheritacne. A possible hypothesis for diabetes. Diabetes 13, 462 (1964)

60. Soret, M.G., Dulin, W.E., Gerritsen, G.C.: Early Diabetes, Advances in Metabolic Disorders, Supplement 2. Camerini-Davalos, R., Cole, H.S. (eds.). New York: Academic Press, 1973, p. 291

61. Soret, M.G., Dulin, W.E., Mathews, J., Gerritsen, G.C.: Morphologic abnormalities observed in retina, pancreas and kidney of diabetic Chinese hamsters. Diabetologia 10, 567 (1974)

62. Stein, S.P., Charles, E.: Emotional factors in juvenile diabetes mellitus: a study of early life experience of adolescent diabetics. Amer. J. Psychiat. 128, 700 (1971)

63. Tattersall, R.B., Pyke, D.A.: Diabetes in identical twins. Lancet 2, 1120 (1972)

64. ThenBerg, H.: The genetic aspect of diabetes mellitus. J. Amer. Med. Assoc. 112, 1091 (1939)

65. Wall, J.R., Pyke, D.A., Oakley, W.G.: Effect of carbohydrate restriction in obese diabetics: relationship of control to weight loss. Brit. Med. J. 1, 577 (1973)

19. Diabetes in the Offspring of Conjugal Diabetic Parents

R. TATTERSALL

Fertile marriages between two diabetic parents, although rare, have
considerable theoretical importance; firstly, because they form the
cornerstone of any theory of the inheritance of diabetes, and secondly,
because the classification of an offspring of such a marriage as a "prediabetic" is only valid if all, or the majority, later develop diabetes. In addtion there is a practical aspect, the need for empirical
data as a basis for genetic counselling.

In this paper four aspects of the marriage of two diabetic parents will
be reviewed: (1) the cross-sectional prevalence of diabetes in the offspring of two diabetic parents (OODP); (2) the ultimate prevalence;
(3) the familial distribution as an index of possible heterogeneity of
diabetes among the parents; (4) the type and severity of diabetes in
OODP and their parents.

Prevalence of Diabetes among OODP

There is considerable disagreement about the prevalence of "the diabetic genotype" among OODP. One reason for this situation is that, since
the basic defect (or defects) in diabetes is unknown, different markers of diabetes have been used by different investigators (Table 1).
There is fairly good agreement that the prevalence of overt or symptomatic diabetes is relatively low, in most series between 3 and 12%
(3,7,8,17,19,21,23) although in the largest series from Roumania the
prevalence was more than double that in any other series (15). In the
latter series an exact definition of the criteria is not given and it
may be that some latent diabetics have been included.

After exclusion of overt diabetics, glucose tolerance tests on the
remaining asymptomatic OODP have shown a variable prevalence of carbohydrate intolerance (latent or chemical diabetes); a single glucose
tolerance test has shown asymptomatic diabetes in 10-35% of OODP although
it has been claimed by Kahn *et al.* (8) that this proportion would be
doubled if each offspring had four or more glucose tolerance tests.
This was not confirmed by Tattersall and Fajans (21) who found that of
17 offspring (mean age 44 years) who had had four or more glucose tolerance tests, 12 (71%) had all normal results.

Attempts to make the glucose tolerance test more sensitive by using
either cortisone or triamcinolone have yielded further conflicting results. Some studies have shown a significantly higher frequency of
abnormal cortisone than standard oral G.T.T.'s in offspring of two diabetic parents (10,20,23), although the Joslin Clinic group found that
both intravenous glucose tolerance and oral cortisone-primed tests
were less sensitive than the standard OGTT. The use of the triamcinolone GTT is even more controversial. In the series of Navarette and
Torres (12) 67% of young OODP had an abnormal test compared to only

Table 1. Diabetes and carbohydrate intolerance in offspring of conjugal diabetics

Author	Criteria	No. of couples	No. of Offspring Studied	% Abnormal
West (23)	Clinical	10	67	7.5
Post (17)	Clinical	17	94	8.5
Simpson(19)	Clinical	-	173	3.0
Cooke et al. (3)	Clinical	164	362	4.5
Pieptea and Pavel (15)	Clinical	484	1173	28.0
Kahn et al. (8)	Clinical	80	274	9.0
Tattersall and Fajans (21)	Clinical	37	199	11.5
Jackson et al. (7)	Clinical	152	899	6.5
Pincus and White (16)	OGTT		137	24
Taton et al. (20)	OGTT		83	35
Kahn et al. (8)	Single OGTT		23	26
	Multiple OGTT		23	57
Navarette and Torres (12)	OGTT		61	10
Jackson et al. (7)	OGTT		332	13
Lozano-Castaneda et al. (11)	OGTT		139	19
Tattersall and Fajans (21)	OGTT		123	23
Taton et al. (20)	CGTT		38	24
Kahn et al. (8)	CGTT		132	13
Navarette and Torres (12)	TGTT		55	67
Jackson et al. (7)	TGTT		76 (Durban Indians)	36
			20 (Cape Indians)	10

OGTT = oral glucose tolerance test; CGTT = cortisone glucose tolerance test;
TGTT = triamcinolone glucose tolerance test.

36% and 10% respectively in Durban Indian and Cape Indian OODP of similar ages (7).

Apart from the use of differing criteria there are other possible reasons for the discrepant results reviewed above:

1. Studies have been carried out in different races and in one case the same investigator using the same test and criteria found different results in two racial groups (7).

2. The ways in which the OODP were ascertained may have differed from series to series. To avoid bias families must be ascertained through the parents. If ascertainment is through a diabetic offspring a bias will be introduced in favour of an excess of diabetics, and if through a nondiabetic offspring the bias will be towards a relative deficiency of diabetics. These factors are more important if the series is small and if there is heterogeneity of diabetes among the parents. Many authors do not state how their families were ascertained and

in some series it is known that this was not exclusively through the parents (17,21).

3. The various series have different distributions of obese and non-obese and of old and young offspring which might have affected the results; it is well recognized that carbohydrate tolerance decreases with advancing age in the general population (1,14,24), so that as many as one-sixth of a "normal" population over the age of 50 years may be abnormal by comparison with standards derived from the test-ing of healthy young nonobese adults without a family history of diabetes. A similar phenomenon would be expected among OODP, although here again the evidence is far from clear. Lozano-Castaneda *et al*. (11) found abnormal glucose tolerance in 40% of offspring aged bet-ween 40 and 50 years and Goto *et al*. (4) in all older than 50 years. By contrast, in the series of Tattersall and Fajans (21), 58% of offspring in the sixth decade had normal glucose tolerance and the prevalence of diabetic glucose tolerance tests did not increased progressively with age. Two other groups (3,8) found a similar pre-valence of overt diabetes and abnormal glucose tolerance tests in young and old offspring and Jackson (6), studying the offspring of Indian diabetic couples in Natal, found that the excess of diabetes in offspring over the general population diminished with age and concluded that if the trend continued to 70 years of age diabetes would have been no more frequent in his group of OODP than in the general population.

4. The effects of obesity on glucose tolerance in OODP are not in dis-pute; three groups (8,11,21) have all concluded that obesity is a more important predisposing cause for diabetes among OODP than is age, although none of these series have included a weight-matched control group.

Ultimate Prevalence of Diabetes among OODP

Many authors have accepted as a fact the hypothesis that diabetes is a homogenous condition with autosomal recessive inheritance, concluding that all offspring of two diabetic parents will develop the disease and are ipso facto "prediabetics." Attempts have been made to test the "single locus" recessive theory of the inheritance of diabetes using data from series of OODP. Both Post (17) and Simpson (19) concluded that their data, derived from questionnaires, were compatible with the suggestion that all OODP would develop overt diabetes if they lived long enough. Others using equally large series have concluded that only 25-40% will develop overt diabetes by the age of 80-90 years (3,8,15). In their series Tattersall and Fajans (21) using a life table procedure, estimated that 36% of OODP would have had "diagnosed" diabetes by the age of 60 years, but that if glucose tolerance tests had been done on all offspring 60% would have been diabetic by the age of 60 years.

Age correction involves a number of assumptions and uncertainties and will remain controversial until better longitudinal data are available (13). Estimates of the ultimate prevalence of diabetes and abnormal carbohydrate tolerance in OODP must be regarded with caution. For example, the data of Post (17) and Simpson (19) would also be statistic-ally compatible with a prevalence of diabetes well below 100%; it may be that by the age of 60 the prevalence of diabetes in OODP reaches a plateau so that age correction with standards derived from a general population is not applicable; furthermore, standards of abnormality of glucose tolerance derived from the testing of young healthy individuals are unrealistically strict and it would be better to judge the degree of abnormality in middle-aged OODP by comparison with age, sex, and weight-matched controls.

Heterogeneity of Diabetes in the Parents

Rimoin (18) has emphasized that in all series no more than 50% of OODP have been found to be affected at the time of study regardless of the parameter used and he suggests that the conflicting results obtained by different investigators might be reconciled if diabetes mellitus were a syndrome comprising a number of distinct disorders due to different gene mutations. In this case it would not be expected that all offspring of two parents with different types of diabetes would themselves be affected. A presumption of heterogeneity would be raised if there were some marriages of two diabetic parents which produced all normal offspring. Unfortunately only five of the published series have analyzed the offspring in terms of families (3,12,17,21,23 and Table 2). In the two series in which glucose tolerance tests were not done

Table 2. Interfamilial distribution of diabetes in families of conjugal diabetics

Author	No. of families	Families with no diabetic offspring	Criteria
Cooke et al. (3)	127	114	Clinical
Post (17)	17	12	Clinical
West (23)	10	4	Fasting Blood sugar
Tattersall and Fajans (21)	37	10	Glucose tolerance test

on offspring (3,17) only 5 of 17 and 13 of 127 fertile marriages produced any overtly diabetic offspring. In another series (21) where glucose tolerance tests were done on the majority of offspring, 10 of 37 families had no diabetic offspring and these families were neither smaller nor younger than families with all diabetic (6 of 37 families) or a mixture of diabetic and nondiabetic offspring (21 of 37 families). It was concluded that these findings suggested a degree of heterogeneity of diabetes among the parents, as suggested by Rimoin. So far it is not known whether there are differences in the diabetic phenotype, in terms of complications and insulin or glucagon secretion, in conjugal diabetic parents with no diabetic offspring compared to those with diabetic offspring, and this needs to be examined.

The Type of Diabetes in Parents and Offspring

The vast majority of conjugal diabetic marriages reported in the literature are marriages of two maturity-onset diabetics. In one representative series both parents were over 40 years at diagnosis of diabetes in 85% of marriages (3) and in another the mean ages of the fathers and mothers at diagnosis were 56 and 53 years respectively (21). Cooke et al. (3) reported a greater frequency of diabetes in OODP, one or both of whose parents became diabetic under the age of 40 years, although their conclusions have not been confirmed (6,19). Phenotype is a more satisfactory criterion than age for classifying diabetic patients for genetic analysis (22) and it is to be regretted that as yet there are no data on the prevalence of diabetes in the offspring of two classical juvenile-onset, ketosis-prone diabetics. Since there appears to be heterogeneity between the classical juvenile-onset and maturity-onset types of diabetes (9,22) the findings in marriages of maturity-onset diabetics cannot be used for counselling conjugal juvenile-onset diabetics.

Little attention has been given to the type and severity of diabetes in OODP. Since OODP carry a greater "genetic load" one might expect both earlier onset and more severe diabetes. In the series of Cooke *et al.* (3) this appeared to be true since 13 of 16 diabetic offspring were taking insulin. However, Tattersall and Fajans (21) found that only four of 170 offspring at risk had presented with symptoms of diabetes before the age of 20. All four, three of whom came from one sibship, were classical juvenile-onset, ketosis-prone diabetics. This finding does not support the hypothesis that maturity-onset diabetics are heterozygous for a gene which in the homozygous state produces juvenile-onset type diabetes (2,5). The remaining 53 diabetic OODP in this series had a mild maturity-onset type of diabetes and this should be emphasized in genetic counselling. Although the diabetes is mild in terms of carbohydrate tolerance and long-term treatment without insulin, it is not known whether the prevalence of complications, especially cardiovascular disease, is similar to or greater in OODP than in other groups of diabetics.

In conclusion: A knowledge of the ultimate prevalence of diabetes in children of two diabetic parents has important theoretical implications for an understanding of the inheritance of diabetes mellitus. Disagreement results from the different methods used to select offspring of two diabetic parents (OODP), different criteria of diabetes, variation in the age and body weight of offspring studied and the lack of longitudinal data.

At least a third of fertile marriages of two diabetic parents do not produce any diabetic offspring, the most likely explanation being that the parents have aetiologically different types of diabetes.

Genetic counselling of diabetics wishing to marry another diabetic is rarely needed in practice. One juvenile-onset type diabetic hardly ever wishes to marry another and there are no data on which to base an estimate of the risk of diabetes in their children. Any advice given ought to be based on the life expectancy of the partners. Where the partners are maturity-onset diabetics, marriage and procreation have already taken place so that the question of genetic counselling does not apply. The risk of overt diabetes in children of such a marriage is not great, the diabetes appears to be mild, and avoidance of obesity is the most important preventative measure.

It cannot be assumed that OODP are necessarily 'prediabetics' and the finding of metabolic abnormalities in offspring of the marriage of two maturity-onset diabetics is unlikely to be relevant to the pathogenesis of juvenile-onset type diabetes.

References

1. Andres, R.: Aging and Diabetes. Med. Clin. N. Amer. 55, 835 (1971)

2. Braunsteiner, H., Hansen, W., Jung, A., Sailer, S.: Latent diabetes mellitus in the parents of juvenile diabetics. Germ. Med. Monthly 11, 227 (1966)

3. Cooke, A.M., Fitzgerald, M.G., Malins, J., Pyke, D.A.: Diabetes in Children of Diabetic Couples. Brit. Med. J. 2, 674 (1966)

4. Goto, Y., Takayoshi, T., Karuhama, Y., Fukyhara, N., Sato, S., Chiba, M., Sato, Y.: Abnormalities in Prediabtes. Proc. 7th Congress of the IDF, Buenos Aires. Rodriguez, Vallance-Owen (eds.). Excerpt. Med. Int'l. Congress Series 23, 240 (1971)

5. Harris, H.: The familial distribution of diabetes mellitus: a study of the relatives of 1241 diabetic propositi. Ann. Eugen. 15, 95 (1950)

6. Jackson, W.P.U.: A Clinician Looks at Genetic Problems in Diabetes. Proc. 7th Congress of the IDF, Buenos Aires. Rodriguez, Vallance-Owen (eds.). Excerpt. Med. Int'l Congress Series 231, 379 (1971)

7. Jackson, W.P.U., Campbell, G.D., Marine, N., Major, V., Seedat, Y.K.: Triamcinolone - augmented glucose tolerance in offspring of diabetic couples. Metabolism 21, 807 (1972)

8. Kahn, C.B., Soeldner, J.S., Gleason, R.E., Rojas, L., Camerini-Davalos, R.A., Marble, A.: Clinical and chemical diabetes in offspring of diabetic couples. New Eng. J. Med. 281, 343 (1969)

9. Köbberling, J.: Untersuchungen zur Genetik des Diabetes Mellitus. Diabetologia 5, 392 (1969)

10. Lambert, T.H., Johnson, R.B., Paul, G.R.: Glucose and cortisone-glucose tolerance in normal and prediabetic humans. Ann. Int. Med. 54, 916 (1961)

11. Lozano-Castaneda, O., Quibrera, R., Garcia-Viveros, M., Rull, J.A.: Metabolic studies in prediabetic subjects. Early Diabetes. In: Advances in Metabolic Disorders, Suppl. 1. Camerini-Davalos, R.A., Cole, H.S. (eds.). New York: Academic Press, 1970, p. 315

12. Navarette, V.N., Torres, I.H.: Triamcinolone provative test in offspring of 2 diabetic parents. Diabetes 16, 57 (1967)

13. Neel, J.V., Fajans, S.S., Conn, J.W., Davidson, R.T.: Genetics and the epidemiology of Chronic Diseases. U.S. Pub. Health Serv. 1163, 105 (1965)

14. O'Sullivan, J.B., Mahan, C.M., Freedlender, A.E., William, R.E.: Effect of age on carbohydrate metabolism. J. Clin. Metab. 33, 619 (1971)

15. Pieptea, R., Pavel, I.: Le Role Protecteur de l'Allèle Non-Porteur dans le Diabète Héréditaire. Acta Diabet. Lat. 6, 76 (1969)

16. Pincus, G., White, P.: On the inheritance of diabetes mellitus. Amer. J., Med. Sci. 186, 1 (1933)

17. Post, R.H.: An approach to the question, does all diabetes depend on a single genetic locus? Diabetes 11, 56 (1962)

18. Rimoin, D.L.: Inheritance in Diabetes Mellitus. Med. Clin. N. Amer. 55, 307 (1971)

19. Simpson, N.E.: Multifactorial inheritance. A possible hypothesis for diabetes. Diabetes 13, 462 (1964)

20. Taton, J., Pometta, D., Camerini-Davalos, R.A., Marble, A.: Genetic determination to diabetes and tolerance to glucose. Lancet II, 1360 (1964)

21. Tattersall, R., Fajans, S.S.: Diabetes and carbohydrate tolerance in 199 offspring of 37 conjugal diabetic parents. Diabetes 24, 452 (1975)

22. Tattersall, R.B., Fajans, S.S.: A difference between the inheritance of classical juvenile-onset and maturity-onset diabetes of young people. Diabetes 24, 44 (1975)

23. West, K.M.: Response to cortisone in prediabetes. Glucose and steroid-glucose tolerance in subjects whose parents are both diabetic. Diabetes 9, 379 (1960)

24. Working Party Appointed by the College of General Practitioners: Glucose tolerance and glycosuria in the general population. Brit. Med. J. 2, 655 (1963)

20. Diabetes Mellitus in Identical Twins

D. A. PYKE and P. G. NELSON

Studies of twins have a long history. Forty or fifty years ago they were thought to be likely to distinguish the genetic and environmental factors in the etiology of several diseases and therefore were widely pursued. However, after a time they became less popular and in recent years relatively few studies on twins have been done.

There are probably two reasons for the decline in popularity of twin studies. (1) It has come to be realised that the fact that identical twins resemble each other in respect of a given disease does not prove that that disease is genetic in origin. Identical twins share a similar environment, particularly in the early years of their lives, and the fact they suffer from the same disease could as well be due to an environmental as to a genetic cause. (2) Many of the early twin studies were done by psychiatrists and psychologists in an attempt to determine the extent of genetic and environmental causes for intelligence, neurosis, and other psychologic features. They inevitably suffered from the disadvantage that measurement of these factors is often difficult· and causation nearly always complex. Too often great weight was attached to single expressions of multiple features.

Concordance rates are not only of uncertain significance but they are difficult to determine accurately. This difficulty springs from limitations of ascertainment. It is seldom possible to define a population precisely and to be certain that one has ascertained all the identical twin pairs in that population. Since identical twins are relatively uncommon - approximately 1 in 250 births - a large population must be searched for twins in order that a reasonable number shall be ascertained. There is a tendency for concordant pairs to be more frequently ascertained than discordant. As each pair contains two affected individuals, instead of one in the discordant pairs, there is a greater chance that observers will notice that they have the disease in question and that they are in fact identical twins.

The authors started their twin study 9 years ago (8). About a quarter of the twins are from their own clinic. Assuming that the population at present attending the clinic is approximately 5000, one would expect to find about the number of identical twins that one does in fact find,

Table 1. Sources from which twins were collected

	KCH clinic	Other physicians	Radio & T.V.	B.D.A.
Total No. of pairs	26	37	21	22
Concordant	19	21	18	13
Discordant	7	16	3	9

namely, 26 pairs, and, assuming a double chance of those being concordant as opposed to discordant we should expect that two third of the individuals would be concordant pairs and one third from discordant pairs. In fact the figures are 19 and 6 respectively. The authors have also been notified of twins by colleagues in other hospitals, through the British Diabetic Association, and through programs on radio and television. There is a striking difference in the concordance/discordance ratio in the twins from these various sources (Fig. 1). Among those referred by other colleagues and through the British Diabetic Association (B.D.A.) there are approximately equal numbers of concordant and discordants, but those who come through radio and television programs are almost all concordant. There are several possible reasons for this and one cannot be sure which is correct. The point is that the ratios are very different and therefore invalidate any firm conclusions that could be drawn from the overall concordance/discordance ratio in this series.

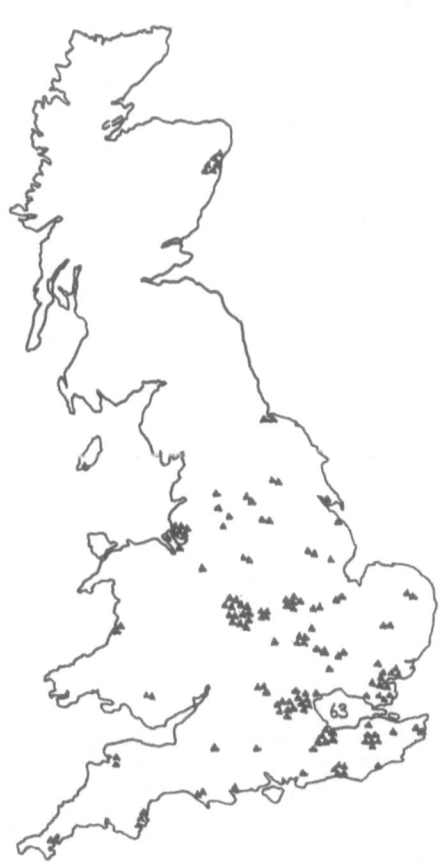

Fig. 1. Map of Britain showing uneven distribution of twins, indicating that there must still be many unascertained pairs

It is clear therefore that concordance rates do not necessarily indicate the degree of hereditability of a condition and that they are influenced by extraneous factors.

The authors have been more interested in discordance rates, i.e. in those pairs of twins in which one is diabetic and the other is not.

This gives much more solid information about what is <u>not</u> inherited in a condition than concordance rates do about what <u>is</u> inherited.

The authors have collected 106 pairs of identical twins, one or both of whom has diabetes. They have been helped in several ways in collecting this relatively large number. It is widely known amongst their colleagues that they are interested in the subject. Many diabetics are members of the British Diabetic Association and also know of their interest; whenever diabetics write with personal enquiries and mention that they know of identical twins, the B.D.A. passes this information on to the authors. The fact that England is a small country with a very high density of population, and that under the National Health Service there are no economic barriers to one doctor notifying another about his patients has also helped. The authors are willing to go anywhere at any time to see twins. As Figure 1 shows, the twins are scattered all over the United Kingdom.

The success of this study has depended greatly on the patients' motivation. The twins are examined and tested as soon as the authors are notified of their existence and thereafter they are kept under observation indefinitely; some of the twins have already been retested over a period of 9 years. It is therefore essential to get, and retain, their full cooperation and that of their doctors. Whenever the authors hear of twins, their full approval and that of their family doctor is secured. The authors have been gratified by the high degree of cooperation and help they have received. In the whole series only 3 individuals out of about 200 have refused to collaborate.

The total series consists of 106 pairs of identical twins. This seems a large number, and indeed is greater than any previously published series. Nevertheless, a simple calculation shows that we have ascertained only a small minority of the total number of identical twin pairs with diabetes (Table 2).

Table 2. Ascertainment of identical twins with diabetes

Population of U.K. (approx)	= 50 million
No. of identical twin pairs (1:250 births)	= 200,000
No. with diabetes (1% of population)	= 2,000
Allowing for increased mortality, say	1,000
of which, number expected aged	<40 = 200
	40+ = 800
This study has 106 pairs: Number diagnosed	<40 = 64 = 32% of estimated total
	40+= 42 = 5% " " "

The population of the United Kingdom is about 50 million. There should therefore be about 200,000 pairs of identical twins. If one assumes a prevalence of diabetes of 1% one would expect 2000 pairs with diabetes; making allowance for increased mortality and other factors one might halve that figure and reduce the number to 1000. If this is correct, only about 10% of the total number of identical twin pairs with diabetes have been ascertained. This figure is different for young-onset and old-onset twins. Of the 1000 pairs of twins with diabetes that one assumes there are in Britain one would expect, assuming that the age of onset of the twins was approximately the same as that for diabetics generally, that there would be about 800 older-onset and 200 with onset under the age of 40. Among twins in this study there are 64 pairs with early onset and 42 with onset over the age of 40. Thus about one third of the cases of diabetes in identical twins under the age of 40 has been ascertained, but only about 5% of those over this age. It is not

immediately clear why the ascertainment of young-onset pairs is so much
better than other cases; perhaps twins of early-onset are more aware
of the fact they are identical twins and therefore more easily ascertained.

Another reason for thinking that ascertainment of the identical twins
with diabetes in the country is far from complete can be seen from a
map showing an uneven distribution of the twins in the country (Fig. 1).
There are several clusters, for example in London, Leicester, Birmingham, and Liverpool, but in other centers of population there are no
twins represented in this study.

It is essential to be sure that the twins are identical. Although in
all possible cases detailed blood grouping has been undertaken this is
really unnecessary. The story that the twins give of being mistaken
for each other and being "alike as two peas in a pod" is characteristic.
Whenever there has been clinical doubt as to the twins being identical,
blood grouping has disproved that they were and, on the contrary, whenever the authors have thought clinically that they were identical,
blood grouping has never disproved it. The error in establishing mono-
zygosity is likely to be very small, certainly no more than 3% (1).

The series consists of 106 pairs of whom 71 are concordant and 35 discordant (Table 3). There is no doubt about the diagnosis of diabetes in
the affected twins. Nearly all had presented with symptoms and were
already under treatment at the time the authors saw them, and verifica-
tion was obtained from hospital records. In the concordant pairs the
second twin was discovered to be diabetic on clinical grounds in the
great majority. Of the remainder, half had been diagnosed on the basis
of a routine test and the other half were discovered to have diabetes
on glucose tolerance testing on apparently unaffected twin (using the
criteria of the British Diabetic Association). In these cases the pair
has been classified as concordant. Of the twins diagnosed under the
age of 40 all but six (3 pairs) were treated with insulin. Amongst those
diagnosed over this age 21 were on insulin. 41 on tablets, and 17 on
diet alone.

Table 3. King's College Hospital twin series

Total No. of monozygotic twin pairs	106
Concordant (both diabetic)	71
Discordant (only one diabetic)	35

The numbers of twins who are concordant and discordant for diabetes
varies greatly with age (Table 4). Before the age of 40 there are equal

Table 4. Concordance and discordance for diabetes among 106 pairs of identical twins
in relation to age at diagnosis in index twin

Age at onset	Number of pairs	
	Concordant	Discordant
<40	32	32
40-49	13	3
50+	26	0
All	71	35

numbers of concordant and discordant pairs; over the age of 50 all are concordant. The authors have still not seen a pair of identical twins in whom diabetes appeared in one twin after the age of 50 when the other twin was not also diabetic, or discovered to be so on testing. This finding that early-onset diabetic twin pairs are more often discordant than older-onset pairs may seem surprising but is in keeping with the published results of other workers (Table 5), particularly those of Then Berg (9) and Gottlieb and Root (4). The series of Harvald and Hauge (6) consisted largely of older-onset pairs and it is perhaps for this reason that they suggested that all twin pairs would eventually become concordant (5).

Table 5. Concordance/Discordance Rates in Monozygotic Twins (published series)

	Total	Discordant	"Juvenile-onset"	
			Number	Discordant
Then Berg (9)	47	16 (34%)	12	6 (50%)
Harvald & Hauge (6)	53	21 (40%)	6	No. GTT's
Gottlieb & Root (4)	30	19 (63%)	20	15 (75%)
Present series	106	35 (33%)	64	32 (50%)

It might be argued that in the discordant pairs the unaffected twin would eventually become diabetic and the reason for the pairs being discordant was simply that there had not yet been time for the second twin to develop diabetes. This is an unlikely explanation for two reasons.

Table 6. Lenght of Discordance

	Number of twin pairs	
	Concordant[a]	Discordant
3 years or less	50	2
4-10 years	16	14
Over 10 years	3	19

[a] In three concordant pairs the interval between diagnosis of diabetes in the first and second twin was not known.

(1) As shown in Table 6, among the concordant pairs the second twin has become diabetic within 3 years of the index twin in the majority of cases; in only 3 pairs was the gap longer than 10 years. However, among the discordant pairs over half are still discordant after more than 10 years. (2) Repeated glucose tolerance testing of the unaffected members of discordant pairs shows no sign of deterioration in their glucose tolerance or of insulin secretion (Fig. 2). For these reasons therefore is unlikely that many of the twins who are at present unaffected will become diabetic. In the whole series there is, to the authors knowledge, only one individual who, having been tested when his cotwin developed juvenile-onset diabetes and having had at that time an almost normal glucose tolerance, after episodes of apparent spontaneous hypoglycaemia himself developed acute insulin-requiring diabetes 5 years later.

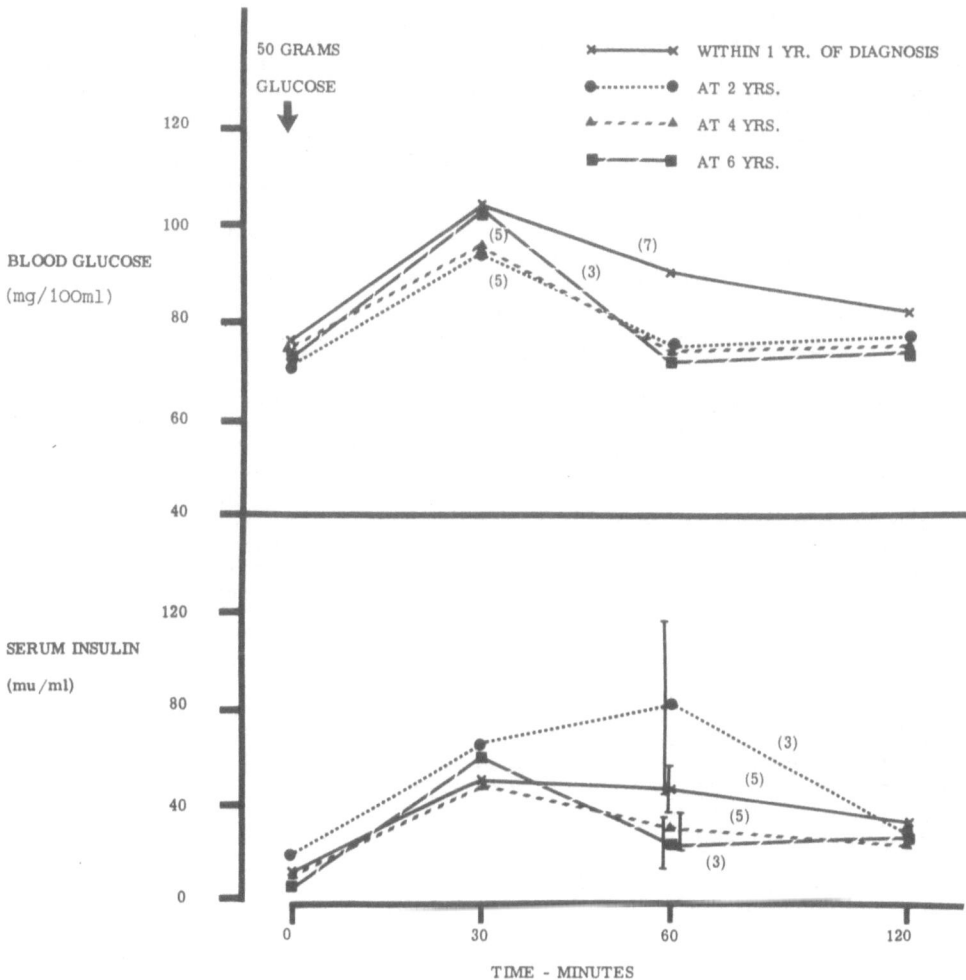

Fig. 2. Repeated glucose tolerance tests with serum insulin in twins tested over 6 years showing no significant deterioration

If one accepts that the discordant pairs are genuinely discordant and that most are likely to remain so, one needs to look for factors to explain their discordance. A family history of diabetes is found more often in the concordant (45%) than the discordant (17%) twins (Table 7), which might suggest that the concordant twins have "genetic" and

Table 7. Number of twin pairs with diabetic first degree relative

Twins	Concordant	Discordant
All ages	32/71	6/35
<40	6/32	4/31
40+	26/39	2/4

the discordant twins "acquired" diabetes. However, the division of the
twins by age of onset shows that among young-onset cases the frequency
of a first degree family history of diabetes is low and is about the
same in concordant and discordant pairs, but that in older-onset cases
which are nearly all concordant, a positive family history is found
in nearly 70%. Thus family history does not distinguish between concordant and discordant twins but rather between young and old. It is in
the older twins that genetic factors seem to be more important. Obesity
appears not to be an etiologic factor since the affected twins were
not heavier than the unaffected ones. If an exogenous or environmental
cause is responsible for the diabetes in the affected twin one might
expect that discordant pairs would be, at the time of diabetes appearing
in the affected twin, living apart more frequently than was the case
in the concordant pairs, but this is not so. Numbers are too small to
draw any conclusions about parity; the evidence does not suggest this
is an explanation for diabetes appearing in the affected twin. A virus
infection may be responsible for some cases of juvenile-onset diabetes
(3) and Coxsackie B4 and other virus titers have been observed in the
twins. No conclusive evidence that virus infection has been the cause
of diabetes has been found; on the other hand, this is not surprising
since in most cases the twins have been examined some years after diabetes first appeared, and at this stage an elevated virus titer might
well have fallen to normal. Only 7 juvenile-onset discordant pairs from
the time of diagnosis of diabetes have been seen; none has shown evidence of recent Coxsackie B4 virus infection.

Recently, great interest has been aroused by the reports of Nerup and
his colleagues of an increase of certain histocompatibility antigens
in juvenile-onset, but not in maturity-onset, cases of diabetes (7).
They found a significantly increased frequency of HL-A8 and W15 antigens in their cases, and calculated the relative risk for juvenile
onset diabetes of slightly over 2 for those with these antigens. So
far 48 pairs of twins with juvenile-onset diabetes have been examined
by the authors and they too show an increase of HL-A8 and, more significantly, of W15 (Table 8). If relative risks from the twin data are
calculated, it becomes clear that there is greater risk for those with
W15 than those with HL-A8 (Table 9).

Table 8. HL-A antigens in diabetic twin pairs (age<40)

	Percent	
	HL-A8	W15
Twins (48)	46	35
Nondiabetic controls (300)(2)	31	10
	P<.1	P<.0001

Table 9. Relative risks for (juvenile-onset) diabetes in relation to HL-A antigens

	HL-A8	W15
Combined published series (2)	2.1	2.6
Identical twins (Present series)	2	5

There is an interesting difference in the HL-A antigen frequency in
the concordant and discordant twins. There is an increase of W15 antigen in both types but of HL-A8 only in the concordant pairs (Table 10).
Previous series have shown an approximately equal increase in preva-

lence of both antigens in diabetics; however, the present results are
based on small numbers and do not achieve statistical significance
(p =.11). More data must be collected before a true genetic heteroge-
netity can be determined. On their present data the authors can cal-
culate the relative risks of diabetes separately from the data for concordant and discordant twins and it becomes clear that although the
risks for HL-A8 and W15 are approximately the same for the concordant
twins they are widely different for the discordant, a sevenfold increase of risk for W15 but no increase for HL-A8 (Table 11).

Table 10. HL-A antigens in concordant and discordant twin pairs

	Total	Number HL-A8	W15
Concordant	25	15	7
Discordant	23	7	10

Table 11. Relative risks in relation to HL-A antigens calculated from concordant
and discordant twins

	HL-A8	W15
Concordant	3.3	3.5
Discordant	1.0	7.1

The authors conclude from these studies (1) that genetic factors cannot
be entirely responsible for diabetes of juvenile-onset but may be the
main cause of older-onset diabetes. This is at variance with previous
suppositions that early-onset diabetes was more dependant upon genetic
factors. (2) Identification of an external factor which might have
caused diabetes in the young-onset discordant pairs was not possible
but virus infection has not been excluded as a cause, at least in some
cases. (3) There may be an increased risk of developing juvenile-onset
diabetes for those possessing HL-A8 or W15 antigens. It is not possible
to say whether they are significant or indicate an altered state of
immunologic resistance which might be related to susceptibility or resistance to infection.

References

1. Cederlöff, F.R., Friberg, L., Jonsson, E., Kaij, L.: Studies of similarity diagnosis in twins with the aid of marked questionnaires. Acta genet. statist. med.
   11, 338 (1961)

2. Cudworth, A.G., Woodrow, J.C.: HL-A antigens and diabetes mellitus. Lancet II,
   1153 (1974)

3. Gamble, D.R., Taylor, K.W., Cumming, H.: Coxsackie viruses and diabetes mellitus.
   Brit. Med. J. 4, 260 (1973)

4. Gottlieb, M.S., Root, H.F.: Diabetes mellitus in twins. Diabetes 17, 693 (1968)

5. Harvald, B.: Genetic perspectives in diabetes mellitus. Acta Medica Scand. 476,
   17 (1967)

6. Harvald, B., Hauge, M.: Selection in diabetes in modern society. Acta Medica
   Scand. 173, 459 (1963)

7. Nerup, J., Platz, P., Andersen, O.O., Christy, M., Lyngsøe, J., Poulsen, J.E., Ryder, L.P., Nielsem. L.S., Thomsen, M., Svejgaard, A.: HL-A antigens and diabetes mellitus. Lancet II, 864 (1974)

8. Tattersall, R.B., Pyke, D.A.: Diabetes in identical twins. Lancet II, 1120 (1972)

9. Then Berg, H.: Die Erbbiologie des Diabetes Mellitus. Arch. Rass. u. Ges. Biol. 32, 289 (1938)

21. Microangiopathy in Diabetics of Different Etiologies

R. ØSTERBY

The long-term diabetic syndrome, as described in the early 1950s by Lundbaek (48), is to a large extent dominated by vascular complications, often in combination with symptoms of neuropathy. Today these late clinical manifestations of widespread vascular involvment, affecting both the large vessels and the capillary system constitute the most serious problem for the patient with diabetes mellitus, threatening his well-being and his life.

Current methods of treatment of the metabolic disorder, available to diabetics in many areas of the world has not abolished these serious complications. Their contribution to the greatly increased mortality in patients with diabetes mellitus makes further investigations in this field very urgent.

Etiology of Diabetic Microangiopathy - Genetic Versus Metabolic Factors

Many fundamental questions about the nature of the vascular disease remain unanswered.

There is not complete agreement as to whether the vascular complications are dependent on genetic factors, or if they develop in diabetic patients solely as a consequence of the disturbed metabolic state.

If the latter were true, it should be possible to prevent the angiopathy by appropriate metabolic control. Many attempts have been made to evaluate the effect of good control. Although the bulk of evidence points to an advantageous effect clearcut proof has never been obtained (36, 40).

It is therefore still relevant to try and clarify the role genetic and metabolic factors play.

One approach to this question is to determine the time relationship between the development of microangiopathy and the metabolic disturbance. Should the angiopathy be a consequence of metabolic factors these must of necessity be present prior to any alterations in the vessels.

Another clearcut approach is to see what happens with the vasculature in cases where the metabolic derangement is present without the genetic trait.

Finally, some valid information might be obtained by studying the natural history of the capillary abnormalities in different populations of diabetics who presumably have different genetic backgrounds.

Development of Basement Membrane Thickening in Relationship to the Metabolic Disorder

The diabetic microangiopathy is a widespread disorder of the small vessels, affecting nearly all capillary areas that have so far been studied. The morphologic appearance of the lesion is primarily a thickening of the capillary wall, seen on light microscopy as a strongly PAS-positive structure. With electron microscopy, it is revealed to be due to thickening of the basement membrane.

For the evaluation of the extent of the microangiopathy the appropriate parameter therefore is the thickness of the basement membrane, and as such it has been used in several studies in recent years.

The thickness of the glomerular basement membrane was employed in the author's study (reported below in short) to determine the time relationship between the onset of microangiopathy and of the metabolic disorder (69). For this purpose it is obviously necessary to investigate diabetic patients in whom the onset of diabetes is well defined, i.e. young patients with juvenile diabetes of acute onset. Secondly, the morphologic parameter must be accurately estimated with a randomized quantitative technique.

Figure 1 shows a section of a glomerular tuft. The basement membrane in the capillary wall is clearly demarcated by cell membranes on both sides. Due to the great variation in thickness a large number of systematically randomized measurements were required. These were obtained from total glomerular cross sections, produced as photomontages of electron micrographs, measuring only at places of perpendicular sectioning. The distribution of measurements from each cross section was markedly right-skewed. With a transformation of reciprocal type, normal distributions were obtained (24) and the mean values of these were employed for the statistical analysis.

Applying the described procedures in a group of young diabetics with newly diagnosed disease and a comparable group of nondiabetics, it was found that the basement membrane thickness is normal at the acute onset of juvenile diabetes, and therefore also, by implication, in prediabetes.

The initial basement membrane lesion was then sought in diabetics with a few years' duration of disease. It was found, that already after about 2 years the basement membrane had thickened (Fig. 2). This conclusion was drawn from paired comparison of results obtained in patients who were followed with repeated biopsies, at the onset of the disease and again 2 years later. In another group of patients with about 3-5 years' duration, basement membrane thickening was found to be even more pronounced (Fig. 2).

Analogous results were obtained by measuring the mesangial regions: they are normal at the onset of diabetes, both as regards the relative size and content of basement membranelike material. The relative mesangial size remained normal within the first 5 years of diabetes. On the other hand, it was shown by a paired comparison of repeated biopsies that the amount of basement membranelike material within the mesangial regions had increased after 2 years of diabetes.

These results have been confirmed in quantitative studies published from other laboratories (31,38,44). Some authors, however, had arrived at different conclusions, but their results were mostly based on nonquantitative investigations or on casual nonrandomized measurements.

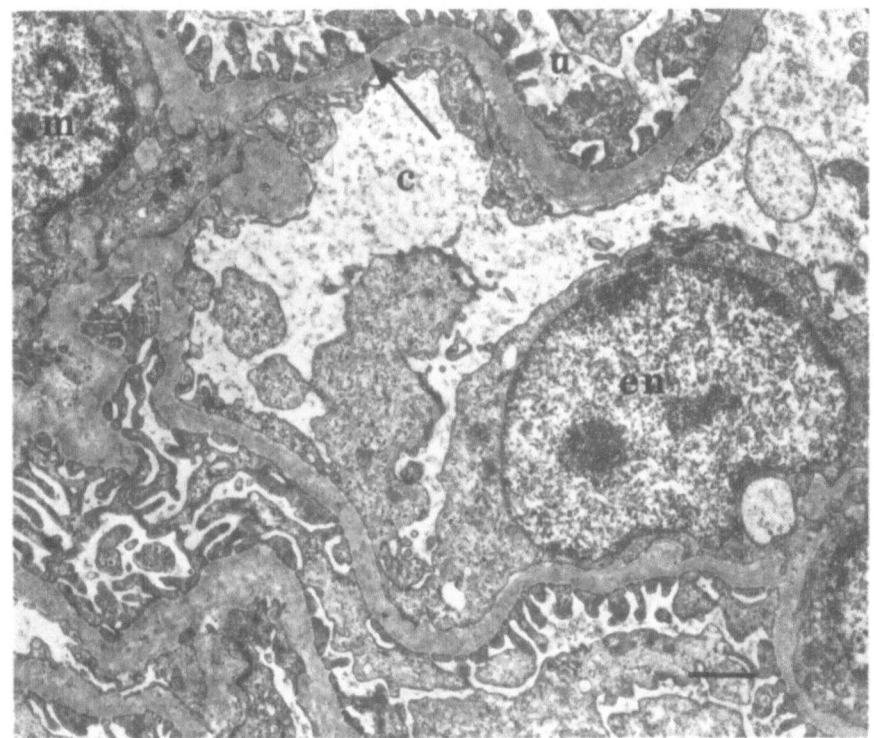

Fig. 1. Electron micrograph showing section of glomerular tuft. Kidney biopsy from newly diagnosed diabetic. The peripheral basement membrane (arrow), which constitutes central layer of the capillary wall, is clearly delineated by endothelial cell at capillary side and by epithelial cell towards urinary space. A small section of solid mesangial area is seen at upper left. en:nucleus of endothelial cell. m:nucleus of mesangial cell. c:capillary space. u:urinary space. Horizontal bar:1μ

Conflicting views have been held regarding muscle capillary basement membrane (62). In recent, well-documented studies, however, it has been concluded that the basement membrane of muscle capillaries is normal in prediabetic subjects (66) and in young, juvenile diabetics at the onset of disease (12,55,67).

It seems by now to be accepted that the basement membrane thickness is normal at the acute onset of juvenile diabetes mellitus. The study of sequential kidney biopsies showed that the initial thickening is very closely connected in time with the clinical onset of metabolic abnormalities. The findings therefore strongly suggest that metabolic factors play an important role in this development.

Development of Microangiopathy in Secondary Diabetes

Proof of metabolic factors alone being sufficient for the development of microangiopathy would be obtained if the angiopathy were to occur in cases without the genetic trait.

Noninherited diabetes occurs, for instance, in patients with pancreatitis, pancreatic cancer, or hemochromatosis, when a sufficiently high

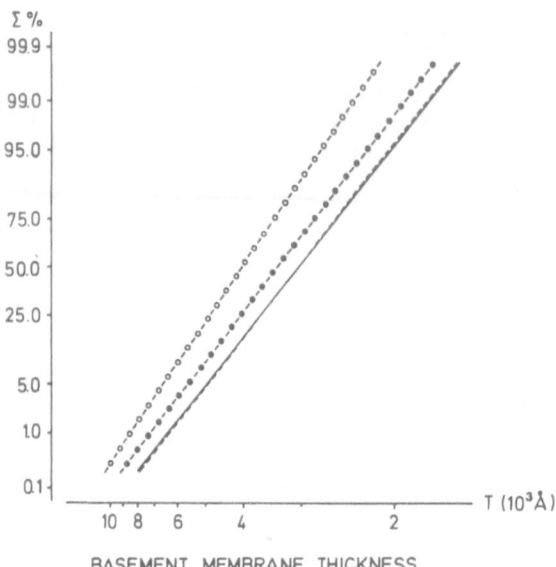

Σ%
99.9
99.0
95.0
75.0
50.0
25.0
5.0
1.0
0.1

T (10³Å)

10 8   6   4   2

BASEMENT MEMBRANE THICKNESS

———   CONTROLS
-----   DIABETICS, recent onset
-•-•-   DIABETICS, 1½-2½ years' duration
-◦-◦-   DIABETICS, 3½-5 years' duration

Fig. 2. The thickness of peripheral glomerular basement membrane in 4 different
goups of subjects is illustrated. From transformed distributions (see text) group
means and SD have been calculated and plotted. The graph illustrates similarity
between controls and recent onset diabetics as well as increase in basement membrane
thickness with increasing duration of diabetes

proportion of the islet tissue is damaged and has ceased to function.
In so far as an idiopathic diabetes may be left out of account, the
pancreatogenic diabetes represents a metabolic disorder, in many ways
similar to that in diabetes mellitus but without the genetic trait.
If a diabetic microangiopathy develops in such patietns it goes very
strongly against the theory that hereditary predisposition is the
decisive factor. It is therefore of great theoretical interest to establish the presence or absence of microangiopathy in cases of secondary diabetes. In the following a brief review of the literature on the
subject is given.

Somewhat divergent conclusions have been drawn by different investigators. In some of the earlier papers, diabetic microangiopathy in secondary diabetes was considered to be extremely rare or nonexistent
(4,47).

Opposing these statements a number of case reports with positive findings appeared.

In Table 1 individual cases are shown that have been reported in the
bibliography. Other cases have been mentioned but without detail.

In the patients reported by Burton (7) and Doyle (15) a total pancreatectomy had been performed. In one of these patients (15) a typical

nodular and diffuse glomerulosclerosis was found at the postmortem examination.

Table 1. Cases with Secondary Diabetes and Microangiopathy

	Duration of diabetes, years	Retinopathy	Glomerulo-sclerosis
Burton *et al.*, 1957 (7)	10	+	
Duncan *et al.*, 1958 (16)	29	+	+
Deckert 1960 (13)	12	+	
Doyle *et al.*, 1964 (15)	14	+	+
Shapiro *et al.*,1966 (61)	9		+
Caird *et al.*, 1968 (8)	16	+	

·The patients with chronic pancreatitis and microangiopathy (Table 1) had a more than 8 years duration of diabetes. The glomerular involvment in 2 of the cases was described and illustrated as Kimmelstiel-Wilson lesions, presumably the most characteristic picture of diabetic microangiopathy.

The conclusions that can be drawn from individual cases are of course limited; but these reports drew attention to the subject, and additional publications have appeared which deal with series of patients with secondary diabetes studied with the purpose of determining the frequency of vascular complications. Results of such studies are shown in Table 2. Evidently the frequency of microangiopathy is not comparable in the different series, since account must be taken of the composition of the patient groups with respect to cause and severity of the pancreatic disorder, duration of the diabetic state etc. Several of

Table 2. Microangiopathy in Series of Secondary Diabetes

	no. of patients studied	duration of diabetes in the series, years.	cases with microangiopathy no., and type of microang.	duration of diabetes, years
Sprague, 1947 (63)	24	?	1,retinopathy	9
Ireland *et al.*, 1967 (30)	10	1/4-15	8,thickening of glomerular basement membrane	1/4=15
Siperstein, 1968 (62)	13	?	1,thickening of muscle cap. basement membrane	?
Derot *et al.*, 1970 (14)	29	<6-18	1,retinopathy 2,retionp. + nephropathy[a]	9 13,18
Sevel *et al.*, 1971 (60)	27	1-15	2,retinopathy	6,21

[a] Albuminuria and lowered creatinine clearance.

the patients included had a mild, asymptomatic diabetes and in most of
the cases the duration of diabetes was less than 5 years. In Sevel's
series the frequency of retinopathy was compared with that in control
groups of diabetics matched for age and duration of diabetes. However,
since most of the patients were over 40 years of age, they may have
had diabetes longer than was estimated from the clinical data. Therefore, the higher frequency of retinopathy among the diabetics (30%
versus , 10% in the cases with secondary diabetes) probably cannot
be ascribed to the different types of diabetes.

Attention should also be drawn to the fact that the diagnostic criteria
used for the assessment of microangiopathy are quite different in the
different series. Ireland *et al.*(30) employed the thickness of the
glomerular basement membrane to characterize the microangiopathy. They
found a statistically significant increase in basement membrane thickness in the patients with secondary diabetes. With light microscopy
one of the patients was furthermore found to have specific nodular
lesions.

In the critical evaluation of these studies it is important to know
whether or not the patients with pancreatic disease were also suffering
from genetically determined diabetes. Here the relatively high frequency of diabetes in the general population causes a problem. However,
the high prevalence of diabetes among the patient groups with secondary diabetes probably indicates that the great majority of the cases
are not genetically determined.

Patients with diabetes due to viral infection of the pancreas may represent a similar type of secondary diabetes. The frequency of this
condition is not known at present, and consequently, there are no data
as to their risk of angiopathy compared to that of other diabetics.

The mechanism which leads to a diabetic state in hemochromatosis is
not entirely clear. Although damage of pancreatic endocrine tissue must
be the cause in many cases this is probably not always the sole factor
(4,10,17,43). This condition is therefore more heterogenous, and the
reported results more difficult to interpret.

The results concerning the occurrence of microangiopathy in hemochromatosis are, in fact, also quite heterogenous. Some authors deny this
coexistence (4,47) and others point out that it does exist (3,17,22,
23,43,56). Some have stressed that the frequency is somewhat lower
than in idiopathic diabetes (10,56).

The sum of observations that have been made indicate that the very
specific elements of diabetic microangiopathy are observed in a number
of patients with diabetes following pancreatic damage.

Whether there is a real difference in frequency or severity from that
in comparable groups of genetic diabetics cannot be firmly estimated.

Development of Microangiopathy in Experimental Diabetes

The situation in animal studies is more clearcut, since populations
are available devoid of genetic predisposition to diabetes. In such
studies in which a diabetic state is experimentally produced by selec-
tively destructing the islet tissue, it has repeatedly been demonstrated that abnormalities develop in the small blood vessels, which
are analogous to those described in human diabetes.

The studies have concerned morphologic abnormalities primarily in glomeruli and retina, and to a lesser extent in other capillaries. It has
been argued against the usefulness of the experimental model, that the
entire picture of diabetic microangiopathy was not observed in such
animals, e.g. retinopathy was frequently absent, as was also the nodular
lesion of diabetic glomerulopathy. However, absolute morphologic identity with the human lesion was hardly to be expected. A glomerular lesion
very similar to human diabetic glomerulosclerosis has been shown to
develop in rats (27,50,53,68), dogs (5), and monkeys (6). Several aspects of diabetic retinopathy have also been found in experimentally
produced diabetes (6,19,41,46). Thickening of capillary basement membranes has been demonstrated in quantitative electron-microscopic studies of glomeruli (9,28), retina, and striated muscle (5).

After insulin treatment (29), pancreatic islet transplantation (54),
and after transplantation of the kidney into nondiabetic animals (45)
some morphologic abnormalities have been seen to be reversed and this
has certainly very important implications. These results await docu-
mentation with precise quantitative morphometric techniques.

The conclusion to be drawn from studies of animals with experimental
diabetes is that metabolic factors alone are sufficient to produce
capillary abnormalities very much like those of diabetic microangiopathy. These results are of great interest, although, of course, they
do not unequivocally prove whether metabolic factors alone are responsible in human diabetes.

Diabetic Microangiopathy in Different Clinical Types of Diabetes Mellitus

In the following some facts about the microangiopathy in different diabetic populations in which presumably the genetic background varies
are enumerated.

The above-mentioned indications about time of onset of angiopathy was
based exclusively on findings in juvenile diabetes. Are there any
principal differences in the nature of microangiopathy in various types
of diabetes?

It is obvious from clinical experience that the microangiopathy in individual patients may develop quite differently. Among a population of
long-term diabetics there may be a few patients who have done extraor-
dinarily well, being practically devoid of signs of microangiopathy
after many years' duration. What may condition this course we do not
know. Other patients, on the other hand, show a rapid progression to
state of gross functional impairment after a few years.

One difficulty in obtaining clear answers is that we do not know the
relevant way to subdivide the diabetics except for the most extreme
cases, for example classical juvenile versus mild maturity-onset type.

The morphologic picture of the angiopathy, e.g. the retinopathy and
the glomerulosclerosis, is basically the same in the two different types
of diabetes, perhaps with slight differences in the frequency of individual elements, e.g., the nodular glomerular lesion being a little
more frequent and the preretinal proliferations perhaps being somewhat
more rare in elderly than in young people.

A typical diabetic microangiopathy occurs also in patients with very
mild disease.

When large groups of patients are studied at the time when the diagnosis of diabetes is made, 5-7% are found to have diabetic retinopathy (42, 49,57). Such cases are nearly always very mild, and occur only in old persons, i.e., some degree of metabolic derangement may have been present for any number of years before the patient found reason to visit the doctor. Similarly, histologic demonstrations of diabetic glomerulosclerosis have been made in old patients with very mild diabetes (2, 18,37).

Some recent data are available on the occurrence of microangiopathy in the peculiar type of asymptomatic diabetes found in some young patients (20,34). Tattersall (see Chapter 10) and Fajans (see Chapter 8) have reported on the rare occurrence of retinopathy. In the series of Fajans *et al.* (21) muscle biopsies were performed and it was found that the group as a whole showed thickening. The degree of basement membrane thickening was found to correlate with the known duration of diabetes.

Diabetic Microangiopathy in Different Ethnic Groups

The study of microangiopathy in different ethnic groups is very relevant to the question of the influence of differences in heredity.

The prevalence of diabetes seems to be quite different among different populations. A very low prevalence has been reported among for example Eskimos and some American Indians, whereas other American Indians and East Indians are found to have a very high prevalence (33,58,59,65). It has been held that the classical juvenile type of diabetes is uncommon in a number of populations, e.g. in the East. It is clear, however, that epidemiologic studies are extremely difficult to carry out in many areas of the world. The prevalence of an acute, rapidly progressive disease may well be greatly underestimated.

It is also difficult to estimate the incidence of vascular disease among different populations. It has been claimed that e.g., nephropathy is more frequent in Japan where it also constitutes a more frequent cause of death than in Europe (26). A relatively high frequency of vascular complications has also been reported in Indian diabetics and among the Pima Indians (32,35). It is, however, impossible to prepare statistics for prevalence, severity, etc., which could be compared between these different groups. The difficulties in carrying out epidemiologic studies in many areas have already been mentioned. Furthermore, "environmental" differences are hard to evaluate, due to the many varieties in diet, the incidence of obesity, various infections, degree of physical activity, etc.

Diabetic Microangiopathy in Different Syndromes Associated with Diabetes

Finally, there are the different syndromes associated with impaired glucose tolerance (58) (see also Chapter 7). Since such patients represent a metabolic disorder considered to be different from that of diabetes mellitus, it is of theoretical interest to see whether such patients develop the same type of microangiopathy as diabetics.

The available amount of information, however, is rather scanty, probably due to the fact that such cases rarely survive long enough for angiopathy to develop. Retinopathy or glomerulosclerosis have been reported to occur in a few individual cases representing some of the different syndromes, e.g. lipoatrophic diabetes (1,25,51), Werner's syndrome (52), and Prader-Labhart-Willi's syndrome (64).

In various neuromuscular disorders, some of them associated with glucose intolerance, thickening of muscle capillary basement membrane
has been described (11,39). However, the morphologic findings did not
correlate with the glucose intolerance.

The conclusions that can be drawn from the finding of a few microaneurysms in a few patients of these categories are obviously very
limited.

The present survey of available information about the microangiopathy
in diabetes of different etiologies has covered fields in which exact
investigations have been possible as well as other fields which are
very difficult to evaluate.

In the opinion of the author the best information available about human
and experimental diabetes strongly suggests that vascular disease in
diabetes mellitus is due in some way to the metabolic disturbance which
we estimate in daily clinical practice by parameters such as blood
glucose level, excretion of glucose, ketone bodies, etc.

References

1. Aarseth, S.: Lipoatrophic diabetes (abstract). Diabetologia 3, 535 (1967)

2. Arnold, J.D., Tarlov, A.R., Spargo, B., Brewer, G.J.: Subclinical diabetes mellitus in patients presenting with clinical chronic "glomerulonephritis". Trans.
   Assoc. Am. Phys. 71, 186 (1958)

3. Becker, D., Miller, M.: Presence of diabetic glomerulosclerosis in patients with
   hemochromatosis. New Eng. J. Med. 263, 367 (1960)

4. Bell, E.T.: Relation of portal cirrhosis to hemochromatosis and to diabetes
   mellitus. Diabetes 4, 435 (1955)

5. Bloodworth, J.M.B., Jr., Engerman, R.L.: Spontaneous and induced diabetic micro-
   angiopathy. In: Acta Diabetologica Latina, Suppl. 1. Blood Vessel Disease in
   Diabetes Mellitus. Lundbaek, K., Keen, H. (eds.). Milano: The Publishing House
   "Il Ponte", 1971, Vol. VIII, p. 263

6. Bloodworth, J.M.B., Jr., Engerman, R.L., Anderson, P.J.: Microangiopathy in
   experimentally diabetic animal. In: Advances in Metabolic Disorders: Vascular
   and Neurological Changes in Early Diabetes, Suppl. 2. Camerini-Davalos, R.A.,
   Cole, H.S. (eds.). New York, London: Academic Press, 1973, p. 245

7. Burton, T.Y., Kearns, T.P., Rynearson, R.H.: Diabetic retinopathy following total
   pancreatectomy. Proc. Mayo Clin. 32, 735 (1957)

8. Caird, F.I., Pirie, A., Ramsell, T.G.: Diabetes and the eye. Edinburgh: Blackwell
   scientific publications, 1968, p. 78

9. Cameron, D.P., Amherdt, M., Leuenberger, P., Orci, L., Stauffacher, W.: Microvascular alterations in chronically streptozotocin-diabetic rats. In: Advances
   in Metabolic Disorders: Vascular and Neurological Changes in Early Diabetes,
   Suppl. 2. Camerini-Davalos, R.A., Cole, H.S. (eds.). New York, London: Academic
   Press, 1973, p. 257

10. Creutzfeldt, W.: Der Diabetes des pancreaslosen Menschen. In: Handbuch des Dia-
    betes Mellitus. Pfeiffer, E.F. (ed.). München: Lehmanns Verlag, 1971, Vol. II,
    p. 239

11. Danowski, T.S., Khurana, R.C., Gonzalez, A.R., Fisher, E.R.: Capillary basement
    membrane thickness and the pseudodiabetes of myopathy. Am. J. Med. 51, 757 (1971)

12. Danowski, T.S., Fisher, E.R., Khurana, R.C., Nolan, S., Stephan, T.: Muscle
    capillary basement membrane in juvenile diabetes mellitus. Metabolism 21, 1125
    (1972)

13. Deckert, T.: Late diabetic manifestations in pancreatogenic diabetes mellitus. Acta Med. Scand. <u>168</u>, 439 (1960)

14. Derot, M., Bour, H., Tutin, M., Guy-Grand, B.: Diabète sucré et pancréatite chronique. Le Diabète <u>18</u>, 93 (1970)

15. Doyle, A.P., Balcerzak, S.P., Geffrey, W.L.: Fatal diabetic glomerulosclerosis after total pancreatectomy. New Eng. J. Med. <u>270</u>, 623 (1964)

16. Duncan, L.J.P., Mac Farlane, A., Robson, J.S.: Diabetic retionpathy and nephropathy in pancreatic diabetes. Lancet <u>I</u>, 822 (1958)

17. Dymock, I.W., Cassar, J., Pyke, D.A., Oakley, W.G., Williams, R.: Observations on the pathogenesis, complications and treatment of diabetes in 115 cases of hemochromatosis. Am. J. Med. <u>52</u>, 203 (1972)

18. Ellenberg, M.: Diabetic nephropathy without manifest diabetes. Diabetes <u>11</u>, 197 (1962)

19. Engerman, R.L., Bloodworth, J.M.B., Jr.: Experimental diabetic retinopathy in dogs. Arch. Ophthal. <u>73</u>, 205 (1965)

20. Fajans, S.S., Conn, J.W.: Tolbutamide-induced improvement in carbohydrate tolerance of young people with mild diabetes mellitus. Diabetes <u>9</u>, 83 (1960)

21. Fajans, S.S., Wiliamson, J.R., Weissman, P.N., Vogler, N.J., Kilo, C., Conn, J.W.: Basement membrane thickening in latent diabetes. In: Advances in Metabolic Disorders: Vascular and Neurological Changes in Early Diabetes. Camerini-Davalos, R.A., Cole, H.S. (eds.). New York, London: Academic Press, 1973, p. 393

22. Galton, D.J.: Diabetic retinopathy and haemochromatosis. Brit. Med. J. <u>1</u>, 1169 (1965)

23. Griffiths, J.D., Dymock, I.W., Davies, E.W.G., Hill, D.W., Williams, R.: Occurrence and prevalence of diabetic retinopathy in hemochromatosis. Diabetes <u>20</u>, 766 (1971)

24. Gundersen, H.J.G., Østerby, R.: Statistical analysis of transformations leading to normal distribution of measurements of the peripheral glomerular basement membrane. J. Microsc. <u>97</u>, 293 (1973)

25. Hamwi, G.J., Kruger, F.A., Eymontt, M.J., Scarpelli, D.G., Gwinup, G., Byron, R.: Lipoatrophic diabetes. Diabetes <u>15</u>, 262 (1966)

26. Hirose, K.: Clinical and pathological features of diabetic nephropathy in Japanese diabetic patients. In: Diabetes Mellitus in Asia, 1970. Tsuji, S., Wada, M. (eds.). Amsterdam: Excerpta Medica, 1971, p. 177

27. Hägg, E.: Renal lesions in rats with long-term alloxan diabetes. Acta Path. Microbiol. Scand. Section A. <u>82</u>, 199 (1974)

28. Hägg, E.: Glomerular basement membrane thickening in rats with long-term alloxan diabetes. Acta Path. Microbiol. Scand. Section A. <u>82</u>, 211 (1974)

29. Hägg, E.: Influence of insulin treatment on glomerular changes in rats with long-term alloxan diabetes. Acta Path. Microbiol. Scand. Section A. <u>82</u>, 228 (1974)

30. Ireland, J.T., Patnaik, B.K., Duncan, L.J.P.: Glomerular ultrastructure in secondary diabetics and normal subjects. Diabetes <u>16</u>, 628 (1967)

31. Ireland, J.T.: Diagnostic criteria in the assessment of glomerular capillary basement membrane lesions in newly diagnosed juvenile diabetics. In: Advances in Metabolic Disorders: Early Diabetes, Suppl. 1. Camerini-Davalos, R.A., Cole, H.S. (eds.). New York, London: Academic Press, 1970, p. 273

32. Jackson, W.P.U., Goldberg, M.D., Major, V., Campbell, G.D.: Vascular and other diabetes-related disorders among natal Indian diabetics and nondiabetics. S. Afr. Med. J. <u>44</u>, 279 (1970)

33. Jackson, W.P.U.: Diabetes mellitus in different countries and different races. Prevalence and major features. Acta Diabet. Lat. <u>7</u>, 361 (1970)

34. Johansen, K.: Plasma insulin in diabetes mellitus and obesity. A review. FADL's forlag. Copenhagen: Arhus, Odense, 1975

35. Kamenetzky, S.A., Bennett, P.H., Dippe, S.E., Miller, M., LeCompte, P.M.: A clinical and histologic study of diabetic nephropathy in the Pima Indians. Diabetes 23, 61 (1974)

36. Kaplan, M.H., Feinstein, A.R.: A critique of methods in reported studies of long-term vascular complications in patients with diabetes mellitus. Diabetes 22, 160 (1973)

37. Kimmelstiel, P., Kim, O.J., Beres, J.: Studies on renal biopsy specimens with the aid of the electron microscope. I. Glomeruli in diabetes. Am. J. Clin. Pathol. 38, 270 (1962)

38. Kimmelstiel, P., Osawa, G., Beres, J.: Glomerular basement membrane in diabetics. Am. J. Clin. Pathol. 45, 21 (1966)

39. Kniffen, J.C., Quick, D.T.: Carbohydrate abnormalities in amyotrophic lateral sclerosis. In: Muscle Disease. Walton, J.N., Cenal, N., Scarlato, G. (eds.). Amsterdam: Excertpa Med., 1970, p. 345

40. Knowles, H.C.: Control of diabetes and the progression of vascular disease. In: Diabetes Mellitus. Theory and Practice. Ellenberg, M., Rifkin, H. (eds.). New York: McGraw-Hill, 1970, p. 666

41. Kojima, K.: Electron microscopic studies on the retina and choroid in alloxan-rats. Acta Societatis Ophth. Japonicae 75, 1698 (1971)

42. Kornerup, T.: Studies in diabetic retinopathy. An investigation of 1000 cases of diabetes. Acta Med. Scand. 153, 81 (1955)

43. Kreines, K., Kim, O., Knowles, H.C.: Glomerulosclerosis, hemochromatosis, and diabetes mellitus. Am. J. Clin. Path. 54, 47 (1970)

44. Lazarow, A.: Glomerular basement membrane thickening in diabetes. In: Diabetes. Proc. 6th Cong. Internat. Diab. Fed. Östman, J., Milner, R.D.G. (eds.). Stockholm, Amsterdam: Excerpta Med. Found., 1969, p. 301

45. Lee, C.S., Mauer, S.M., Brown, D.M., Sutherland, D.E.R., Michael, A.F., Najarian, J.S.: Renal transplantation in diabetes mellitus in rats. J. Exp. Med. 139, 793 (1974)

46. Leuenberger, P., Cameron, D., Stauffacher, W., Renold, A.E., Babel, J.: Ocular lesions in rats rendered chronically diabetic with streptozotocin. Ophthal. Res. 2, 189 (1971)

47. Lonergan, P., Robbins, S.L.: Absence of intercapillary glomerulosclerosis in the diabetic patient with hemochromatosis. New Eng. J. Med. 260, 367 (1959)

48. Lundbaek, K.: Long-term diabetes. Copenhagen: Munksgaard, 1953

49. Lundbaek, K.: Diabetic retinopathy in newly diagnosed diabetes mellitus. Acta Med. Scand. 152, 53 (1955)

50. Lundbaek, K., Steen-Olsen, T., Ørskov, H., Østerby-Hansen, R.: Long-term experimental insulin-deficiency diabetes. A model of diabetic angiopathy? Acta Med. Scand., Suppl. 476, 159 (1967)

51. Marcus, R.: Retinopathy, nephropathy, and neuropathy in lipoatrophic diabetes. Case report and discussion. Diabetes 15, 351 (1966)

52. Matras, A., Kohler, J.: Ein Beitrag zum Werner-syndrom. Wien Med. Wschr. 106, 437 (1956)

53. Mauer, S.M., Michael, A.F., Fish, A.J., Brown, D.M.: Spontaneous immunoglobulin and complment deposition in glomeruli of diabetic rats. Lab. Invest. 27, 488 (1972)

54. Mauer, S.M., Sutherland, D.E.R., Steffes, M.W., Leonard, R.J., Najarian, J.S., Michael, A.F., Brown, D.M.: Pancreatic islet transplantation. Effects on the glomerular lesions of experimental diabetes in the rat. Diabetes 23, 748 (1974)

55. Pardo, V., Perez-Stable, E., Alzamora, D.B., Cleveland, W.W.: Incidence and significance of muscle capillary basal lamina thickness in juvenile diabetes. Am. J. Pathol. <u>68</u>, 67 (1972)

56. Pirat, J., Barbier, P.: Effet protecteur de l'hémochromatose vis-à-vis des lésions vasculaires séniles ou diabétiques. Diabetologia <u>7</u>, 227 (1971)

57. Pyke, D.A., Roberts, D.St.C.: Retinopathy in early cases of diabetes mellitus. Acta Med. Scand. <u>163</u>, 489 (1959)

58. Rimoin, D.L.: The genetics of diabetes mellitus. In: Diabetes Mellitus: Theory and Practice. Ellenberg, M., Rifkin, H. (eds.). New York: McGraw-Hill, 1970, p. 564

59. Rosenbloom, A.L.: The natural history of diabetes mellitus. Pub. Health Reviews <u>2</u>, 115 (1973)

60. Sevel, D., Bristow, J.H., Bank, S., Marks, I., Jackson, P.: Diabetic retinopathy in chronic pancreatitis. Arch. Ophth. <u>83</u>, 245 (1971)

61. Shapiro, F.L., Smith, H.T.: Diabetic glomerulosclerosis in a patient with chronic pancreatitis. Arch. Intern. Med. <u>117</u>, 795 (1966)

62. Siperstein, M.D.: Capillary basement membranes and diabetic microangiopathy. Adv. Intern. Med. <u>18</u>, 325 (1972)

63. Sprague, R.G.: Diabetes mellitus associated with chronic relapsing pancreatitis. Proc. Staff Meet. Mayo Clin. <u>22</u>, 553 (1947)

64. Steiner, H.: Das Prader-Labhart-Willi-Syndrom. Eine morphologische Analyse. Virchows Arch. <u>345</u>, 205 (1968)

65. West, K.M.: Diabetes in American Indians and other native populations of the New World. Diabetes <u>23</u>, 841 (1974)

66. Williamson, J.R., Vogler, N.J., Kilo, C.: Basement membrane thickening in muscle capillaries. Observations on diabetics and nondiabetics with both parents diabetics. In: Endocrinology. Proc. 4th Internat. Congr. Endocrinol., Wash. D.C., 1972. Internat. Congr. Series no. 273. Srow, R.O., Ebling, P.I.G., Henderson, I.W. (eds.). Amsterdam: Excerpta Med., 1973, p. 1122

67. Williamson, J.R., Vogler, N., Kilo, C.: The natural history of basement membrane disease in diabetes mellitus. In : Diabetes. Proc. 8th Congr. Internat. Diab. Fed. Brussels, 1973. Internat. Congr. Series no. 312. Malaisse, W.J., Pirart, J. (eds.). Amsterdam: Excerpta Med., 1974, p. 424

68. Ørskov, H., Olsen, T.S., Nielsen, K., Rafaelsen, O.J., Lundbaek, K.: Kidney lesions in rats with severe long-term alloxan diabetes. I. Influence of age, alloxan damage, and insulin administration. Diabetologia <u>I</u>, 172 (1965)

69. Østerby, R.: Early phases in the development of diabetic glomerulopathy. A quantitative electron microscopic study. Acta Med. Scand., Suppl. <u>574</u> (1975)

22. Diabetic Complications in Concordant Identical Twins

P. G. NELSON and D. A. PYKE

Introduction

The cause and prevention of the long-term complications of diabetes remain a major puzzle. It is still unclear whether the microvascular lesions of diabetes are a genetically determined and integral component of the disorder, or the secondary outcome of abnormal metabolism. There is no conclusive evidence of histologic changes, in particular capillary basement membrane thickening, in so-called prediabetics, potential diabetics, or diabetics examined soon after diagnosis. Capillary basement membrane thickening has been reported in potential diabetics, i.e., offspring of conjugal diabetics (9) but these findings have not been confirmed (12). Similarly, thickening of the glomerular capillary basement membrane has been reported in recently diagnosed and prediabetic patients (8,12) but Østerby Hansen in a careful study, (6) found no difference in glomerular capillary basement membrane thickness between recently diagnosed diabetics and nondiabetics.

In the King' College Hospital series of identical twins no sign of retinopathy has been found in the unaffected twin of the discordant pairs, a group which, theoretically, should have a strong genetic predisposition (7).

As evidence that microangiopathy may be the result of the metabolic abnormalities in diabetes, the appearance of typical small vessel lesions in diabetes secondary to hemochromatosis and chronic pancreatitis is often quoted (3,4,11).

This argument concerning the genesis of the microangiopathy of diabetes has naturally led on to the question of the influence of diabetic control on the incidence and rate of progression of the microvascular lesions. Knowles (5), in an exhaustive analysis of over 300 publications on this subject, was unable to reach a conclusion and the matter is still unresolved.

A study of complications in identical twins concordant for diabetes may help to elucidate the relative roles of hereditary and exogenous factors in their development. While similarities within pairs may be due either to genetic factors alone or to the effects of a shared environment, any differences in complications must be environmentally determined, as the twins are genetically identical. "Environment", in this context, includes the effects of diabetic control and treatment.

The aim of the present study was to define the prevalence of retinopathy, neuropathy, and nephropathy in a group of monzygotic twins concordant for diabetes. Attention was concentrated on those pairs in which there was a marked difference between the cotwins in the severity

of complications and an attempt has been made to identify the factors
which might account for the differences.

Materials, Methods, and Results

The King's College Hospital series consists of 106 pairs of identical
twins, one or both of whom has diabetes (10) (see also Chapter 20).
Fifty-three pairs concordant for diabetes are included in this study.
There are 31 female and 22 male pairs. In 31 pairs both twins are
insulin-dependent and in 22 pairs, one or both twins receive oral therapy alone. The ages at diagnosis and duration of diabetes in the twins
of each group are shown in Table 1. In both groups the mean interval
between diagnosis in the cotwins was 3 years. As might be expected, in
the older-onset noninsulin-dependent group the mean duration of diabetes
was somewhat shorter than in the insulin-dependent pairs.

Table 1. Concordant twins (53 pairs)

	No. of pairs	Mean Age at Diagnosis (yrs)		Mean Duration of Diabetes (yrs)	
		1st Twin	2nd Twin	1st Twin	2nd Twin
Insulin dependent	31	20 (1-59)	23 (2-60)	18 (1-46)	15 (1-44)
Noninsulin dependent	22	52 (29-71)	55 (30-76)	11 (3-18)	8 (2-16)

Ranges of age at diagnosis and duration of diabetes are given in brackets.

In the non insulin-dependent group there are 2 pairs (K.C.H. pair Nos.
68 and 86) in which the index twins are insulin-dependent but their
cotwins have mild diabetes controlled by tablets. They are of some interest. In each pair the first twin presented with severe thirst, poly-
uria, and weight loss at ages 45 and 58. After the unusually long intervals of 8 and 11 years their cotwins developed mild diabetes and
remain well controlled on oral therapy. In each case there is a family
history of diabetes in first degree relatives. However, no obvious
environmental factor could be identified which might have precipitated
the onset of more severe clinical disease in the index twins.

All the twins were interviewed and examined either at home or at the
hospital. In most, both members of a pair were seen at the same time.
Diabetic control was assessed from medical records. It was adjudged
satisfactory if less than 50% of urine tests showed 2% glycosuria and/
or less than 50% of blood sugar estimations were over 200 mg/100 ml.
The number of admissions for diabetic ketosis were also taken into account.

Retinopathy

All the twins had their fundi examined after pupillary dilatation.
The fundal appearances were classified as follows:
(a) Normal (b) Background retinopathy - this included microaneurysms,
dot and blot hemorrhages, and exudates (c) Proliferative retinopathy.

The results in the insulin-dependent cases and the rest are shown in Table 2. In 17 out of the 31 insulin-dependent pairs both twins had normal fundi, in 6 both had background changes and in 3 pairs, both twins were blind from retinitis proliferans.

Table 2. Retinopathy in Concordant Pairs

	Both Normal	Both background	Both proliferative	Different type of retinopathy
Insulin dependent	17 (12yrs)	6 (21yrs)	3 (26yrs)	5 (22yrs)
Noninsulin dependent	13 (8yrs)	7 (10yrs)	1 (15yrs)	1 (12yrs)

Figures in brackets show mean duration of diabetes.

The figures for the 22 noninsulin dependent pairs were: 13 pairs both normal, 7 pairs both background changes, and in only one pair did both have proliferative changes.

In both groups the more severe degrees of retinopathy were seen with increasing duration of disease. In none of the pairs was there evidence that the twins with retinopathy had been less well controlled than those without.

Five of the insulin-dependent pairs and one of the non insulin-dependent pairs showed a difference in severity of retinopathy between the co-twins. In four of the five insulin-dependent pairs this was striking; one twin was blind from proliferative retinopathy while the other had only background changes and normal vision. These 4 pairs are Nos. 1-4 in Table 6 and their case histories are summarized in relation to that table. In the other 2 pairs with different types of retinopathy, one twin had background changes and the other normal fundi.

One of the three insulin-dependent pairs (K.C.H. pair No. 105), in which both twins had severe retinitis proliferans, is especially interesting. The course of diabetes in this pair is summarized in Table 3. The index

Table 3. K.C.H. Pair No. 105

	Twin 1	Twin 2
Age at diagnosis	24 yrs.	44 yrs.
Discovery	Glycosuria, no symptoms	Glycosuria, no symptoms (No glycosuria aged 36)
Treatment	None for 9 yrs. then S.I. + P.Z.I.	N.P.H. from diagnosis
Retinopathy		
Background	33 yrs.	At diagnosis
Proliferative	34 yrs.	45 yrs.
Neuropathy	33 yrs.	45 yrs.
Nephropathy	37 yrs. Died renal failure aged 38	None

twin was discovered to have glycosuria at a routine medical examination aged 24. His fasting blood sugar was 241 mg/100 ml. He received no specific treatment during the next 9 years. At the end of that period, at the age of 33, he was referred to hospital and a random blood sugar was found to be 450 mg/100 ml. On examination he had bilateral retinal hemorrhages and exudates, absent ankle jerks, and a blood pressure of 190/130. He was started on a single daily injection of a mixture of soluble and Protamine Zinc insulin. The following year there was new vessel formation in both eyes and 4 years later extensive neovascularization and heavy proteinuria. One year later, aged 38, he died in renal failure.

His cotwin was discovered to be diabetic, aged 44, also as a result of a routine urine test. He was known not to have had glycosuria 8 years earlier. The interval between the onset of diabetes in the two twins was therefore at least 12 and may have been 20 years. At the time of diagnosis the second twin was found to have hemorrhages and exudates in one eye and to have a blood pressure of 190/110. Treatment with Isophane insulin was started at once. One year later there was extensive neovascularization in both eyes and both ankle jerks were absent. After another year, i.e. two years after diagnosis, he was almost completely blind. There was no evidence of renal impairment.

This pair had lived apart from the age of 20 years. As the duration of diabetes seems to be so different in the two twins, the accelerated development of severe retinopathy in the second twin suggest a genetic influence.

Neuropathy

Absent ankle jerks and/or diminished vibration sense were the minimal requirements for the diagnosis of peripheral neuropathy. Those twins who first developed neurologic signs over the age of 60 years were discounted in view of the knwon effects of age on peripheral nerve function.

Table 4. Neuropathy in concordant pairs

	Both normal	Both neuropathy	One normal/One neuropathy
Insulin dependent	17 (11yrs)	9 (23yrs)	4 (20yrs)
Noninsulin dependent	8 (7yrs)	1 (8yrs)	0

Figures in brackets show mean duration of diabetes.

Table 4 shows the prevalence of neuropathy. Seventeen out of the 30 insulin-dependent pairs had normal reflexes and peripheral sensation and in 9 pairs both twins had evidence of neuropathy. Neuropathy was found in only one of the 9 noninsulin dependent pairs under the age of 60.

In four pairs, the index twin had evidence of neuropathy and the second none. Three of these 4 are included in the description of 5 pairs in which the cotwins had the most striking differences in complications (see Nos. 1, 2, and 4, Table 6).

In all but one of the twins neuropathy was associated with retinopathy.

Nephropathy

A twin was classified as having diabetic nephropathy if there was persistent or intermittent proteinuria or a raised blood urea nitrogen without evidence of nodiabetic renal disease. There were only four pairs in which one or both twins had nephropathy by these criteria (Table 5).

In the only pair in which both twins had evidence of nephropathy, (K. C.H. Pair No. 54) the cotwins had followed remarkably similar courses. They developed diabetes aged 49 and 50 years respectively and 14 years later were both found to have bilateral background retinopathy and absent ankle jerks. At that time the index twin was also noted to have proteinuria and a blood urea of 62 mg/100 ml. Her cotwin developed proteinuria a year later.

One year later they both died of myocardial infarction within six months of each other.

In 3 pairs one twin had undoubted nephropathy but the second had none. One of these three pairs is described in detail in Table 3 and the other two are included in Table 6 (Pair Nos. 1 and 5).

Table 6 gives the clinical findings in the 5 pairs in which there were the most marked differences between cotwins in severity of complications. These 5 pairs offer the best opportunity for the identification of possible environmental factors responsible for the differences. In view of the potential importance of these pairs a brief clinical summary follows.

Pair No. 1. (K.C.H. No. 74)

Twin 1 was diagnosed at the age of 10 and treated with soluble insulin. For the first 8 years of his diabetic life control was strict, his mother ensuring that he kept to his diet and that he tested his urine frequently. Between the ages of 18 and 25 he stopped attending a diabetic clinic and ignored his diabetes. There are no medical reports of that period; diabetic control, however, seems to have been very bad. By the time he reattended the clinic at the age of 25 he had developed glaucoma secondary to rubeiosis iridis and one eye had to be removed. Six years later he had retinitis proliferans in the remaining eye and when seen by the authors 11 years later was blind, when he had been diabetic for 31 years. Three years later he became chair-ridden as a result of severe combined motor and sensory neuropathy and had proteinuria with blood urea of 52 mg/100 ml.

In contrast, Twin 2 had normal sight after 27 years of diabetes. Diabetes was diagnosed at the age of 17 and he has always been treated with soluble and Protamine Zinc insulin. He has been consistently more conscientious than his twin regarding his diet and urine testing and has remained a healthy, active man with no evidence of peripheral neuropathy or renal disease. He was noted to have a small patch of flat new vessels in his right eye in 1968 and again in 1971, but these have since disappeared. There are now only a few dot hemorrhages in the right eye and some microaneurysms in the left.

Table 5. Nephropathy in concordant twins

	KCH nos.		Age	Duration	Treatment	Other complications
Both twins	54	Twin 1	66	17	0	Background retinopathy, neuropathy
		Twin 2	66	16	0	Background retinopathy, neuropathy
One twin only	74	Twin 1	44	34	I	Retinitis proliferans, severe neuropathy
		Twin 2	44	27	I	Background retinopathy only
	18	Twin 1	54	11	0	Background retinopathy, neuropathy
		Twin 2	54	11	0	Neuropathy only
	105	Twin 1	38	14	I	Retinitis proliferans, neuropathy
		Twin 2	47	3	I	Retinitis proliferans, neuropathy

Twin with nephropathy underlined
0 = oral; I = insulin.

Table 6. Twins with striking differences in complications

KCH Pair No.		Present age	Duration of diabetes	Retinopathy	Neuropathy	Nephropathy	Family History
1.	Twin 1	44	34	R.P.,blind	Severe	Yes	Brother
	Twin 2		27	Background	No	No	
2.	Twin 1	32	22	R.P.,blind	Yes	No	None
	Twin 2		13	Background	No	No	
3.	Twin 1	41	22	R.P.,blind	Yes	No	None
	Twin 2		20	Background	Yes	No	
4.	Twin 1	65	23	R.P.,blind	Yes	No	Niece
	Twin 2		23	1 microan.	No	No	
5.	Twin 1	65	11	Background	Yes	Yes	Father
	Twin 2		11	None	Yes	No	

All pairs are on Insulin therapy except Pair No. 5.

The twins' eldest brother, aged 52, has been an insulin-requiring diabetic for 33 years. His diabetic control has always been poor and he also is blind as a result of proliferative retinopathy.

The main difference between these two twins appears to be the period of total self-neglect of the first twin between the ages of 18 and 25.

Pair No. 2. (K.C.H. No. 64)

The twins are both insulin-dependent diabetics, now aged 32. They were diagnosed at the ages of 10 and 19. Twin 1's control has never been satisfactory and he developed proliferative eye changes 16 years after diagnosis. He is now blind and has absent ankle jerks. Twin 2, after an initial one year of poor control, appears to have stabilized his diabetes satisfactorily. After 13 years of diabetes he has only background changes in the eyes and no neuropathy. The 9 year interval between diagnoses in this pair may be a factor accounting for the differences in their eyes. The course of the second twin over the next few years will be observed to see if his eyes show a similar deterioration.

The last three pairs provide a better natural experiment, as in each pair the twins have developed diabetes within a short time of each other.

Pair No. 3. (K.C.H. No. 28)

Twin 1 became diabetic at the age of 19 years and Twin 2 two years later. Twin 1 did not attend a diabetic clinic during the first 16 years of his diabetes; by then he had new vessel formation in both eyes. We know nothing of the quality of diabetic control during that period. Twin 2 was a regular clinic attender but his urine tests frequently showed heavy glycosuria. Now, after 20 years of diabetes, he has only background fundal changes. Both twins have severe peripheral and autonomic neuropathy with impotence, postural hypotension, and gustatory sweating. Thus, in this pair of twins the difference in the severity of their diabetic complications is mainly in their retinal appearances.

Pair No. 4. (K.C.H. No. 87)

These twins show the most startling dissimilarities. Their clinical course has been reported in detail elsewhere (7). Both developed diabetes aged 42, within months of each other. They have been treated with very similar insulin regimes with apparently satisfactory control in each case. Yet, now after 23 years of diabetes Twin 1 is totally blind as a result of proliferative retinopathy and Twin 2 has normal fundi except for a single microaneurysm in one eye only. There is no obvious reason for the striking difference in this pair.

Pair No. 5. (K.C.H. No. 18)

These are the only twins in this dissimilar group not on insulin. Both are mild hemophiliacs. At the time they were diagnosed in 1962 Twin 1 was living in Toronto and Twin 2 in London. Their diagnoses were made quite independently at the age of 54 within months. The London twin is a regular clinic attender. He has been treated with Chlorpropamide since diagnosis, to which Phenformin was later added, and his control has usually been excellent. Apart from absent ankle jerks and reduced vibration sense in the lower legs, which may not be significant in a 66 years old man, he has no evidence of diabetic complications.

The Canadian twin was treated with Tolbutamide for the first 10 years and thereafter Chlorpropamide and Phenformin. He did not attend a clinic regularly and was in his own words "rather neglectful regarding his health". He visited his twin in London on several occasions and the authors took the opportunity to examine him. In 1968 he had normal fundi but by 1971 had developed widespread background retinopathy. In

1972 there was proteinuria. One year later extensive acute background
retinopathy with many hard and soft exudates and hemorrhages had developed. By then he had heavy proteinuria, a blood urea nitrogen of
42 mg/100 ml, a blood pressure of 150/90 and diminished tendon reflexes
in the legs. He looked aged and ill beside his twin brother and died
in July 1974 of massive intracerebral hemorrhage.

The index twins who were the more severely affected by complications
did not appear to have had more severe clinical disease than their
cotwins, as judged from the acuteness of symptoms at diagnosis, their
intensity, and insulin dosages. In four out of five of these pairs
there was some suggestion that diabetic control was less satisfactory
in the more severely affected twin; however, the authors think that
it is unlikely that diabetic control was the only factor accounting
for their differences, but no other cause could be identified.

Conclusion

The outstanding feature of this study is the remarkable similarity of
complications in most of the cotwins. This similarity is more likely
to be the result of shared genes rather than the fact that both are
diabetic, for the following reasons:

1. In 19 out of 25 pairs in which both twins had complications, the
   cotwins have lived apart all their diabetic lives. This often meant
   that they attended separate diabetic clinics and received different
   types and dosages of insulin or tablets. Therefore, neither their
   external nor internal environments were identical.

2. The frequencies of both the second series histocompatibility anti-
   genes HL-A8 and W15 are significantly increased in the concordant
   pairs. By contrast, in the discordant pairs, W15 alone is increased,
   the frequency of HL-A8 being the same as in the control nondiabetic
   population (see Chapter 12). Although the absolute numbers are too
   small to achieve statistical significance, the trend suggests genetic heterogeneity between the concordant and discordant pairs, with
   stronger hereditary factors operating in the concordant pairs.

It has previously been noted that retinopathy was more frequent and
severe in the concordant than in the discordant twins (7). The complications in the discordant twins are mild. This, when seen in the light
of the HL-A frequencies, is suggestive evidence that the more powerful
genetic component in the concordant pairs is associated with the development of more severe complications.

The few pairs in this study in which there was a marked difference in
the severity of complications indicate that nongenetic factors, including diabetic control, can also modify the appearance and severity
of these complications.

References

1. Daysog, A., Jr., Dobson, H.L., Brennam, J.C.: Renal glomerular and vascular lesions in prediabetes and in diabetes mellitus: a study based on renal biopsies. Ann. Int. Med. 54, 672 (1961)

2. Goetz, F.C., Hartmann, J.F., Lazarow, A.: Electron microscopy of the human glomerulus in early diabetes. J. Clin. Invest. 39, 991 (1960)

3. Griffiths, J.D., Dymock, I.W., Davies, E.W.G., Hill, D.W., Williams, R.: Occurrence and prevalence of diabetic retinopathy in hemochromatosis. Diabetes 20, 766 (1971)

4. Ireland, J.T., Patnaik, B.K., Duncan, L.J.P.: Glomerular ultrastructure in secondary diabetics and normal subjects. Diabetes 16, 628 (1967)

5. Knowles, H.C.: On the Nature and Treatment of Diabetes. Leibel, B.S., Wrenshall, G.A. (eds.). Amsterdam: Excerpta Medica Foundation, 1965, p. 595

6. Østerby Hansen, R.: A quantitative estimate of the peripheral glomerular basement membrane in recent juvenile diabetes. Diabetologia 1, 97 (1965)

7. Pyke, D.A., Tattersall, R.B.: Diabetic retinopathy in identical twins. Diabetes 22, 613 (1973)

8. Rees, S.B., Camerini-Davalos, R.A., Caulfield, J.B., Lozano-Castaneda, O., Catellier, C., Pometta, D., Cervantes-Amezcura, A., Krauthammer, J., Marble, A.: In: Aetiology of Diabetes Mellitus and its Complications. Cameron, M.P., O'Connor, M. (eds.). Ciba Foundation Colloq. on Endocrinol. 15, 315 (1964)

9. Siperstein, M.D., Unger, R.H., Madison, L.L.: Studies of muscle capillary basement membrane in normal subjects, diabetic, and prediabetic patients. J. Clin. Invest. 47, 1973 (1968)

10. Tattersall, R.B., Pyke, D.A.: Diabetes in identical twins. Lancet II, 1120 (1972)

11. Tutin, M., Rathery, M., Rousselie, F.: L'angiopathie spécifique dans les diabètes secondaires à des pancréatites et à des hémochromatoses (61 observation). Jour. Ann. Diabet. Hôtel Dieu 7, 377 (1967)

12. Williamson, J.R., Vogler, N.J., Kilo, C.: Microvascular disease in diabetes. Med. Clin. N. Amer. 55, 847 (1971)

23. Prospective Studies on Patients with Asymptomatic Diabetes

S. S. FAJANS, J. C. FLOYD, JR., S. PEK, and C. I. TAYLOR

In children and adolescents the initial manifestations of symptomatic or overt diabetes mellitus are frequently of sudden or explosive onset. Until recently diabetes in this age group had been assumed to be rarely recognizable at an early or asymptomatic stage and the course had been assumed to be characterized by a rapid and progressive decrease of insulin secretory reserves, leading to the ketosis-prone diabetes. In contrast, it is usually accepted that asymptomatic or latent diabetes of middle age may be characterized by a mild abnormality of glucose tolerance which may remain stable, may show little or slow progression in severity over many years, or may regress, depending on a variety of environmental factors.

As early as 1960 we reported on the latent, asymptomatic or chemical diabetes that also can be recognized in children, adolescents, and young adults by the finding of abnormal carbohydrate tolerance. Such patients are readily found if a search is made among the first-degree relatives of diabetic patients (3-5). We have reported also that such patients may exhibit the nonprogressive course of carbohydrate intolerance characteristic of "maturity-onset type" diabetes (5,6,7,9). Since 1966, others have confirmed that asymptomatic diabetes can be discovered in young people by the use of the glucose tolerance test (1,2,10-17).

It is the purpose of this report to summarize our prospective study of the natural history of asymptomatic or latent diabetes especially in young people.

Levels of blood glucose and plasma insulin were obtained during glucose tolerance test performed in 94 children, adolescents, and young and middle-aged adults who were diagnosed as having latent diabetes. Follow-up observations have been made over periods of up to 22 years in 83 of these individuals. These results extend observations which have been reported previously (6,7,9).

Some characteristics of these patients are given in Table 1. The majority had a strong family history of diabetes. The number of subjects in each group, number of patients with fasting hyperglycemia (fasting blood glucose greater than 120 mg/dl at diagnosis or at some time during follow-up), the mean sum of increments (sum of increments = sum of increases, above fasting levels for all 6 half-hourly intervals during the 3-hour glucose tolerance test) of levels of blood glucose or plasma insulin (initial insulin determinations were made at the time of the diagnostic glucose tolerance test or of the first test after 1961, when the immunoassay for insulin became available), mean increments of plasma insulin at 1/2 hour of the test, are given in Table 1 among other data. Considerable fluctuation in glucose tolerance may occur in some patients when the test is repeated at intervals of months or years, whether such patients receive no treatment, are treated with

Table 1. Characterization of patients with latent diabetes and of control subjects without family history of diabetes or high birthweight

	Patients Age 9–17 (Group I)	Patients Age 18–25 (Group II)	Control Subjects Age 18–25	Patients Age 26–35 (Group III)	Patients Age 36–47 (Group IV)
Number of subjects	25	34	67	19	16
Mean Age (yrs)	13.3	21.6	21.9	31.0	39.6
Fasting blood glucose (FBG) (highest)					
<99 mg/dl	3	13	67	5	5
100–120 mg/dl	10	9	0	9	8
>120 mg/dl	12	12	0	5	3
GTT–sum of increments above FBG mg/dl; mean±SEM					
Initial diagnostic	610±55[a*]	505±32[a*]	119±8	506±68[a*]	431±32[a*]
Highest (before insulin-requiring diabetes)	824±85[a*]	681±60[a*]		624±62[a*]	597±68[a*]
Plasma insulin µU/ml: Nonobese subjects; <116% IBW) Diagnostic GTT (or first test, after 1961)					
Increments at 1/2 hr. Mean ± SEM	30.7±7.1[a*](18)	30.1± 5.2(26)[a]* 24.1±4.4(22) 66.3±12.3(4)	89.7±7.7	62.8± 30(9) 38.1±23(7) 160.5±60(2)	40.3± 8.4[**](8) 32.8±11.5 62.5±5(2)
Sum of increments Mean ± SEM	226±41[a*](18)	357± 6(26) 229±33*(22) 1059±91(4)	464±39	483± 164(9) 247±41(7) 1312±167(2)	670± 276(8) 288±45(6) 1625±388(2)
Obese	4	5	0	9	7
Progression to insulin-requiring diabetes	4	7		1	1
Age at diagnosis (yrs)	11,14,11,17	23,18,18,18,22,24,21		33	39
Initial FBG, mg/dl	125,99,106,77	111,85,60,111,81,102,111		123	134
Time interval from initial diagnosis (yrs)	0.3,0.3,2,2	1.5,2,3.2,4.9,7,8.4,8.8		18.1	15.2
Years of follow-up Mean	1.7–19.5(20) 9.7	1.6–16.7(27) 7.9		4.8–22(15) 14.2	3.2–16.0(12) 11.6

[a] Differences from healthy control subjects without family history of diabetes. All statistical comparisons by Student's t-test *p = <0.01. **p < .C1.

225

diet alone, or with diet and hypoglycemic agents. In the 4 groups of
patients the mean sums of increments of their most abnormal (highest)
glucose tolerance tests (prior to the development of insulin-requiring
diabetes in some patients) are also given in Table 1 (and Figs. 1 and
2). For groups II-IV the sum of increments of plaama insulin are subdivided. The mean results of tests of individuals in which the sum of
increments exceeded the mean sum of increments óf the control subjects
by more than 1 S.D. are given separately. In group II the values of
two patients, and in groups III and IV of one each, exceeded the mean
sum of increments of the controls by more than 2 S.D. (1180 µU/ml).
Ketosis-prone diabetes developed in four patients of group I, and within
1.5 and 7 years in two patients of group II. Five other patients of
group II and one each of groups III and IV have progressed to insulin-
requiring diabetes in 2-18.1 years after diagnosis. Their fasting hyperglycemia can no longer be normalized by diet and oral hypoglycemic
agents (Table 1).

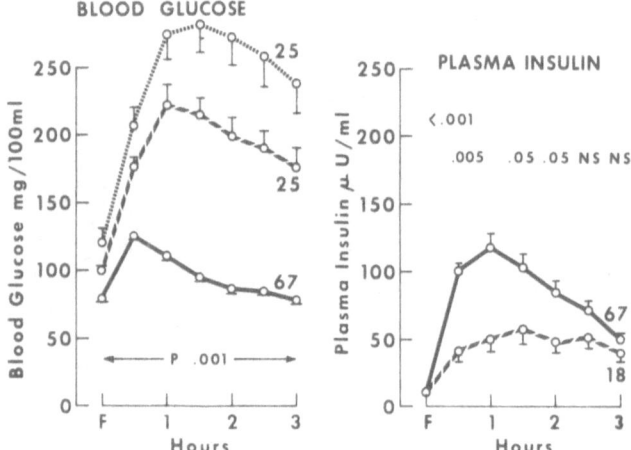

Fig. 1. Initial diagnostic standard glucose tolerance tests (1.75 g glucose orally/
kg ideal body weight) and glucose tolerance tests with highest increases in blood
glucose in patients with latent diabetes (group I, ages 9-17 years at diagnosis)
and glucose tolerance tests in healthy control subjects

In the patients aged 9-17 years at diagnosis (group I), the mean of
the initial fasting and postglucose blood glucose levels were significantly higher than in the control subjects aged 18-25 years (Fig. 1).
Also shown are the results of the highest glucose tolerance tests
observed in these subjects (prior to the development of insulin-dependent diabetes in four of them) (Fig. 1). Plasma level of insulin for
18 of theses patients who were nonobese (percent ideal body weight
<116%, Metropolitan Life Insurance table) are shown also. After the
administration of glucose, the diabetic group exhibited an increase in
plasma insulin which was significantly delayed and subnormal (Fig. 1).

The mean results of the initial diagnostic and highest tests of group
II are shown in Figure 2. For all 26 nonobese patients the mean levels
of plasma insulin after ingestion of glucose were significantly lower

at 1/2 and 1 hour of the test (p < .001 and .005, respectively) than
in the control subjects. Four of the 26 patients had responses which
were greater than the mean +1 S.D. of the sum of increases of the
control subjects (Fig. 2; Table 1) while in 22 mean insulin levels
were subnormal and similar to those of the younger patients.

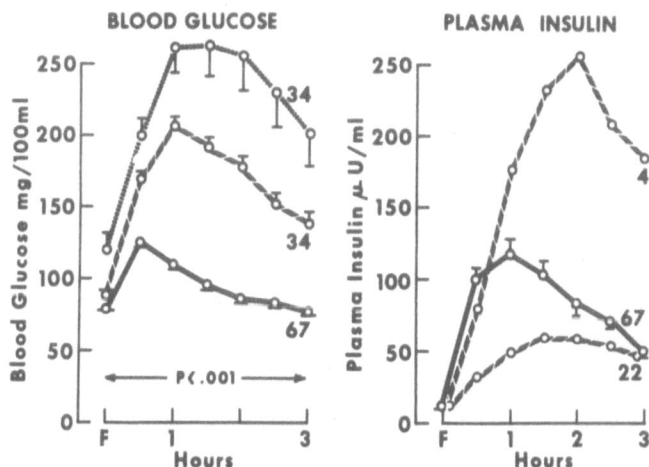

Fig. 2. Initial diagnostic standard glucose tolerance tests (1.75 g glucose orally/
kg ideal body weight) and glucose tolerance tests with highest increases in blood
glucose in patients with latent diabetes (group II, ages 18-25 years at diagnosis)
and glucose tolerance tests in healthy control subjects. Shown separately are (a)
the mean of the insulin responses of four patients whose sum of increments exceeded
the mean of the control subjects by more than 1 S.D., and (b) the mean of the insulin responses of the remaining 22 of 26 patients shown in Fig. 2

Twenty of 21 patients in group I whose carbohydrate tolerance has not
deteriorated to insulin-dependent diabetes have had follow-up tests
for periods of 1.7-19.5 (mean 9.7) years. The patients have been treated
either with diet alone or diet and sulfonylureas. Although the abnormality in glucose tolerance has definitely progressed in two of these
patients, the mean glucose tolerance of this group shows some improvement (fig. 3). The mean plasma insulin response during glucose tolerance tests performed 1.7-11.7 (mean 7.1) years after the one on which
the initial insulin determinations were made has shown no evidence
of deterioration (Fig. 3); on the contrary there has been a small but
significant mean increase in plasma insulin at 1/2 hour of the test.

An example of lack of progression of latent diabetes is shown in Figure
4. This female patient was 16 years old when a diagnosis of latent
diabetes was made in 1958. The patient has been treated with diet and
sulfonylureas. In 1973, 15 years later, glucose tolerance and the
decreased insulin response to glucose (11-year follow-up) are unchanged
after withdrawal of chloropropamide for 2 weeks. While taking chlorpropamide, glucose tolerance is normal. The results are identical to those
obtained in August 1974, 16 years later, which are not shown in Figure

4. This patients is one of seven siblings with latent diabetes (8); she is of a family of three generations of maturity-onset type diabetes.

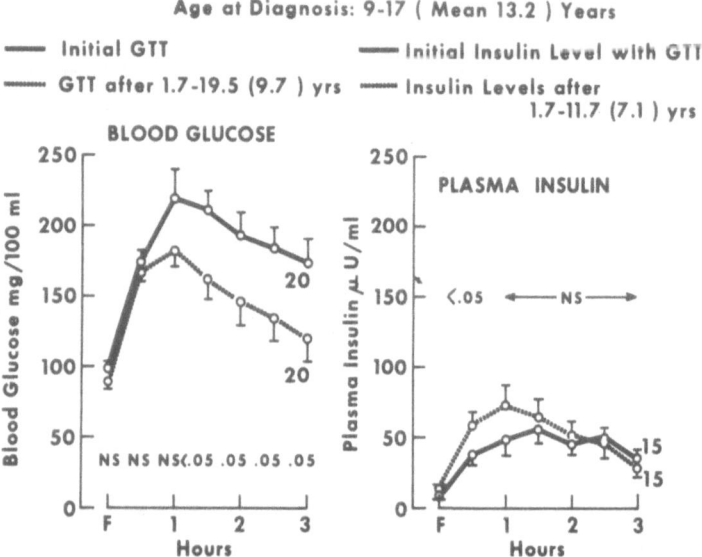

Fig. 3. Initial and last follow-up glucose tolerance tests in latent diabetic patients, ages 9-17 years at diagnosis (group I)

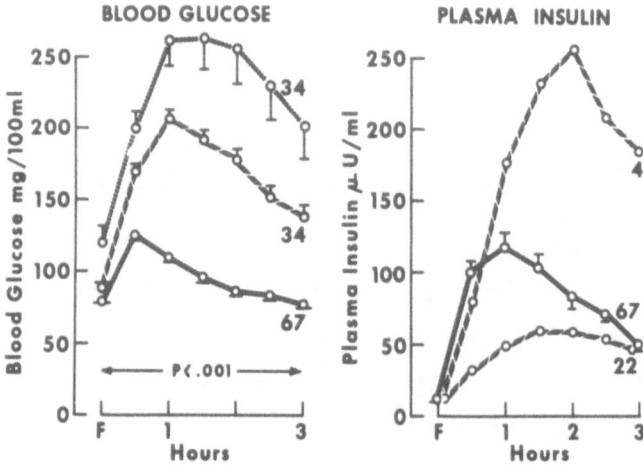

Fig. 4. Lack of progression of latent diabetes for 15 years in a 16-year-old female (see text)

Twenty-three patients of group II who have not progressed to insulin-requiring diabetes have been retested at intervals of 1.6-16.7 (mean 7.9) years. In the 20 patients who had a subnormal insulin response initially, after intervals of up to 12.2 years, there is a significant increase in the mean insulin response to glucose at 1/2 hour of the follow-up tests (Fig. 5). In three of four patients who had an excessive insulin response to glucose initially, and who have been followed for more than 1 year, there has been a decrease in insulin levels subsequently, also associated with improvement in glucose intolerance (Fig. 5).

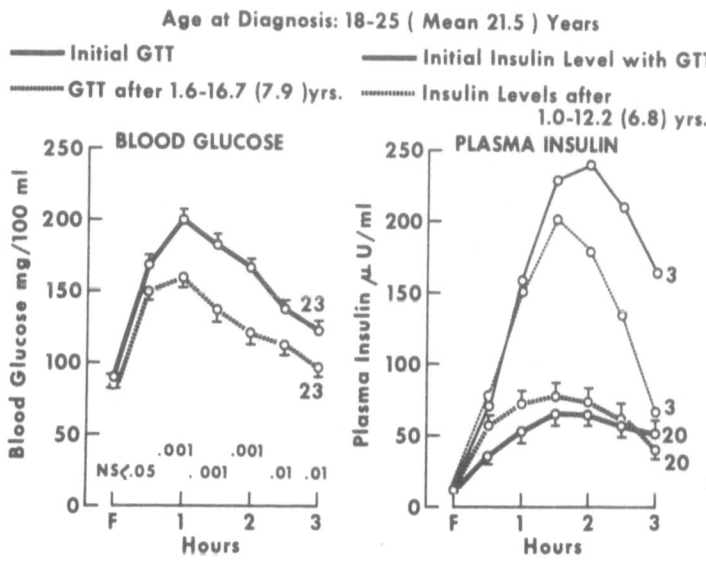

Fig. 5. Initial and last follow-up glucose tolerance tests in latent diabetic patients, ages 18-25 years at diagnosis (group II). Results of insulin levels separated into two groups: Three patients whose initial insulin responses exceeded the mean of the sum of increases of the control subjects by more than 1 S.D., and the remaining 20 patients

In groups III and IV the results of initial glucose tolerance tests, highest glucose tolerance tests (Table 1) and of glucose tolerance tests after follow-up periods of up to 20.7 and 16.0 years, respectively, were similar to those of group II.

Figure 6 shows lack of progression of latent diabetes for 22 years in a family member of the third of four consecutive generations with maturity-onset type diabetes. Diabetes was diagnosed at the age of 31 years when she had fasting hyperglycemia. Glucose tolerance is essentially unchanged between 1952 and 1974, and the plasma insulin response is subnormal (Fig. 6). This patient has thickening of the basement membrane of muscle capillary by the Williamson technique (19).

As stated above, considerable fluctuation in glucose tolerance occurs in some patients when the test is repeated at intervals of days, months, or years. Fluctuations may occur also in the insulin response to glucose. On repetitive tests in an individual patient with low insulin response there may be no consistent relationship between glucose tol-

erance and the accompanying plasma insulin response in peripheral
blood as measured by levels of insulin by conventional radioimmunoassay (6,7). There may be (1) the expected inverse relationship between changes in glucose tolerance and the associated insulin response,
or (2) glucose tolerance may vary while the insulin response remains
unchanged, or (3) the insulin response may vary while glucose tolerance remains constant. Examples of these findings have been reported
previously (6,7). However, a low insulin response and a supernormal
insulin response are not observed in the same patient on repetitive
testing. These findings suggest that factors in addition to an abnormal pancreatic insulin response to glucose may determine normality
or abnormality of glucose tolerance and other changes.

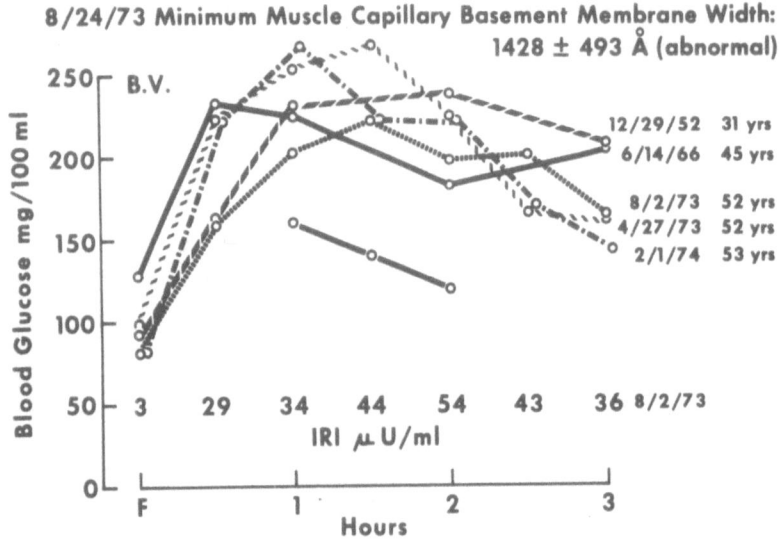

Fig. 6. Lack of progression of latent diabetes for 22 years. B.V., female: diagnosis
age 31; FBS 152 mg/dl. Family history of diabetes mellitus (age at diagnosis): Father (age 76), FBS 243 mg/ml, on oral agent; paternal grandfather (age 76), on insulin; paternal uncle, on insulin; paternal aunt (age 83), on oral agent; mother (age
68), FBS 250 mg/dl, on oral agent; brother (age 54), myocardial infarction at age
50; son (age 17), abnormal GTT for 10 years; son (age 17), abnormal GTT for 7 years

The implications of these findings are that: (1) Although latent diabetes may progress to overt, insulin-requiring diabetes in some children, adolescents, and young adults, in 80% of young patients studied,
it does not, nor does glucose intolerance necessarily advance in severity over periods of up to 22 years. In many of these patients asymptomatic diabetes might remain undiscovered if they had not been tested
as first-degree relatives of diabetic patients. (2) In 90% of latent
diabetic patients under age 25 years at diagnosis, mean insulin responses to glucose are delayed and subnormal, but the insulin responses
may not deteriorate over periods of up to 12 years. Johansen (11) has
confirmed that in the majority of young people with asymptomatic maturity-onset type diabetes the disease does not progress to insulin-requiring diabetes and that abnormal carbohydrate tolerance and the delayed and decreased insulin response to glucose remain unchanged 1-1/2
to 2 years after the initial study. (3) The slow progression to insulin-
requiring diabetes in some, or lack of evident progression of latent
diabetes in many children, adolescents, and young adults, suggests that
230

early detection should allow time for the institution of possible pro-
phylactic procedures which would be more effective than those presently available, and that might arrest or reverse abnormalities of insulin
secretion and glucose tolerance.

Finally, we wish to propose a tentative classification of diabetes in
young people (Table 2), based on the degree of carbohydrate intolerance,
which takes into consideration: (1) the prospective studies reported
above, (2) phenotypic differences in diabetes, (3) heterogeneity of
diabetes as expressed in terms of inheritance (19), and as discussed
earlier by Tattersall (Chapter 10), (4) heterogeneity of insulin responses in latent diabetes (Chapter 8), and (5) the insulin response
to glucose in terms of prognosis with regard to progressin to insulin-
requiring diabetes (Chapter 8).

Table 2. Classification of diabetes in young people on basis of carbohydrate
intolerance

I. Classical juvenile-onset type (JOD): ketosis-prone
   a. Explosive onset; no previously known abnormality
   b. Previously recognized abnormality of carbohydrate tolerance by prospective
      testing

II. Insulin-requiring, nonketotic D.M. (insulin for correction of fasting
    hyperglycemia)
   a. Within 2 years of diagnosis (JOD)
   b. More than 2 years after diagnosis (MODY)

III. Non insulin-requiring, maturity-onset type (MODY)
      with follow-up for up to 22 years
   a. "Low" insulin responders or insulin responses below mean of control
      subjects (progressive and nonprogressive to insulin-requiring diabetes)
   b. "High" insulin responders or insulin responses above mean of control
      subjects (nonprogressive)

In the first category we place classical juvenile-onset type diabetes
(JOD) with susceptibility to ketosis (Ia). This type of diabetes is
characterized by a fairly abrupt clinical onset, severe symptoms, and
tendency to ketoacidosis. Since children and young people are not tested
routinely there is usually no previously known abnormality of carbohydrate tolerance. The loss of insulin secretory capacity appears to
be a relatively rapid event. In the siblings of juvenile-onset type of
diabetic patients, by frequent prospective testing, occasionally one
can find a recognizable abnormality of carbohydrate tolerance (Ib).
Usually it deteriorates rapidly, and almost always within 2 years, to
fasting hyperglycemia, symptomatic diabetes, and proneness to ketosis.
In our experience such individuals have had delayed and decreased insulin responses to glucose.

The second category of diabetic patients among the young are individuals
who require insulin but do not have proneness to ketosis. Insulin is
necessary for correction of fasting hyperglycemia; diet or oral hypoglycemic agents are not able to achieve this therapeutic goal. If
insulin is required within 2 years of diagnosis these patients (IIa)
are classified arbitrarily as juvenile-onset type diabetic patients
(JOD), although the defect in insulin secretory capacity is less severe
than that of the classical juvenile-onset type (I). If insulin is required for correction of fasting hyperglycemia more than 2 years after

diagnosis, these patients (IIb) show, in general, the pattern of inheritance of the maturity-onset type diabetes of the young (MODY, 19)
placed in the third category (III). Most affected individuals in the
families of these propositi have the nonprogressive, noninsulin-requiring type of disease. It their insulin response to glucose is "low"
or below the mean of the control subjects (IIIa), we cannot differentiate at the present time between those who will retain the mild nonprogressive form of the disease in which hyperglycemia can be normalized without insulin and those who will progress to need insulin in
the future. We have followed young individuals with extremely low insulin responses who could regain or retain fasting euglycemia without
insulin for periods of up to 19.5 years. Others, approximatels 20%,
have progressed to insulin-requiring diabetes within 2-18 years (Table
1). To date, none of the patients with maturity-onset type diabetes
whose insulin responses were above the mean of these of control subjects have progressed to insulin-requiring diabetes (IIIb).

References

1. Burkeholder, J.M., Pickens, J.C., Womack, W.N.: Oral glucose tolerance test in
   siblings of children with diabetes mellitus. Diabetes 16, 156 (1967)

2. Chiumello, G., DelGurcio, M., Carnelutti, M., Bidone, G.: Relationship between
   obesity, chemical diabetes, and beta pancreatic function in children. Diabetes
   18, 238 (1969)

3. Fajans, S.S., Conn, J.W.: Tolbutamide-induced improvement in carbohydrate tolerance of young people with mild diabetes mellitus. Diabetes 9, 83 (1960)

4. Fajans, S.S., Conn, J.W.: The use of tolbutamide in the treatment of young people with mild diabetes mellitus - a progress report. Diabetes (Suppl.) 11, 123
   (1962)

5. Fajans, S.S., Conn, J.W.: Prediabetes, subclinical diabetes and latent clinical
   diabetes: interpretation, diagnosis and treatment. In: On the Nature and Treatment
   of Diabetes. Excerpt. Med. Int. Cong. Series 84. Leibel, B.S., Wrenshall, G.S.
   (eds.). Amsterdam: 1965, p. 641

6. Fajans, S.S., Floyd, J.C., Jr., Pek, S., Conn, J.W.: The course of asymptomatic
   diabetes in young people, as determined by levels of blood glucose and plasma
   insulin. Trans. Assoc. Amer. Phys. 82, 211 (1969)

7. Fajans, S.S., Floyd, J.C., Jr., Pek, S., Conn, J.W.: Studies on the natural
   history of asymptomatic diabetes in young people. Metabolism 22, 327 (1973)

8. Fajans, S.S.: The definition of chemical diabetes. Metabolism 22, 211 (1973)

9. Fajans, S.S., Taylor, C.I., Floyd, J.C., Jr., Conn, J.W.: Some aspects of the
   natural history of diabetes mellitus. Excerpt. Med. Intern. Cong. Series 312,
   1974, p. 329

10. Johansen, K., Lundbaek, K.: Plasma insulin in mild juvenile diabetes. Lancet I,
    1257 (1967)

11. Johansen, K.: Mild diabetes in young subjects. Clinical aspects and plasma insu-
    lin response pattern. Acta Med. Scand. 193, 23 (1973)

12. Kahn, C.B., Soeldner, J.S., Gleason, R.E., Rojas, L., Camerini-Davalos, R.A.,
    Marble, A.: Clinical and chemical diabetes in offspring of diabetic couples.
    N. Eng. J. Med. 281, 343 (1969)

13. Lister, J.: The clinical spectrum of juvenile diabetes. Lancet 1, 386 (1966)

14. Poulsen, E.P., Richenderfer, L., Ginsberg-Fellner, F.: Plasma glucose, free
    fatty acids, and immunoreactive insulin in 66 obese children. Diabetes 17, 261
    (1968)

15. Rosenbloom, A.: Insulin responses of children with chemical diabetes mellitus. N. Eng. J. Med. <u>282</u>, 1228 (1970)

16. Rosenbloom, A., Drash, A., Guthrie, R.: Chemical diabetes mellitus in childhood - report of a conference. Diabetes <u>21</u>, 45 (1972)

17. Sisk, C.W.: Application of one-hour glucose tolerance test to genetic studies of diabetes in children. Lancet <u>1</u>, 262 (1968)

18. Williamson, J.R., Vogler, N.J., Kilo, C.: Estimation of vascular basement membrane thickness. Theoretical and practical considerations. Diabetes <u>18</u>, 567 (1969)

19. Tattersall, R.B., Fajans, S.S.: A difference between the inheritance of classical juvenile-onset and maturity-onset type diabetes of young people. Diabetes <u>24</u>, 44 (1975)

Supported in part by USPHS Grants AM-00888, AM-02244, and TI-AM5001 from the National Institute of Arthritis, Metabolism, and Digestive Diseases and by grants from the Upjohn Company, Kalamazoo, Michigan, and Charles Pfizer, Inc., New York.

24. Problems in Genetic Counselling for Diabetes Mellitus

W. FUHRMANN

There appear to be two sets of problems in counselling diabetics - the first concerning the unsolved problem of the genetic basis of diabetes mellitus per se, and the second concerning the inherent multifaceted problems of genetic counselling in general, which become particularly obvious in the case of diabetes. Family studies, twin studies, and the general question of the genetic and environmental background of diabetes mellitus have been treated in several foregoing chapters. As far as genetic counselling is concerned, it ought to be emphasized again that diabetes is a heterogeneous disease, and therefore, no definite risk figures applying to all cases can be given. The first step must be to make a precise diagnosis of the type of diabetes present and to identify or exclude special forms on the basis of clinical and bio-chemical data and personal and family history. In fact, each case deserved a detailed family analysis. Only on this basis can risk figures be calculated. Even now, sufficiently large series are not available to give information on empiric risk figures for each special type and each single constellation.

The most important single criterion to be considered is the age of onset in the index patient. The most recent available risk figures based on this differentiation alone may be those given by Darlow, Smith, and Duncan (1) (Table 1). If the risks for second and third degree relatives of an index patient are sought, the risk figures of the table should be halved.

Table 1. Risk figures for first degree relatives of patients with diabetes mellitus by age of onset (according to Darlow, Smith, and Duncan, 1973) (Percent)

	25	45	65	85
Population	0.2-0.3	0.5-0.9	1.7-3.8	1.4-9.2
First degree relatives Proband onset				
under 25	8	13	17	25
over 25	(1)	(2)	9	21

The data are derived empirically from a large sample collected in Scot-land, and in the strict sense, apply only to this population under the given circumstances. More generally applicable may be data which take in consideration the incidence of diabetes in the particular age group of the general population. Simpson (8) calculated from her data the risk figures given in Table 2. All figures presented should only be taken as a crude general estimate, and a careful search into the his-

tory of the particular family to be counselled should be undertaken
to unveil possible further facts that might call for adjustments.
Further affected members in the family indicate a higher risk, and
application of a factor between 1.5 and 4 was found appropriate depending on the age of onset and the degree of relationship of further affected relatives. Other factors to be considered are the severity of
diabetes in the proband and the relatives, whether it is insulin dependent or not and whether obesity runs in the family. One might thus
arrive at a considerably higher or lower estimate than the general
figures suggested.

Table 2. Increased risk for clinical diabetes in first degree relatives of diabetics
as compared to the general population (after Simpson, 8)

Age of onset of diabetes in proband	Increased risk of clinical diabetes over that in the general population		
	siblings	offspring	parents
0-19 years	x 10 - 14	x 18 - 41	x 2 - 3
20-39 years	x 4 - 5	x 6 - 13	x 2 - 3
40+ years	x 2 - 4	x 1 - 3	x 2 - 3

The most important family factor in counselling a diabetic who inquires
concerning risks to children will be a diabetes-positive history in
the spouse and his or her relatives, as well as information about the
type of diabetes present in either family. If further affected relatives can be found in the family of both spouses, on theoretical grounds
in a multifactorial disease, as diabetes is, the risk should be considerably higher than in a case, where the same number of affected relatives is known in the family of only one spouse, and the higher genetic
predisposition may also reflect itself in an earlier onset and more
severe manifestation. Empirical data in this regard are however again
missing.

The greatest risk, of course, is to be expected, if both spouses themselves suffer from diabetes. Under the assumption of an homogenous
autosomal recessive inheritance of diabetes in these cases, 100% involvment of children should be expected, except for possibly reduced
penetrance or later manifestation. The fact that in the offspring of
conjugal diabetics only between 3 and 9% of the children were found to
be overtly diabetic, and estimated life-time risks not exceeding 50%
were calculated, was one of the major arguments against this mode of
transmission, although the figures given were based on a very limited
number of observations (1,2,6,9).

What then are the consequences of this rather unsatisfactory state of
knowledge? Should diabetics be encouraged at all to seek genetic counsel? And if they ask for advice, what could and should they be told?

To the first question the answer must be definitely yes, in spite of
the fact that at many counselling services diabetics are rarely or
never seen. These patients are troubled by so many uncertainties, problems, and anxieties that a clear and responsible genetic counselling
can do much to relieve them and help them to a clear decision in this
important matter. Counselling, of course, may well be done at a diabetic clinic, if a competent counsellor is available, who is familiar
with the genetic problems involved, but it is mandatory to offer these
patients the best empiric risk estimate that can be derived, considering all the clinical and genetic facts mentioned.

At the same time it must be made clear that any such estimate can only be a crude guideline and probably must be reconsidered, should diabetes occur in the future in children or other relatives, at first thought to be unaffected. One should not forget that diabetes is not recognized in many individuals until late or when specifically sought for. Since usually no special screening of family members will have been carried out, anamnestic data given in good faith may be misleading.

The decision to have or not to have children will usually depend not so much on a few percent of risk more or less, but on other considerations as well. It will, therefore, suffice to give a certain range of risks and point out the probable age of manifestation in the offspring considered. Severity of the expected manifestation will be another very important factor which might be estimated to some degree from the family history.

Most of the time the risk will not be so great as to deter patients from having children, and the recommendations found in most publications agree that a diabetic patient married to a nondiabetic may have children. On the other hand, the opinion predominates that a marriage between two diabetics should remain childless, the latter as much on medical as on genetic grounds. Both statements should be qualified. In the first case, although in general the risk of diabetes in each child may not appear formidable if only one parent is diabetic, further family anamnesis may lead to a much higher estimate. Furthermore, one should consider carefully, which type of diabetes could most likely be expected and which consequences this may have for this particular child. In the lay press, and unfortunately also even among nonclinical genetic counsellors, the late sequelae of diabetes mellitus tend to be underrated.

Understandably, diabetic patients, particularly of the younger age group, are quite often unaware of the persistent danger of neurovascular complications even in well-controlled diabetes. It is, of course, in general, desirable to cause patients as little worry as possible. However, they must be sufficiently concerned to ensure close observation of the given dietary and drug prescriptions. If, however, the founding of a family is at stake, the dangers to the working and earning capacity or even the shortened life expectancy of the diabetic patient cannot be kept secret from him and his spouse, if he is to make a responsible decision. The same holds true in regard to the danger of late complications in potential children.

For the diabetic woman, in addition, the increased risk involved for the metabolic state of the mother and for the child in each pregnancy is a point to be discussed. Even under the best care the risk for each pregnancy has remained higher than average in regard to perinatal morbidity, mortality of the child, and incidence of congenital malformations. It is still controversial, whether near ideal control of the diabetes may help to prevent most of these sequelae. The general vascular status of the mother may be of critical importance, but may be difficult to classify.

No definite rules can be set as to where the balance is to be set between sufficient and complete information for the patient, and the physician's desire to save his patient from possibly depressing knowledge. Genetic counselling must be more than just the calculating and offering of risk figures, it means guiding of individual patients in a field of central importance to their life, their family, and their future. In any case, the physician has to search for possible risk factors before he gives reassuring advice. Such factors, among others, may be cardiovascular problems or hyperlipoproteinemia.

In deciding about advising a diabetic parent about children, it may be remembered that, even if a child becomes diabetic, the fact that he has a diabetic parent ensures that he will probably have an early diagnosis, better understanding of his problems, and more effective treatment and diet control than average. A possible way out of the dilemma is to restrict the number of offspring to one or two.

Deciding against children usually means to decide for contraception. The choice of the best means again deserves some consideration, since the method should be acceptable and safe. However, on theoretical grounds the most reliable method, hormonal contraception, may carry an increased risk for the diabetic woman, since it possibly increases the risk of vascular thrombosis and, by increasing blood lipids, presumably could promote atherogenesis (5,10). Since hormonal contraception simulates pregnancy to some degree an unfavorable influence on the glucose tolerance could also result.

Provided the decision not to have any further children is definite, tubal ligation might be the better solution. An alternative temporary method would be the intrauterine device. Surgical sterilization of males, again, might be more apt to lead to complications in diabetic males and in addition, since impotentia coeundi is a frequently found symptom in diabetic men, the surgical procedure might be wrongly blamed.

Genetic counsel should always be given with the interest of the counselee and his family in mind, but what about diabetes and the genetic quality of mankind? Many articles have been written on the possible effects of modern treatment on the increase of genes for diabetes or of the effect of modern civilization in bringing the trait to manifestation, thus strengthening selection against it, and shifting the balance against the assumed advantageous effects of diabetic genes in previous times. No matter what genetic theory one applies, particularly, however, under the most likely assumption of multifactorial inheritance of diabetes, the wide distribution of genes contributing to diabetes ensures that even the exclusion of all diabetics from procreation could decrease the number of such genes only very slowly, even if other possibly balancing factors are neglected. Marriage of diabetics with normals will help to just maintain the frequency, if it becomes true that diabetics in such a marriage are just as fertile as other people. What, however, about the widely given advice endorsed among others by an expert comittee of the WHO, that diabetics should not marry each other or not produce children?

It certainly is true that a marriage between two diabetics makes diet, treatment, and the general adjustment of the way of life to the rules dictated by their disease easier for both of them. It also holds that potential diabetic children of such a couple find circumstances most suitable to them. Again, such a marriage is endangered by the fragile health of both partners, and the danger of diabetes mellitus appearing in children is considerably higher than in any other type of marriage. In addition, more severe expression and possibly earlier manifestation must be feared.

And what about eugenics? Do not such marriages help to spread genes for diabetes to a most undesirable degree? The concern could be real, because summer camps for diabetic children, diabetic clinics, and special office hours for diabetics bring patients of both sexes together and presumably may promote such unions. In fact this problem rarely comes up and for this simple reason alone would not be a eugenic problem. Furthermore, Edwards (Chapter 5) has taken issue with the statements given by the expert comittee cited above. He argues convincingly that, if diabetics marry at all and have children, from a eugenic point of view it makes no difference, whether they marry normals or marry each other, as long as the second type of marriage does not carry more than twice the risk for affected children than the first type. Empirical data from Simpson (Chapter 3) gave the risk in the first case with about 1% and in the second type of marriage close to 3%. As Edwards concludes, at the expense of a "rearrangement" of about 100 potential marriages, involving about 400 individuals, the birth of about 2 diabetic children might be prevented, and he proceeds, even this is not true, because the lowered fertility of diabetic couples has not been considered. Figures of other authors may modify the picture, but the main point remains unchanged: preventing diabetics from having children at all would probably slightly decrease the frequency of responsible genes in the population, but advising against the union of two diabetics and suggesting they seek other partners will not have any such effect and hardly any effect on the number of manifest diabetics. The fact that such couples most probably will restrict their number of children far below the average figure of the normal population, would in reality act against the further spread of diabetic genes.

It is, of course, quite another matter, if the advice not to have children or to restrict their number is given for purely personal reasons of the individuals involved. Counselling in diabetes as in general counselling is not an affair of population genetics or eugenics, but mainly a physician-patient relationship, designed to relieve personal anxiety and prevent a genetical burden on the single family (4). To the extent that such measures can be proved to be effective, counselling should also include advice on preventive measures to be observed in children and relatives known to be at risk to develop clinical disease.

Counselling of diabetics in regard to offspring is only in part genetic counselling. As with most genetic counselling, it requires genetic and clinical experience. When both are not available in a single person, some sort of cooperation between a medical geneticist and a clinician will have to be worked out.

References

1. Darlow, J.M., Smith, C., Duncan, L.J.P.: A statistical and genetical study of diabetes. III. Empiric risks to relatives. Ann. Hum. Genet. (Lond.) 37, 157 (1973)

2. Edwards, J.H.: Should diabetics marry? Lancet I, 1045 (1969)

3. Falconer, D.S., Duncan, L.J.P., Smith, C.: A statistical and genetical study of diabetes. I. Prevalence and morbidity. Ann. Hum. Genet. (Lond.) 34, 347 (1971)

4. Fuhrmann, W., Vogel, F.: Genetische Familienberatung. Heidelberger Taschenbücher. Berlin, Heidelberg, New York: Springer-Verlag, Bd. 42, 2. Aufl., 1975

4a. Fuhrmann, W., Vogel, F.: Genetic counseling. Heidelberg Science library, Vol. 10, 2nd ed.. Berlin, Heidelberg, New York: Springer, 1976

5. Hazzard, W.R., Spiger, M.J., Bagdade, J.D., Bierman, E.L.: Studies on the mechanism of increased plasma triglyceride levels induced by oral contraceptives. New Eng. J. Med. 280, 471 (1969)

6. Rimoin, D.L.: Genetics of diabetes mellitus. Diabetes 16, 346 (1967)

7. Rimoin, D.L.: Inheritance of diabetes mellitus. Med. Clin. N. Amer. 55, 807 (1972)

8. Simpson, N.E.: Diabetes in the families of diabetics. Can. Med. Assoc. J. 98, 427 (1968)

9. Simpson, N.E.: Heritabilities of liability to diabetes when sex and age at onset are considered. Ann. Hum. Genet. (Lond.) $\underline{32}$, 283 (1969)

10. Wynn, V., Doar, J.W.H., Mills, G.L., Stockes, T.: Fasting serum triglyceride, cholesterol, and lipoprotein levels during oral-contraceptive therapy. Lancet $\underline{II}$, 756 (1969)

25. Towards a Better Understanding of the Genetic Basis of Diabetes Mellitus

J. V. NEEL

Fathered by intuition, born of frustration, the concept of the heterogeneity of diabetes has finally been legitimized. Much of the attention in this volume has centered upon the recently recognized, differing associations of the ketosis-resistant and ketosis-prone diabetes
of relatively early onset. Within the next several years we will surely see efforts to determine whether the associations which have been
established for each of these two types will hold up for diabetes of
late onset. The necessary data for a first step in this direction are
to some extent undoubtedly already at hand in those centers with a
long-standing interest in the genetics of diabetes mellitus; one has
only to separate the "idiopathic" diabetics of onset in the fifth and
sixth decade into ketosis-prone and ketosis-resistant and scrutinize
the pedigrees and the results of glucose tolerance tests on close relatives in the same fashion as was done for early-onset diabetes.

We will probably also agree that there is already evidence for heterogeneity within the two principal types we now recognize. Thus, among
persons with early-onset, brittle diabetes, by no means do all affected individuals exhibit the statistically significant antibody or HL-A
type (MLC type) associations. While to some extent this may indicate
only that further associations with the same "family" of antibodies
or with HL-A types remain to be discovered, it may also indicate a
fundamental heterogeneity. With respect to the early-onset, more stable
diabetics, on the other hand, I am, with respect to their heterogeneity, especially intrigued by the evidence summarized by Fajans (Chapter 8, p. 71) that some at the time of first, very early detection
by Köbberling's (Chapter 9, p. 85) and Keen's (Chapter 13, p. 120) evidence concerning the different family histories of diabetes obtained
evidence concerning the different family histories of diabetes obtained
from very obese as contrasted to nonobese, adult-onset type diabetics.
At the very least, this suggests a shifting genetic threshold to diabetes according to the strength of the environmental "insult" (i.e.,
overnutrition).

Keen and Pyke have commented on the seeming deemphasis of the role of
heredity in the juvenile-onset type and further emphasis on heredity
in the maturity-onset type. To me the emphasis is the reverse. The fact
that we can relate the juvenile-onset type to a well-characterized
genetic system is the first identification of one of the heretofore
elusive components in the kinds of multifactorial systems we have been
discussing, and is a big plus for the genetic viewpoint. Otherwise
stated, the HL-A association is what multifactorial inheritance is
all about.

Incidentally, with reference to genetic counselling, it seems as if
in counselling sibs of a juvenile-onset type diabetic concerning liability to the disease, HL-A types should now be taken into consideration.
This leads to another thought: As we discover more of these associa-

tions, is it possible that we can learn to predict the predisposed with high accuracy? What preventative measures should then be instituted? Also, what preventative measures are indicated when family or other studies lead us to young, asymptomatic persons with disturbances of sugar metabolism? We will certainly agree that the first target for preventative measures should be those individuals among them who will develop early ophthalmologic, renal, or cardiovascular complications. Can we develop better techniques for identifying and protecting such individuals? It may soon become a routine responsibility of the physician to arrange for family studies when a new case of diabetes is discovered, with the introduction of appropriate measures as pre- or early diabetics are uncovered within the family.

An important point with respect to this emerging heterogeneity is that the evidence is almost all of the indirect type. Thus, etiologically we distinguish between the young brittle and the young stable diabetic because of associations between findings - different family histories, different disease histories, and HL-A types. The closest we come to a primary effect would appear to be the differences in assayable plasma insulin in the two groups, but even here, such is the complexity of insulin metabolism, we usually cannot say when this is a primary and when a secondary effect.

Our efforts to dissect this heterogeneity are greatly handicapped by the very low concentrations in which insulin occurs, so that we study it by its congeners or its effects rather than directly. There is a parallelism between the recognition of a relative lack of insulin and the recognition of tissue anoxia; both are grave disturbances of tissue metabolism. However, fortunately for the physician confronted with tissue anoxia, he can proceed in an orderly fashion to a precise diagnosis of the cause of the anoxia. Once cardiovascular disease has been excluded, central to this precision in diagnosis is the ability to obtain large samples of the chief molecule engaged in oxygen transport, and in the event of either an excess or deficiency in this molecule, move to an analysis of the dynamics of the situation. In diabetes mellitus we can for the individual patient only indirectly assay for circulating insulin, and can do extremely little with reference to analyzing insulin dynamics.

In the opening chapter a very general outline of the various disturbances which might manifest themselves as a relative insulin deficiency was presented.

Returning to that outline we may now consider how the physician - especially the hematologist - presented with a comparable situation, the symptoms of an inadequate oxygen supply to the tissues, is able at present to identify very positively counterparts to situations which are still only vague postulates for diabetes mellitus. Table 1 presents, with some license, "hematological counterparts" to most of the etiologies that can be postulated for a relative insulin deficiency. While I am not prepared to defend some of these analogies in any detail, I will defend the general argument that the hematologist has well-known counterparts for a number of the types of defects we can at present only surmise to be of possible importance in the etiology of diabetes mellitus. Conversely, while the events which ensure our ability to metabolize glucose may not be quite as complicated as those responsible for ensuring adequate oxygen to the tissues, a high degree of complexity does seem reasonable, and until we can define that complexity better, progress in elucidating the genetic basis of diabetes mellitus must be slow.

Table 1. A fanciful comparison of known abnormalities in tissue oxygenation with postulated deficiencies underlying abnormal glucose metabolism

---

1. Decreased output of normal insulin

   a. Decreased number or affinity of B-cell receptor sites to glucose or amino acids, i.e., insufficient stimulus

   DECREASED ERYTHROPOIETIN PRODUCTION IN CONGENITAL OR ACQUIRED RENAL DISEASE

   b. Decreased net synthesis of proinsulin

   THE THALASSEMIAS

   c. Abnormal or deficient "excision enzyme"

   NOT APPLICABLE

   d. Defective release of insulin from beta cell

   NOT APPLICABLE

   e. Degeneration of beta cell

   FANCONI'S APLASTIC ANEMIA

2. Production of abnormal insulin molecule

   THE HEMOGLOBINOPATHIES WHICH RESULT IN ANEMIA

3. Production of insulin antagonist

   a. Antibody in nature

   b. Hormonal in nature

   THE ACQUIRED HEMOLYTIC ANEMIAS

4. Abnormal insulin transport

   THE CONGENITAL NONSPHEROCYTIC HEMOLYTIC ANEMIAS DUE TO AN ENZYME DEFICIENCY

5. Abnormal cellular receptors of insulin (including inability to dissociate insulin complexes)

   a. Decreased number

   b. Decreased function

   FAMILIAL METHEMOGLOBINEMIA DUE TO DEFICIENT NADH-METHEMOGLOBIN REDUCTASE ACTIVITY

6. "Obesity factor"

   ANOXIA SECONDARY TO CHRONIC LUNG DISEASE

7. Abnormal rate of insulin degradation by target cells

   NOT APPLICABLE

As one who spent some time working on the hemoglobin diseases, I am especially intrigued by the possibility of abnormalities in the insulin molecule as one of the causes of diabetes. As you know, one of the developments resulting from the availability of inexpensive electrophoretic techniques has been the demonstration of an unexpectedly large amount of previously hidden variation in a whole series of serum proteins and erythrocyte enzymes. Roughly a third of the proteins examined are characterized by specific variants which affect more than 2% of the population, thus qualifying as genetic polymorphisms. Moreover, in addition to these polymorphisms, almost every protein examined in any depth has also been characterized by rare variants, of the order of 2-3 per 1000, presumably due for the most part to amino acid substitutions. Since the insulin molecule is smaller than most of the molecules studied thus far, one might expect such substitutions to be somewhat less frequent. On the other hand, the conversion of proinsulin to insulin subjects the insulin polypeptide to an event susceptible to genetic modifications of a type to which to the best of current knowledge, the other molecules studied thus far are not subjected, and so might increase the frequency of variants. The most reasonable first step in the search for abnormal insulin molecules would seem to involve the use of large domesticated animals where one might recover enough insulin from a single animal for biochemical studies. It will be important not to work with a single breed, but to sample widely among existing breeds.

Barring unexpected developments which will permit us to characterize the insulin of single humans, perhaps the strongest approach we have at present to unraveling the heterogeneity is to establish cohorts of predisposed - be it on the basis of family history, recency of civilization, a rare syndrome, HL-A types, or disease experience - and measure periodically from an early age onwards those various parameters of glucose metabolism which might help us distinguish subtypes. This is so laborious an undertaking that one can only conclude that there must be a better way. Incidentally, although the rare syndromes of which diabetes mellitus is a component seem to offer an attractive investigative approach to the disease, one wonders to what extent what passes as diabetes in the rare syndromes is not true diabetes mellitus, whatever this is, but rather reflects, as Rimoin (Chapter 7) seems to feel, muscle wastage, inactivity, and poor alimentation.

Finally, I would like to return to an aspect of diabetes of great fascination to the geneticist - its apparently low frequency in primitive man, and relatively high frequency in civilized man. So long as we believe that most diabetes mellitus has the same, relatively simple genetic basis, we must account somehow both for the frequency of that gene and its failure to find expression as diabetes mellitus in primitive man. Sometime ago (1962), I proposed that those predisposed to diabetes mellitus might well under primitive conditions have represented those "thrifty genotypes" who by virtue of an ability to respond to the stimulus of food with rapid insulin production - i.e., a "quick insulin trigger" - had an advantage over those not so endowed, an advantage only occasionally offset by the development of diabetes. It was argued that with civilization and the advent of refined foods, we were overstimulating this mechanism, resulting, in those with the quick insulin trigger, in the development of antiinsulins which eventually led to diabetes mellitus. The force of that suggestion has been considerably weakened by the fall from favor of insulin antagonists and the inability to demonstrate an overproduction of insulin in many very early diabetics, but the circumstances which prompted that suggestion - the high frequency of diabetes mellitus in civilized peoples - remains unchanged. However, the need for some such theory is inversely proportional to the heterogeneity of the disease. Thus, to take an extreme example, if there are 20-30 genes involved in that hypothetical multifactorial complex that results, in the requisite environment, in diabetes mellitus, and thus 20-30 loci sharing the mutation pressure necessary to maintain this phenotypic frequency in the absence of balancing selection, then the need to postulate some type of balancing selection in the past is considerably diminished. The possibility that some diabetes mellitus may be a sequel to infection would also tend to defuse the genetic issue created by the high frequency of the disease. To return to the earlier analogy with anoxia, the acquired anemias do not present the same gentic problem in accounting for their frequency as the congenital. It is clear that we cannot know the need for a "thrifty genotype" kind of hypothesis until we better understand the heterogeneity and pathogenesis of diabetes mellitus. On the other hand, it is difficult not to perceive a remarkable parallelism between the emergence of diabetes mellitus in recently domesticated rodents, as described in Chapter 17 and the emergence of diabetes in such groups as the Amerindian or the Maori, who have undergone just as striking a change in their life style in a comparable number of generations. It may well be that these recently primitive groups will by circumstance be forced to telescope into a very few generations genetic adjustments that our own ancestors spread over very many more generations. It is certainly to be hoped that at the same time the appropriate medical services are rendered these groups, as many of the kinds of observations described above as possible be made on them. Perhaps the "thrifty genotype" hypothesis will eventually be a shining example of the right hypothesis based on the wrong data. And returning again to our discussion of counseling, viewing the problems of overpopulation and diminishing agricultural base, one wonders if we may not need those thrifty genotypes in the future, and question how far we should go to discourage their reproduction in the present.

Reference

Neel, J.V.: Diabetes mellitus: a "thrifty" genotype rendered detrimental by "progress". Am. J. Hum. Genet. 14, 353 (1962)

Subject Index

eskimos 8
etiology 23,33,37,99,106,112,115,134,203
eugenics 237
expression 2

family history 3,80,119,129,234
Fanconi's anemia 242
founder effect 4
free fatty acids 139
Friedreich's ataxia 44,52,53

gastrointestinal diseases 131
Gaussian curve 26
genetic counseling 192,234-240
genetic marker 109
genes, dose of 84
genotype, diabetic 37
glomerulosclerosis 209
glucagon 39,40,45,49,138
glucagonoma 39
glucose receptor 41
glucose tolerance 2,229
--, intravenous 118
glucose tolerance test 2,7,115
glycogen storage disease 44,48
gonadal dysgenesis 126
Grave's disease 106
growth hormone deficiency 44,46
growth rate 100
gynecomastia 125

Hashimoto's disease 106
hemochromatosis 44,46,142,205,208
hepatitis 102
hepatomegaly 147,150
heritability 4,14,15,28,29,79,195
Herrmann's syndrome 44,51
heterocygotes 30
heterogeneity 5,7,86,147,191,240,241
-, etiological 6
-, genetic 1,13,17,23,54,79,83,84,222
high density lipoprotein 140
Hippel-Lindau disease 47
histocompatibility 65
-, antigens 200
-, system 6,107
HL-A antigens, see histocompatibility
  antigens
HL-A region 30
HL-A system, see histocompatibility
  system
Huntington's chorea 44,51
hyperalaninuria 52
hyperchylomicronemia 140
hyperinsulinemia 49
hyperinsulinism 141
hyperlipidemia 44,49,138-146,150
-, primary 138
-, secondary 138
hyperphagia 167,172,182,184
hyperthyroidism 149

hyperuricemia 117
hypogonadism 45,54,55,56,58,106,125
hypoparathyroidism 45,106
hypopituitarism 58

immunity, cell-mediated 65
impotence 221,237
incidence 81,82,117
infections 134,201
-, congenital 102
inheritance, co-dominant 6
-, dominant 1,2,13,90,92
-, multifactorial 3,4,7,14,22,35,84
-, multigenic 177
-, recessive 1,2,13
-, single-factor 4
-, X-linked 13
insulin antagonist 17
- levels 131,132
- production of 17
-, release of 17,158
- requirement 37
- response 64,71,73,74,75,229,230,231
- resistance 138,147,151
- secretion 132
- sensitivity 141
- transport, abnormal 7
insulitis 45,106
islet cell antibodies 107

JOD 88-93

ketoacidosis 64,89,157
Kimmelstiel-Wilson disease 207
Klinefelter's syndrome 44,125,128
K-ratio 80,81
K value 126,128

laboratory rodents, diabetes in 155-164
Laron dwarfism 47
Lawrence-Moon-Biedl syndrome 6,44,53,54,
  56
Lawrence type of diabetes 147
leucine 49
liability 14,79
-, genetic 177
life expectancy 236
lipid metabolism 138
lipodystrophy, cephalothoracic 151
-, congenital 149
-, generalized 149
-, partial 149,150,151
-, progressive 151
lipoproteinlipase 139,140
liver cirrhosis 39
low density lipoprotein 140

Machado's disease 44,51
malformations 127,134
malnutrition 28
map, genetic 27

ulcer, duodenal 30
units, environmental 28
-, genetic 28

variance, additive genetic 14
-, genetic 79
-, phenotypic 14,79
variation, additive 4
viral infection 6,46,208
virus 40,95-104,112
-, antibodies 95
-, ECHO 98

viruses 12,29,31
-, arthropod-borne 102
-, coxsackie 6,95,116,117
virus infection 39,134
-, EMC 95,106
-, picorna group 98
-, poliomyelitis 102
Von Gierke's disease 48

Werner's syndrome 6,44,55,210

Yemenite Jews 8,117

Related Titles

End-Stage Diabetic Nephropathy

Proceedings of a Symposium on End-Stage Diabetic Nephropathy, Minneapolis, Minn., May 23–24, 1974 (Kidney International, Supplement No. 1, October 1974 to Vol. 6, No. 4)

The newly launched series of supplement issues will present the actual proceedings of conferences, symposia, workshops, etc., carefully selected to appeal to a broad segment of the journal's readership. The theme of the first supplement is exceedingly timely in view of the current controversy on the suitability of the advanced diabetic patient for kidney transplantation.

A. Labhart

Clinical Endocrinology

This comprehensive textbook of clinical endocrinology includes gynecological and pediatric endocrinology and diabetology. The author's successful combination of the clinical-morphological and biochemical-pathogenic points of view places the emphasis firmly on the clinical treatment. The very full and up-to-date select bibliography makes this a valuable reference work of the handbook type.

Monographs on Endocrinology

Vol. 1: S. Ohno: Sex Chromosomes and Sex-linked Genes

An excursion into the phylogenetic past of mammalian sex chromosomes and X-linked genes which gives an insight to an unique dosage compensation mechanism for X-linked genes possessed by man and other mammals.

Vol. 6: K. Federlin: Immunopathology of Insulin

After reviewing the antigenicity of insulin and the methods developed for the demonstration of antibodies, the author reports his own work on cellular and humoral antibodies in patients with insulin allergy, both delayed and immediate, and discusses animal experiments to study the process of anti-insulin antibody formation.

Vol. 7: E. W. Horton: Prostaglandins

The book emphasizes micromethods of identification and estimation, pharmacological actions, physiological roles, and clinical implications of prostaglandins.

Vol. 8: E. Gurpide: Tracer Methods in Hormone Research

This monograph presents the theoretical foundations necessary for the design and interpretation of tracer experiments in hormone research. Such experiments enable the researcher to follow the dynamics of steroid hormones from their formation and distribution through a range of reversible metabolic reactions to their degradation or elimination.

Springer-Verlag Berlin Heidelberg GmbH

Methods in Human Cytogenetics

Editors: H. G. Schwarzacher, U. Wolf

This comprehensive compilation of modern methods in mammalian cytogenetics includes chromosome banding, the culture of cells obtained from amniotic fluid, and the preparation of cell cultures for biochemical analysis. The various methods are described and discussed and presented in a form convenient for laboratory use.

A. Jacquard

The Genetic Structure of Populations
(Biomathematics, Vol. 5)

Population genetics involves the application of genetic information to the problems of evolution. Since genetics models based on probability theory are not too remote from reality, the results of such modeling are relatively reliable and can make important contributions to research. This textbook was first published in French; the English edition has been revised with respect to its scientific content and instructional method.

Comparative Aspects of Reproductive Failure

An International Conference at Dartmouth Medical School, Hannover N.H., July 25–29, 1966. Editor: K. Benirschke

Comparative Mammalian Cytogenetics

An International Conference at Dartmouth Medical School, Hannover N.H., July 29-August 2, 1968. Editor: K. Benirschke

W. Fuhrmann, F. Vogel

Genetic Counseling

A Guide for the Practicing Physician. 2nd revised edition. (Heidelberg Science Library, Vol. 10)

Diabetes mellitus A

Herausgeber: K. Oberdisse. (Handbuch der Inneren Medizin, Band 7, Teil 2A)

Diabetology has links with almost all branches of internal medicine and many of its marginal areas, so that 48 experts were called upon to contribute to this comprehensive treatise. Basic research and applied diabetology receive equal attention and this work will appeal to those with scientific interests as well as to the practicing physician. Reference is made to all the relevant literature.

Springer-Verlag Berlin Heidelberg GmbH